MW00533208

Nutrivore Testimonials

"The health and wellness world can feel like a maze that I can't get out of, and it ends up becoming a place of stress for me. I *love* Dr. Sarah's liberating, nutrient-focused approach to food, which allows me to feel informed and free from the shackles of confusing and contradictory information."

—Allison B., Monroe, CT

"I was diagnosed with celiac disease about ten years ago, and rheumatoid arthritis and Sjogren's syndrome were added to the list three years ago. Lots of pain and fatigue over here! Figuring out how to eat has been challenging . . . and at times has led to disordered eating and fear of food. Dr. Sarah's Nutrivore concept has made such a positive impact on my life. Looking at food in terms of what I can add instead of what I can't have is life changing!"

—Juliet F., Houston, TX

"I have always struggled to 'eat healthy,' and still do. The mindset shift from restrictive eating to nutritious eating is something that would *never* have occurred to me without Dr. Sarah's Nutrivore philosophy. Thank you!"

—Georgios K., Sunnyvale, CA

"In the storm of nutritional misinformation that is typically espoused in the quest to sell a product and profit from the unaware, I'm thankful for Nutrivore, as it serves as a beacon that guides and informs me through the decision-making process when it comes to food selection."

—Charlie M., Cockeysville, MD

"I can't tell you how much Nutrivore has changed the way I look at food. I used to think 'Why bother?' feeling like that extra carrot or some iceberg lettuce wouldn't make much of a difference. Now my whole diet has changed, because it's fun to add to my Nutrivore Score!"

—Mary N., Anaheim, CA

"Dr. Sarah presents nutritional information in such a unique and interesting way that my brain is extra happy. I'm making much more considered choices about what I add to my food intake and cutting myself a bit more slack on the treat stuff (which has actually moderated my intake of sugary items, since I know how much won't impact my health, which keeps me out of the deprived/binge loop)."

—Simone B., Sydney, Australia

"As a registered dietitian, I've been searching for something like the Nutrivore approach to eating to help clarify that what we include in our meals is much more important than what we take out."

—Amy S., RDN, Evansville, IN

"I'm just geeking out on Nutrivore, so thank you! Importantly for me, I can focus more on the nutrients in a meal, which takes away all my food phobias. Plus, it's kind of fun and satisfying to play around with new/old recipes that I can make more nutrient dense and yummy."

—Shelly S., San Jose, CA

"I thought I knew quite a bit about nutrition, but learning about Nutrivore has opened up a whole new world. I think about it whenever I'm shopping, cooking, or eating, and I find it fascinating."

—Sara C., Fort Wayne, IN

"I treat Nutrivore as my bible for diet and lifestyle. When in doubt in terms of my diet, I head over to Nutrivore.com for guidance. The knowledge and vibe of Dr. Sarah help me feel sane and centered."

—Olivia L., Brooklyn, NY

NUTRIVORE

The Radical New Science for Getting the Nutrients You Need from the Food You Eat

SARAH BALLANTYNE, PhD

SIMON ELEMENT
New York London Toronto Sydney New Delhi

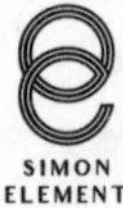

An Imprint of Simon & Schuster, LLC
1230 Avenue of the Americas
New York, NY 10020

This publication contains the opinions and ideas of its author. It is intended to provide helpful and informative material on the subjects addressed in the publication. It is sold with the understanding that the author and publisher are not engaged in rendering medical, health, or any other kind of personal professional services in the book. The reader should consult his or her medical, health, or other competent professional before adopting any of the suggestions in this book or drawing inferences from it.

The author and publisher specifically disclaim all responsibility for any liability, loss, or risk, personal or otherwise, that is incurred as a consequence, directly or indirectly, of the use and application of any of the contents of this book.

First Simon Element hardcover edition May 2024

SIMON ELEMENT is a trademark of Simon & Schuster, LLC

Simon & Schuster: Celebrating 100 Years of Publishing in 2024

For information about special discounts for bulk purchases, please contact Simon & Schuster Special Sales at 1-866-506-1949 or business@simonandschuster.com.

The Simon & Schuster Speakers Bureau can bring authors to your live event. For more information or to book an event, contact the Simon & Schuster Speakers Bureau at 1-866-248-3049 or visit our website at www.simonspeakers.com.

Interior design by Renato Stanisic

Manufactured in the United States of America

10 9 8 7 6 5 4 3 2 1

Library of Congress Cataloging-in-Publication Data has been applied for.

ISBN 978-1-6680-3161-2
ISBN 978-1-6680-3163-6 (ebook)

For my amazing daughters and fellow storytellers,
Adele and Mira.

Contents

NUTRIVORE

Introduction

An herbivore eats plants. A carnivore eats animals. An omnivore eats both plants and animals. So, what is a Nutrivore? Nutrivore is the revolutionary yet simple dietary concept: Get all the nutrients our bodies need from the foods we eat. Or, if you're looking for a sound bite: A Nutrivore eats nutrients.

If this seems like an incredibly basic concept, well, I admit, it is! And yet, Nutrivore represents a completely new lens through which to view foods.

How do you think about food? You might think of food as satiating—when you're hungry, you eat until you're full. You might think of food in terms of celebration, the social bonding that comes with Sunday brunch, sharing a birthday cake, or snacks at a Super Bowl party. You might be a foodie, chasing the dopamine rush that decadent foods can provide. Or you might be a food addict, needing ever more sugar, salt, and fat to satisfy that craving. You might reach for food when you're stressed or sad or alone. You might eat to keep yourself awake when you're feeling tired and unfocused. You might think of food in terms of athletic performance, measuring macros to fuel recovery. You may think of food in terms of allergies, avoiding those foods that trigger a reaction. Or you might not even think of food at all, eating mainly while distracted, food as a matter of routine. Whether you resonate with one or all of these, most people nowadays additionally, if not fundamentally, think of food in terms of diet and weight loss. And that's where the problem lies.

Open most any other diet book on the store shelf and you'll read promises that by applying the simple changes prescribed within its pages, you'll lose weight, thereby gaining self-confidence and happiness. All you have to do is cut out . . . Well, what exactly you're supposed to cut out will depend on which book you're reading. You might be asked to reduce or eliminate completely calories or carbs or fats or protein; gluten or dairy or soy; FODMAPs or sugar or starch or yeast; phytates or oxalates or lectins; plant foods or animal foods. You might be asked to obsessively measure the quantities or relative ratios of allowed foods. Even a more enlightened book that focuses on health rather than weight—perhaps promising to fix leaky gut, reduce inflammation, improve your memory, or help you kill it at the gym—will typically present food restrictions as its purported solution.

Instead of explaining what to eat and why (which is what I'll do in this book), most diets are defined by what you eliminate, reduce, restrict, or measure. To state the obvious: It's just not possible for all of these diets to work as advertised. Between them, every food, food group, and macronutrient is demonized; if you bought into every diet's claims, there would be nothing left to eat. And these diets are more likely marketed to you with a compelling narrative—the quest for the best diet as a culture war—rather than a strong scientific foundation. I can say this because scientific studies actually have compared the efficacy of different diets, and concluded that while there are some dietary patterns that are really important for overall health, there is no clear winner in terms of dietary templates.[1]

I'm going to change how you think about food. You will stop seeing one food as good and the other as bad, and by extension, that you're good if you eat this "good food" and bad if you eat that "bad food." Instead, we're going to focus on actual nutrition.

Almost everyone's diet is falling short of the mark in terms of meeting their nutritional needs—and not just a small differential that can be easily made up with a multivitamin. The high rates of nutrient deficiency and insufficiency we see today are the result of the confluence of the convenience of delicious and affordable ultraprocessed foods that offer little nutrition, with confusion over what foods are healthy and how much of them we should eat—the latter driven by both dietary guidelines and the messaging from the diet industry and weight-loss gurus. Basically, it's harder than ever to choose healthy foods, and most people are unsure about which foods those even are. You're not alone and it's not your fault—the amount of conflicting recommendations out there is dizzying.

This is why Nutrivore is so important—we learn about what nutrients do in the body, how much of those nutrients we need, and which foods supply those nutrients. We stick with the facts: Everything you're about to learn is based on scientific consensus with a wealth of evidence to support it. With this knowledge, you'll find it easy to choose foods to meet your body's nutritional needs. Even better, there are many ways to do so, which means you can apply the Nutrivore philosophy to however you eat now.

Diet culture has led many people to develop encyclopedic knowledge of the calories, carb grams, and fat grams per serving of foods (I know because I am one such person—I've been there!). But as Nutrivores, we're looking to understand much more meaningful nutritional information while embracing a less calculated and rigid way to choose foods. You generally don't need to count, measure, weigh, or log your foods, but will instead improve your nutrient awareness so you can choose nutritionally complementary, health-promoting, and satisfying foods more often. You'll be able to use rough estimates for serving guides and diversify your diet by trying new foods. Being a Nutrivore helps you focus your food choices on the most nutritionally important foods that align with your preferred diet or anti-diet.

The aim of a Nutrivore diet is to thoughtfully select foods each day so the sum of their nutrients fulfills or safely surpasses our daily needs for all essential and nonessential (yet crucial) nutrients while adhering to our caloric requirements. A key tool for identifying those foods that supply ample nutrients and thus help us achieve this goal is the Nutrivore Score, which is a measurement of the total amount of nutrients per calorie in a food.

The Nutrivore Score is an objective way to measure how nutritious a food is to inform your decision making as you peruse the grocery store shelves. This simple number helps us to appreciate the nutrients inherent in most foods while feeling empowered by the knowledge that we're making the right choice in the right way with the right balance. Plus, the Nutrivore Score facilitates a focus on what you can *add* to your diet to get the nutrients you're lacking, rather than a dietary ethos centered on what to remove. The Nutrivore Score is an invaluable weapon in your arsenal to fight back against food value judgments and restrictive mindsets.

You still get to enjoy food, whether thanks to social experiences or epicurean pleasures. In fact, by ditching the fear and guilt triggered by eating "bad foods," you may find yourself enjoying food even more, all while improving the quality of your diet. Win-win!

This book is divided into three parts, with the broad themes of why, what, and how.

In part 1 (why), I'll explain what nutrients are; what's behind the incredible prevalence of nutrient insufficiencies; how not getting enough nutrients drives both the high rates of disease and the common symptoms that erode quality of life; and why Nutrivore is the solution you've been waiting for. We'll dig into the Nutrivore philosophy, but I won't leave you hanging—in this first part, I'll also share all the basics of how to choose foods to up your Nutrivore game right off the bat, including how to use the Nutrivore Score to identify the most nutrient-dense options.

In part 2 (what), we'll build a solid knowledge foundation of nutrients, what they do in the body, and what foods contain them, by highlighting a curated collection of relevant effects of nutrient shortfalls that are contributing to your health complaints. We'll also review some of the history of discovery of nutrients in order to uncover the origins of many of the most pervasive and damaging diet myths today. I've written this part like a series of short stories, so while I hope you'll read through all four chapters, you can also jump around and read about just those nutrients known to improve your particular symptoms or diagnoses, or peruse the handy-dandy cheat sheets just to get an overview.

In part 3 (how), I'll build a veritable toolbox of practical resources to help you implement Nutrivore principles. We'll summarize the foundational foods on Nutrivore, those foods that have something unique to offer us nutritionally, along with serving guidelines for each, with a flexible and simple-to-use weekly checklist to track your nutrient density. We'll highlight the most valuable foods and food groups, review the science on taste adaptation, discuss tips for eating a Nutrivore diet on a budget, and break a bunch of food myths that might be holding you back. This part will culminate in a dozen mix-and-match-style recipes—like a choose your own adventure of a delicious nutrient-dense meal—and fifteen nutrient-dense snack suggestions.

So, without further ado, let's jump in!

Part 1

WHY NUTRIVORE?

Fad diets have a storied history. The first fad diet promising rapid weight loss for minimal effort was started in 1820 by Lord Byron (yes, that Lord Byron), who was by all accounts obsessed with dieting and staying thin.[1] Byron's weight fluctuated drastically, with periods of extreme starvation dieting—often combined with chewing tobacco or cigars to reduce appetite and woolen layers to induce sweating—and what Byron himself referred to as his "morbid propensity to fatten." His most famous crash diet included drinking large amounts of vinegar mixed with water as well as dousing the little food he ate in vinegar. And as the celebrity Romantic poet, philanderer, and politician that he was in England, he inspired many young Regency ladies to follow suit, hoping to attain a fashionable level of thinness.

In 1824, Lord Byron died tragically at the age of thirty-six of a fever—perhaps a malarial relapse or neurosyphilis, and certainly not helped by the leech and blood-letting treatments he received. Some medical historians believe the wear and tear on his body from years of malnourishment contributed to his extreme susceptibility to illness. Certainly, his postmortem revealed a brain that looked like that of an octogenarian, and a damaged liver and intestines.[2] And yet, Byron's influence on beauty standards persisted for decades after his death.

I'd like to think that nowadays we'd recognize that Lord Byron had an eating disorder (anorexia and bulimia), and we wouldn't follow his advice. But it's hard not to be intrigued by the diet recommendations of any person conforming to conventional beauty standards who guarantees dramatic results with little effort; after all, it worked for them.

A 2017 study estimated that 42 percent of adults globally are on a diet with the goal of losing weight, and an additional 23 percent of adults are on a diet with the goal of maintaining their weight.[3] In the United States, nearly half of adults are on a weight-loss diet.[4] A 2010 study of dieting women showed that calorie restriction increased the stress hormone cortisol, but that simply monitoring food and calorie intake also increased perceived stress.[5] What's the result of this increased stress? Studies show that dieting is a risk factor for food obsession, cravings, emotional eating, disordered eating, eating disorders, and weight-regain cycles (yo-yo dieting). According to a 1995 study, 35 percent of "normal dieters" progress to pathological dieting, and 20 to 25 percent of those individuals develop eating disorders.[6]

In a word, yikes. And this is why Nutrivore is different. First of all, it's a permissive structure—on Nutrivore, there are no foods you have to cut. Instead, we focus on eating more of those foods that supply us with ample nutrition and that are known to improve our health. By doing so, Nutrivore supports a healthy relationship with food, ending restrictive dieting leading to disordered eating. Second, instead of your health being something to be sacrificed for the sake of a diet, Nutrivore is all about supplying your body with the nutrients it needs to support health and reduce risk of disease. It's a balanced approach that fosters sustainability, a way of eating for lifelong health that additionally mends our relationship with our own bodies.

In this part, we're going to look at the incredibly high prevalence of nutrient deficiencies and insufficiencies that are driving health problems, and in what ways the multibillion-dollar weight loss and diet industry shares the blame with other culprits. We'll talk about how dietary shortfalls of certain nutrients are linked to specific diseases and symptoms, and how increasing your nutrient intake can improve your health and alleviate symptoms. And I'll provide you with an overview of the solution, the Nutrivore framework and its key tenets, as well as its most practical resource, the Nutrivore Score. We'll also talk about the simple changes you can make today to make your first steps toward Nutrivore and improve the quality of your diet.

CHAPTER 1

You're Not Getting Enough Nutrients

I have some bad news: You're not getting all the nutrients that your body needs. How can I say this with such certainty? Studies evaluating not just the average American's diet but also people following various diets billed for their health-promoting effects show rampant nutrient shortfalls. For at least ten essential nutrients, more than half of the US population is falling short of dietary requirements; and for at least four essential nutrients, more than 90 percent of us aren't getting enough from the foods we eat.[1]

Sure, there's a statistical possibility that you're the magic rainbow unicorn with the perfect nutrient-dense diet. But I'm going to hedge my bets based on a wealth of scientific studies that demonstrate that even people who are incredibly intentional about every bite still end up falling short of essential nutrients. For example, a 2006 analysis of seventy detailed food logs from twenty healthy subjects—half male and half female, and including fourteen athletes—showed that each of them had dietary shortfalls of between three and all seventeen essential vitamins and minerals evaluated in the study.[2] A variety of other studies show widespread nutrient shortfalls across dietary templates, from low-carb to vegetarian, from gluten-free to the DASH (Dietary Approaches to Stop Hypertension) eating plan.

"But I eat so healthy!" I hear you shout, ready to hurl this book across the room. Please know that I completely understand how frustrating it is to put so much effort into choosing, preparing, and paying the premium price for foods you've been told are good for you, only to find out that your diet is still not meeting your nutritional needs.

It's not your fault.

Over the last seven years, I have been on a mission to unlearn all the erroneous value judgments of foods that I myself had bought into, by diving deep into the scientific literature to objectively understand how to actually get all the nutrients our bodies need from the foods we eat: how to be a Nutrivore. That knowledge, and the practical tools I've created to help you implement it, is what I'm sharing with you in this book.

So let's start at the beginning: What is a nutrient, exactly?

WHAT ARE NUTRIENTS AND WHY DO THEY MATTER?

Nutrients are those substances within the foods we eat that provide nourishment essential for growth and the maintenance of life. You can think of nutrients as raw materials. They are the building blocks for every part of every cell and all the awesome stuff that holds our cells together. They are necessary for the ways our cells work together and communicate with each other, from electrical impulses to hormones. And they are both the reagents and catalysts for all the life-sustaining chemical reactions happening inside and outside of every cell—by some estimates, 370 sextillion (that's 370,000,000,000,000,000,000,000) of them in our bodies every single second![3]

We broadly categorize nutrients into two categories. *Macronutrients*—protein, fat, and carbohydrates—are the nutrients we need in large quantities. They supply the energy that fuels the complex functions of life along with being basic building blocks for cellular structures. *Micronutrients*—vitamins, minerals, phytonutrients, and other compounds—are those we need in smaller quantities. They can also be incorporated into cellular structures, but more commonly are necessary resources that facilitate or get used up in cellular chemical reactions.

While macronutrients are all deemed essential, micronutrients can be categorized as either essential or nonessential.

Essential nutrients are those that our bodies can't make—we'll develop a disease of deficiency and eventually die without them. Because diseases of deficiency can be studied in detail, it is easy to establish recommended dietary allowance (RDA) levels of essential nutrients, the minimum amount of that specific nutrient needed to meet the nutritional needs of 97.5 percent of the population (the remaining 2.5 percent needing more). Being even slightly deficient in a single essential nutrient can have negative consequences for our health.

In contrast, nonessential nutrients are those for which there is no clearly defined disease of deficiency. Typically, our body can synthesize them to some degree, which is the case for many amino acids, fatty acids, and vitamin-like compounds. Alternatively, their actions may be interchangeable with other nutrients, which is the case for antioxidant phytonutrients. We'll go on living without these nonessential nutrients, though we may not be particularly healthy. Indeed, many nutrients that are considered nonessential are known to improve health the more of them we eat.

Our nutrient stores must be frequently replenished from the foods we eat. When we are short on nutrients, the biological processes that rely on those nutrients can't function like they normally do. This might mean a chemical reaction is less efficient, producing less product than is required; or, an alternate pathway might be necessary, but it creates a product that isn't as good or a by-product that is undesirable or even toxic. It might mean more wear and tear on our cellular machinery, and a hampered ability for our cells and tissues to regenerate, rejuvenate, and repair. When the nutrient shortfalls are ongoing, strain builds up on the biological systems that require them, causing that entire biological system—like the cardiovascular system, the central nervous system, the musculoskeletal system, the digestive system, and the reproductive system, to name a few—not to work quite as well as it's supposed to. This sets the stage for an eventual chronic condition, when enough damage has built up due to lack of nutritional resources.

Daily Value Vocab

Recommended dietary allowance (RDA): Represents the dietary intake level of a specific nutrient considered sufficient to meet the needs of 97.5 percent of healthy individuals. These values should be considered minimum daily targets.

Adequate intake (AI): Represents an amount of a nutrient assumed to ensure nutritional adequacy for everyone in the demographic group when there isn't sufficient information to develop an RDA.

Estimated average requirement (EAR): A nutrient intake value that is estimated to meet the requirement of half the healthy individuals in a particular life stage and gender group.

Percent daily value (% DV): The percentage of the recommended daily intake for each nutrient per serving or amount of food, calculated based on a two-thousand-calorie-per-day diet.

Tolerable upper limit (TUL): The maximum level of daily nutrient intake that is likely to pose no risk of adverse effects. The upper limit differs from toxicity, which is typically only seen in the context of supplementation and not from dietary intake of whole foods.

PREVALENCE OF NUTRIENT DEFICIENCY AND INSUFFICIENCY

Almost all of us are nutrient deficient or insufficient, eroding both our health and our quality of life. Let's look at the statistics.

Nutritional deficiency is defined as inadequate dietary intake of an essential nutrient resulting in a disease of malnutrition, such as iron-deficiency anemia (iron), scurvy (vitamin C), rickets (vitamin D), beriberi (vitamin B_1), pellagra (vitamin B_3), and night blindness (vitamin A).

A 2017 study estimated the prevalence of deficiency in vitamin A, vitamin B_6, vitamin B_9 (folate), vitamin B_{12}, vitamin C, vitamin D, and vitamin E, as well as anemia, based on biochemical markers using data from blood tests taken as part of the 2003 to 2006 National Health and Nutrition Examination Survey.[4] The study showed that 31 percent of Americans are at risk for at least one vitamin deficiency or anemia, 6.3 percent are at risk for two vitamin deficiencies or anemia, and 1.7 percent are at risk for three to five vitamin deficiencies or anemia.

The study authors further identified low dietary intake as the reason for the high prevalence of nutrient deficiencies. Their analysis showed that a paltry 6.4 percent of the study population consumed the estimated average requirement for each of the vitamins A, B_6, B_9, B_{12}, C, and E, and iron. To emphasize just how dire this situation is, the estimated average requirement (EAR) is the amount of a nutrient thought to be sufficient for half of the population, the remainder needing more. So it's possible that even the 6.4 percent of study participants meeting the EAR still aren't really getting enough of those nutrients. And this analysis only looked at eight of the forty-nine essential nutrients![5] This feels like an appropriate time for a whomp-whomp sound effect.

Demographic disparities (including racial, gender, and socioeconomic disparities) have been found in many studies. For example, the CDC's Second Nutrition Report found that menstruating women are more likely to be iron deficient, non-Hispanic Blacks are more likely to be deficient in vitamin D, and women ages twenty to thirty-nine are more likely to be iodine deficient.[6]

Nutrient deficiency isn't the only concern, however. Nutrient insufficiency also contributes to health challenges.

Nutrient insufficiency (or inadequacy) refers to a dietary shortfall of a nutrient that isn't bad enough to cause a disease of deficiency. While that might sound relatively harmless, especially in comparison to a disease like scurvy or rickets, nutrient insufficiencies are increasingly showing up as a major underlying driver of chronic disease, such as increasing risk for cardiovascular disease, type 2 diabetes, obesity, cancer, chronic kidney disease, asthma, allergies, neurodegenerative disease, autoimmune disease, gout, and infection.

A 2011 study evaluated Americans' usual nutrient intake including nutrients that are naturally occurring in foods, from fortified and enriched foods, and from supplements.[7] The results are astounding. The table below shows the proportion of American adults whose usual diet falls short of essential vitamins and minerals.

Prevalence of Nutrient Insufficiencies

Nutrient	Proportion of American adults consuming *less than* the estimated average requirement
Vitamin D	100%
Potassium	97.8%*
Vitamin E	96.2%
Vitamin B9 (folate)	90.2%
Vitamin A	80.1%
Vitamin K	72.4%*
Magnesium	66.3%
Vitamin B1 (thiamin)	56.3%
Calcium	54.9%
Vitamin C	52.0%
Vitamin B6 (pyridoxine)	25.5%
Iron	23.1%
Zinc	16.8%
Vitamin B3 (niacin)	11.7%
Vitamin B2 (riboflavin)	9.6%
Vitamin B12 (cobalamin)	7.2%
Copper	5.4%
Phosphorus	2.0%
Selenium	1.1%

Adapted from V. L. Fulgoni III et al., "Foods, Fortificants, and Supplements: Where Do Americans Get Their Nutrients?" *Journal of Nutrition* 141, no. 10 (2011): 1847–54, doi: 10.3945/jn.111.142257.

*Vitamin K and potassium do not have estimated average requirements established. For these two nutrients, the number in the table above is the percentage of people who are not consuming the adequate intake level.

It should be no surprise that dietary insufficiency of essential nutrients is more prevalent among people living with food insecurity (an inability to consistently access or afford adequate food). A 2020 study found that adults living with food insecurity had a higher risk of micronutrient insufficiency for most of the vitamins and minerals examined when compared with food-secure adults, the only exceptions being for calcium, iron (examined only in men), vitamin B9 (folate), and choline.[8]

About a third of us are nutrient deficient and nearly everyone is nutrient insufficient. Let's look at the biggest contributors to our current nutritional predicament.

EATING HABITS THAT REDUCE NUTRIENTS

Why do almost all of our diets fall short of meeting our body's nutritional needs? The complex reasons include ultraprocessed and hyperpalatable foods displacing more nutritionally valuable options; dietary guideline shortcomings; and weight-loss and fad diets propelling diet myths, healthism, and restrictive eating patterns. Basically, most people are confused about which foods are healthy choices, and less nutritious options are cheaper, tastier, more convenient, and everywhere we look.

Let's go through these points one by one.

Yes, Ultraprocessed Foods Are Addictive

Studies have shown that about 58 percent of the calories consumed in the United States are derived from ultraprocessed foods.[9] Ultraprocessed foods are made mostly from ingredients extracted from foods—such as vegetable oils, cornstarch, high-fructose corn syrup, and table sugar—and contain low amounts of nutrients. Furthermore, it's common for ultraprocessed foods to have many added ingredients, including salt, sugar, fat, flavorings, emulsifiers, food dyes, flavor enhancers, or preservatives, making them *hyperpalatable*, i.e., so addictively delicious that eating that food overrides the body's natural satiety signals and triggers overeating.[10]

Examples of these ultraprocessed, hyperpalatable foods are soft drinks, fast food, pizza, packaged cookies, cakes, and salty snacks like chips and pretzels. Generally, the more a food is manipulated to make it shelf stable, convenient, cheap, and addictively delicious, the fewer valuable nutrients remain in that food.

A 2021 meta-analysis showed that the more ultraprocessed foods a person ate, the lower their intake of fiber, protein, potassium, zinc, magnesium, vitamin A, vitamin B3, vitamin B12, vitamin C, vitamin D, and vitamin E.[11] The only nutrients considered that were not significantly decreased by ultraprocessed food consumption were iron, calcium, phosphorus, vitamin B1, vitamin B2, and sodium. The people who ate the most ultraprocessed foods were only getting about 60 percent of the daily value of fiber, magnesium, vitamin A, and vitamin E, while also falling quite short of potassium, calcium, zinc, and vitamin D. This is the direct result of consuming ultraprocessed food instead of more nutrient-dense options.

While some ultraprocessed foods can absolutely fit into a Nutrivore template, it can be challenging to switch to a whole foods–focused diet while continuing to consume a lot of ultraprocessed foods. The surge in dopamine caused by these foods causes an intense feeling of pleasure, which leads to developing a strong preference for these foods but also addiction-like deficits in brain reward function, meaning we need more and more of these hyperpalatable foods to get that good feeling from eating them.[12] Nutrient-dense whole foods just can't compete when your taste buds are attuned to ultraprocessed foods.

There's another reason to consider reducing them: Studies show that when people eat a diet plentiful in ultraprocessed foods, they tend to eat more. A 2019 study fed participants a diet of 83 percent of calories from ultraprocessed foods or 83 percent of calories from unprocessed foods for two weeks, with a crossover design so each participant ate one diet for two weeks before switching to the other diet for an additional two weeks.[13] The meals the participants were fed were matched for total calories, fat, carbohydrate, protein, fiber, sugars, and sodium, and the participants were told to eat as much, or as little, as they liked. While on the ultraprocessed food arm of the study, participants ate an average of five hundred calories more per day and gained an average of two pounds, whereas they lost two pounds on average while on the unprocessed food arm of the study. Ultraprocessed foods trigger overeating while delivering very little in the way of valuable nutrition.

While no food is off-limits on Nutrivore, it's important to be aware of how ultraprocessed foods are not only displacing more nutrient-dense options but perhaps also making choosing a healthier option feel (and taste) much more difficult. We'll talk more about ultraprocessed foods in chapter 4.

Of course, ultraprocessed foods aren't the only culprit here.

Mixed Messages from Dietary Guidelines

The U.S Dietary Guidelines Advisory Committee has been criticized by experts for being too influenced by the food industry, while failing to protect against bias and partiality in its review of the relevant science, and while accepting weak evidentiary support as adequate justification to construct the USDA Dietary Guidelines for Americans (DGA).[14] As a result, there are many aspects of the dietary guidelines that are wrought with controversy.

There is a large amount of cynicism and apathy toward USDA dietary guidelines, resulting in very few adherents. The Healthy Eating Index (HEI) is a measurement of how well someone's diet follows the USDA Dietary Guidelines for Americans, and analyses show that American adults average a measly score of fifty-eight out of one hundred.[15] A 2022 analysis revealed that only 8.3 percent of Americans try to adhere to the USDA Dietary Guidelines for Americans; indeed, only about one quarter of Americans have even heard of MyPlate, a successor to the food guide pyramid established in 2011.[16]

One of the most important hallmarks of a health-promoting diet is high intake of whole vegetables and fruit. A 2017 meta-analysis showed that consuming 800 grams (equivalent to 1.75 pounds, or 28 ounces) of vegetables and fruits daily reduces all-cause mortality by 31 percent compared to eating less than 40 grams daily.[17] The authors calculated that 2.24 million deaths from cardiovascular disease, 660,000 deaths from cancer, and 7.8 million deaths from all causes could be avoided globally each year if everyone consumed 800 grams of veggies and fruits every day. Wow!

In contrast, a 2019 analysis by the CDC (Centers for Disease Control) revealed that only 10 percent of American adults eat the current recommended intake of vegetables, and only 12.5 percent of adults eat the current recommended intake of fruit.[18] In fact, the average vegetable consumption is a mere 1.64 cup equivalents of vegetables per day. In contrast, Americans consume about double the recommended amount of grains, averaging 6.7 ounce equivalents per day compared to the current MyPlate recommendation of 3 servings of whole grains daily for females and 3.5 to 4 servings for males. In fact, the consumption of grains has increased by 35 percent since 1970 (this increase is mainly driven by a 23 percent increased intake of wheat-based products and a 202 percent increased intake of corn-based products). Yes, swapping out the excess grain servings for fruits and vegetables in the average American diet would be a huge win.

And what about that 8.3 percent of people adhering to MyPlate? The USDA Dietary Guidelines for Americans' own analysis highlights nutrient shortfalls even for those who follow the guidelines perfectly. The 2015–2020 Dietary Guidelines for Americans delivers insufficient amounts of potassium, magnesium (for men over fifty), vitamin D, vitamin E, and choline;[19] and the 2020–2025 Dietary Guidelines for Americans delivers insufficient amounts of iron, vitamin D, vitamin E, choline, and vitamin B9 (folate).[20] That might explain some of the cynicism and apathy toward these guidelines.

Fad Diets, Like Throwing Kerosene onto a Fire

The vast majority of fad diets have restrictive dietary structures, meaning there's a collection of foods or food groups, or certain macronutrients, that are eliminated, reduced, restricted, or obsessively measured. What exactly you're supposed to cut out or cut down on will depend on which diet you're following. But regardless of what foods you're restricting when following these eating plans, the unintended consequence is that you're also reducing your intake of essential nutrients. In many cases, these diets are exacerbating nutrient insufficiencies rather than fixing them.

Just because something is harmful in large quantities doesn't mean it's harmful in any quantity. If truth be told, there is a startling lack of data corroborating the claims of most of popular diets, and in fact, studies have failed to demonstrate superiority of any specific diet. Instead, studies substantiate the benefits of eating patterns that focus on whole and minimally processed foods, emphasize plant foods, and avoid overeating.[21] These are all eating patterns that are reinforced by the Nutrivore philosophy.

Of course, we all have complex reasons for following our preferred diet, and it's absolutely okay if you resonate with a specific dietary philosophy, choose a specific diet for religious or health reasons, or have found success with a specific diet and opt to continue following it simply because it works for you. Nutrivore is not a diet itself nor a substitute for your preferred diet—I'm not here to change how you eat. Instead, Nutrivore is a diet modifier that can be applied to however you eat now to help you avoid common pitfalls from nutrient insufficiencies. Nutrivore will help you make those small changes that can make all the difference in the world.

Wondering how your diet stacks up in terms of nutrients? Here's a summary of the most common nutrient shortfalls among popular diets. (This doesn't mean that you are automatically deficient in all of these nutrients but rather that they are harder to get on your chosen diet.)

Vegan and vegetarian diets are commonly deficient in vitamin A, vitamin B3, vitamin B9, vitamin B12, calcium, chromium, copper, iodine, iron, magnesium, manganese, zinc, and omega-3 fats.[22]

Low-carb diets, such as the Atkins diet and South Beach diet, are commonly deficient in vitamin A, vitamin B2, vitamin B5, vitamin B6, vitamin B9, vitamin C, vitamin D, vitamin E, biotin, choline, calcium, chromium, iodine, iron, magnesium, molybdenum, potassium, zinc, and fiber.[23]

Low-fat diets are commonly deficient in vitamin A, vitamin D, vitamin E, vitamin K, calcium, and omega-3 fats.[24]

Calorie-restriction programs, such as Weight Watchers, Jenny Craig, and intermittent fasting, are commonly deficient in vitamin A, vitamin B_1, vitamin B_2, vitamin B_3, vitamin C, vitamin E, calcium, iron, magnesium, potassium, and zinc.[25]

Gluten-free diets are commonly deficient in vitamin D, vitamin B_3, vitamin B_9, vitamin B_{12}, iron, magnesium, calcium, zinc, and fiber.[26]

Paleo and primal diets are commonly deficient in calcium, chromium, biotin, vitamin B_9, choline, vitamin E, vitamin K, vitamin D, vitamin B_{12}, iron, magnesium, manganese, potassium, iodine, and selenium.[27]

Ketogenic diets are commonly deficient in vitamin A, vitamin B_2, vitamin B_5, vitamin B_6, vitamin B_9, vitamin E, vitamin D, vitamin K, biotin, choline, calcium, chromium, choline, iodine, iron, magnesium, molybdenum, potassium, selenium, zinc, and fiber.[28]

The good news is that you can increase the nutrient density of your current diet by overlaying a Nutrivore emphasis on top of the core dietary structure, selecting a wide variety of foods such that the body's nutrient requirements are met by the diet. And I'll teach you exactly how to do that in this book!

If you follow a diet where all food sources of specific nutrients are eliminated, a Nutrivore approach can still be used to improve the quality of the diet. However, in these cases, it's additionally important to work with a nutritionist, registered dietitian, or your doctor to identify nutrient shortfalls and supplement accordingly.

THE PROBLEM WITH WEIGHT-LOSS DIETS

The entire weight-loss and diet industry—which, by the way, was worth $276 billion in 2022[29]—is based on a false premise: that being overweight or obese is itself a health problem, even classifying obesity as a chronic illness.

Sure, many chronic diseases are associated with obesity, including heart disease, type 2 diabetes, nonalcoholic fatty liver disease, and cancer. But overweight and obesity are, in fact, poor proxies for measuring health and disease risk. A collection of important studies from the past twenty-five years has revealed that overweight and obesity themselves are not the risk factors but instead symptoms of an underlying health challenge (like chronic stress, gut dysbiosis, hypothyroidism, or insulin resistance) and/or are an indicator of poor health-related behaviors (like sedentary lifestyle or poor diet quality).[30] It is actually these factors, and not body weight itself, that increase risk of chronic illness.

It would be much more helpful from a medical perspective to dissociate weight from the risk assessment and instead look directly at health behaviors, like activity. A 2008 study busted the myth that overweight and obese individuals are all unhealthy, and that thin people are healthy by default.[31] This study showed that despite what one might assume, among overweight individuals, 51.3 percent were metabolically healthy; among obese individuals, 31.7 percent were metabolically healthy; and, among normal-weight individuals, 23.5 percent were actually metabolically abnormal. The authors also evaluated risk factors other than weight for poor metabolic health; physical activity was the most protective for all sizes, and the more active, the better.

It's even unclear whether being thin is healthier than being overweight. In 2013, a meta-analysis of 97 studies, including more than 2.88 million individuals and more than 270,000 deaths (can we just get a collective "wow" for what a huge dataset that is?), confirmed that class 1 obesity (defined as a body mass index, or BMI, between 30 and 35) was not associated with overall higher mortality, and that overweight was associated with significantly lower mortality, compared to normal-weight individuals.[32] (Don't get me started on how the BMI was invented to measure populations rather than individuals, and how it's a very flawed metric of our personal health because it doesn't consider body composition and simply reflects the ratio of our height to weight.) Incidentally, this study was published the same year the American Medical Association voted to label obesity as a disease, despite the fact that its own expert panel recommended against it.

Of course, the biggest problem with the diet and weight-loss industry is that it preys upon our insecurities and body dissatisfaction in order to propel sales. Studies show that 70 to 75 percent of women and 54 to 59 percent of men are preoccupied with body weight, leading to dieting and weight cycling; yes, the dreaded yo-yo diet.[33]

Yo-yo dieting is super problematic for our health because during weight loss, the body loses some muscle mass as well as body fat; but during the weight regain phase of yo-yo dieting, fat is regained more easily than muscle. The net effect is that yo-yo dieters have a greater risk for type 2 diabetes, cardiovascular disease, and nonalcoholic fatty liver disease than if they simply remained overweight or obese, in addition to having an increased risk of depression and eating disorders. For example, a 2018 study found that yo-yo dieters had a 1.43 times higher risk for heart attack, 1.41 times higher risk for stroke, and 2.27 times higher risk for all-cause mortality, adjusting for age, sex, smoking, alcohol, regular exercise, income, baseline fasting blood glucose, systolic blood pressure, total cholesterol, and BMI.[34]

All this to say that weight loss is not the primary goal of Nutrivore. I hope to direct your attention to developing habits that are much more meaningful from a long-term health perspective, like choosing more whole foods, eating plenty of vegetables, and eating a wide variety of foods.

Of course, if weight loss is a goal for you, then you'll be keen to learn that many people do experience weight loss when they choose more nutrient-dense whole foods, finding themselves more often satisfied with fewer calories. In fact, obesity is associated with key nutrient deficiencies, and studies show that increasing intake of vitamin A, vitamin B1, vitamin B3, vitamin B5, vitamin B6, vitamin D, biotin, coQ10, iron, carnitine, and creatine each facilitates healthy and maintainable weight loss.[35] I like to think of this as getting healthy to lose weight, rather than losing weight to get healthy. You can find some tips for healthy weight loss with Nutrivore in appendix A.

DON'T WASTE YOUR MONEY ON MULTIVITAMINS

Approximately one third of Americans take a daily multivitamin. Is this doing any good? Scientific studies tell us probably not.

Now, it's important to note that targeted supplementation recommended by a health care provider in response to laboratory test results indicating nutrient deficiency still has a role to play in the overall health equation. There are many situations where nutritional supplements are still indicated; for example, prenatal vitamins have an excellent track record for reducing risk of neural tube defects, like spina bifida. So we're not dissing all nutritional supplements here but instead simply questioning the concept of a multivitamin as nutritional insurance.

An important 2013 meta-analysis showed that multivitamins had absolutely no effect on all-cause mortality, nor on mortality associated with cardiovascular disease.[36] A 2018 meta-analysis showed that multivitamin and multimineral supplements provided absolutely no benefit to cardiovascular disease incidence or outcomes, including coronary heart disease and stroke.[37] And a 2013 systematic review showed no benefit of vitamin and mineral supplements in the prevention of cardiovascular disease or cancer.[38]

An important 2019 study helped to shed some light on this question by comparing the health effect of nutrients from foods versus supplements.[39] This study revealed that consuming sufficient vitamin A, vitamin K, magnesium, zinc, and copper from food—but not from supplements—reduced all-cause mortality and mortality associated with cardiovascular disease. Furthermore, excess calcium from supplements—but not from food—increased risk of mortality from cancer. Supplemental calcium is also associated with calcium oxalate kidney stones, and elevated serum levels of folic acid (a common form of vitamin B_9 found in supplements) have been associated with increased cancer risk and can mask vitamin B_{12} deficiency.[40] This study reinforces the importance of meeting our nutritional needs from food and even highlights some potential harmful effects from supplementation.

Bottom line: Talk to your doctor about whether they recommend a specific nutritional supplement. But in general, you just can't supplement your way out of a nutrient-poor diet.[41]

THE LIMITED BENEFITS OF FORTIFIED FOODS

If you've ever been told to avoid foods with ingredients you can't pronounce, well, that's just silly, because many of those big words on a food label are just vitamins and minerals added to fortify that food, that is, to increase its nutritional value. These are the same vitamin and mineral forms found in supplements, so fortification is a little like sprinkling some multivitamin powder over your breakfast cereal. Let's be clear: There's no reason to avoid fortified foods. But it is good to know the limits of their benefits, as yet more rationale for placing higher value on whole foods.

Food fortification goes way back: The first fortified food was iodized table salt, introduced in the 1920s. In the 1930s, fortification of milk with vitamin D began. The bread and cereal enrichment program started in the 1940s, adding B vitamins and iron to many grain products. And in the 1980s, calcium fortification became popular, adding calcium to everything from orange juice to breakfast cereal to almond milk.[42] In Australia and New Zealand, they even have calcium-fortified chewing gum.

Unfortunately, fortification has only yielded measurable benefit to a few health outcomes. Anemia has reduced 34 percent, risk of goiter has reduced 74 percent, and risk of neural tube defects has reduced 41 percent.[43] It's certainly not nothing, but it's also a drop in the bucket in terms of health challenges faced by the average person.

DITCH THE GUILT

Okay, so we've established the incredible magnitude of this problem, and in the next chapter, we'll get down to the fundamentals of how these nutrient insufficiencies are harming health. But I want to wrap up this particular topic with a really important message: Guilt and blame do not serve our goals.

It doesn't help you to feel shame or guilt about previous food or diet choices, even breakfast this morning! First of all, shame and guilt are strongly associated with disordered eating, from anorexia to binge eating, making these emotions a barrier to creating lasting improvements to diet quality. But second, I implore you to recognize that the reason you feel guilty about a food choice is because of a value judgment placed on that food. Somewhere along the road, you learned that that food was bad, and that you're bad for eating it. Let's transcend this old way of thinking about food.

On Nutrivore, there are no "good foods" or "bad foods"; instead we look at the quality of the whole diet. You can absolutely meet your body's nutritional needs from the foods you eat while choosing some foods that aren't particularly nutrient dense but are just plain tasty. It's okay if some of our food choices are centered around joy rather than nutrient density. One food will not make or break your diet, nor make or break your health.

It's never too late to improve diet quality and see a dividend in terms of health in return, and I'll actually share some statistics on this in the next chapter.

CHAPTER 2

Fix Your Diet (and Health) with Nutrivore

A 2019 systematic analysis showed that each year globally, poor diet quality is responsible for more deaths (about eleven million) and more disability (255 million disability-adjusted life years) than any other factor, including smoking, sedentary lifestyle, and high blood pressure.[1] In fact, approximately 60 percent of Americans have at least one diet-preventable disease, and 40 percent of Americans have two or more diet-preventable diseases.[2]

What does that mean? It means that higher diet quality could have prevented that disease from developing. It means that higher diet quality could save eleven million lives across the globe every year. It means 255 million more people on Earth could live without a disabling chronic illness if their diets were healthier.

The causes of poor diet quality are complex, and none of them are your personal failing. My goal is to empower you with the knowledge you need to improve your diet quality, while ditching the guilt so you can heal your relationship with food and your body. As we dive into the links between nutrition and just about every possible ailment, I want you to remember: This information is about bettering your future, not about relitigating the past.

Most diets and medical providers focus on the dietary excesses that increase risk for chronic and infectious disease: too many calories, too much added sugar, too much sodium, and too much saturated fat. But the much stronger link between diet choices and diet-preventable disease is what's lacking in these same diets: nutrients. To fully appreciate why focusing on adding nutrients to our diets is a far more powerful strategy to improve health than worrying about what to cut back on, let's start by more closely examining the link between nutrient insufficiency and health problems.

HOW NUTRIENT INSUFFICIENCY CONTRIBUTES TO DISEASE DEVELOPMENT

Diseases of nutrient deficiency are well defined. A lack of a single nutrient is behind the disease; we know what low level of intake of that specific nutrient will cause symptoms; and we know how much of that specific nutrient we need to consume to restore levels and reverse the disease. An example of this would be scurvy, where very low intake of vitamin C results in a potentially fatal disease of malnutrition in which collagen production is impaired. Only ten milligrams of vitamin C per day is necessary to prevent scurvy, although the recommended dietary allowance (RDA) of vitamin C is ninety milligrams for adult males and seventy-five milligrams for adult females.

But the effect of nutrient insufficiencies on disease risk is not so cut and dried. Instead, a collection of insufficiencies means that biological systems in the human body don't have the nutritional resources they need to function optimally. Over time, the strain this puts on that biological system gradually increases the risk for chronic diseases of that biological system. Usually, nutrient insufficiencies are not even the sole factor but instead interact with lifestyle—like sleep habits, stress levels, and how active you are—genetics, and the environment.

Even though the causes of these chronic conditions are complex, nutrition is a clear point of intervention. So you can better understand how low levels of a nutrient can increase risk of developing a chronic condition, let's look at one specific example: the link between low vitamin D and type 2 diabetes.

When we consume carbohydrates, our blood sugar increases. In response to that rise in blood sugar, the pancreas releases the hormone insulin, which facilitates the transport of glucose into the cells of the body. When insulin binds to its receptor, a series of biochemical events are triggered within the cell that ultimately result in the glucose transporter moving glucose from outside of the cell to inside of the cell. Insulin further signals to the liver to convert glucose into glycogen for short-term energy storage in liver and muscle tissues and into triglycerides for long-term energy storage in adipose (fat) tissues.

It's a beautifully efficient system . . . until things go wrong. Chronically elevated blood sugar levels stimulate adaptations within cells, rendering them less sensitive to insulin. These adaptations may include decreasing the number of receptors to insulin embedded within the cell membranes, and suppressing the signaling within the cell that occurs after insulin binds with its receptor. The decrease in insulin sensitivity causes the pancreas to secrete more and more insulin to lower the elevated blood glucose levels. This is called *insulin resistance*, when more insulin than normal is required to deal with blood glucose. When normal blood sugar levels can no longer be maintained, you get type 2 diabetes.

Over the past few decades, type 2 diabetes has reached epidemic proportions, skyrocketing from 108 million people worldwide in 1980 to over 422 million people today (according to 2022 World Health Organization data).[3] That includes 37.3 million people with diabetes in the United States alone, which is 11.3 percent of the entire US population (yes, more than one out of nine people in America have diabetes), of which 8.5 million Americans are living with undiagnosed diabetes.[4] And, if we think about all the additional cases of prediabetes and metabolic syndrome out there, those numbers shoot up even higher. In fact, prediabetes is estimated to affect an additional ninety-six million Americans, 38 percent of US adults.

Those are some awfully depressing statistics. The good news? Improving vitamin D levels could have an enormous impact.

There are several ways low vitamin D can contribute to the development of type 2 diabetes.[5] Let's talk about just two of them.

First, vitamin D deficiency results in less insulin being released by the pancreas when we eat carbohydrates. Not enough insulin reduces our capacity to lower high blood sugar levels.

Second, vitamin D affects how all the rest of the cells in our body respond to insulin. Low vitamin D decreases the number of insulin receptors our cells have in their membranes. Fewer receptors for insulin to bind to means fewer glucose transporters, thus reducing the cells' capacity to shuttle glucose into itself. And that's not all. Vitamin D deficiency also lowers glucose transporter activity, so each glucose transporter has a lower capacity to do its job of transporting glucose into the cell. Our cells aren't as responsive to insulin and we're making less of it.

Low Vitamin D Levels? Test, Don't Guess!

Scientists generally agree that the optimum level of vitamin D, as determined by a simple blood test that measures serum 25-hydroxyvitamin D concentration, is between 50 and 70 nanograms per milliliter. Vitamin D deficiency is defined as levels below twenty nanograms per milliliter, and insufficiency is defined as levels between twenty and thirty nanograms per milliliter. And this is shockingly common! Globally, about half of people are vitamin D deficient or insufficient.[6] In the United States, nearly 30 percent of people have vitamin D deficiency, and more than 40 percent of people have vitamin D insufficiency.[7]

Note that if you're deficient or insufficient, it can be very tough to get enough vitamin D from sun exposure and foods to bring levels up to the optimal range. Consider supplementing with vitamin D (2,000 to 5,000 IU daily is a standard dose to address deficiency,[8] but ask your health care provider for a recommendation based on your personal health history) and recheck levels with a blood test every three to six months to make sure both that you are getting enough vitamin D and that you don't overshoot the mark—vitamin D levels in excess of 150 nanograms per milliliter can also cause health problems.

In patients with metabolic syndrome, low levels of vitamin D (under thirty nanograms per milliliter) are linked to a higher risk of becoming fully diabetic,[9] and vitamin D supplementation has been shown to improve insulin sensitivity in people with type 2 diabetes.[10] Even in healthy individuals, vitamin D is positively associated with pancreatic beta cell function, insulin sensitivity, glucose homeostasis, glucose tolerance, and insulin sensitivity.[11] And across a spectrum of prospective studies, people with the highest (versus lowest) circulating vitamin D levels and/or vitamin D intakes have a consistently reduced risk of developing type 2 diabetes over many years.[12] For people already at high risk of the disease, every four nanograms per milliliter increase of serum vitamin D is estimated to reduce progression from prediabetes to diabetes by 25 percent![13]

Yes, the high prevalence of vitamin D insufficiency and deficiency are a major contributor to the high rates of prediabetes and type 2 diabetes. There are other nutrients involved in glucose metabolism and insulin signaling, and addressing low vitamin D is not the only intervention. But it can make a huge difference to type 2 diabetes risk, and the message remains: Upgrading your nutrition has the capacity to greatly improve your health, both today and over the long term.

Phew! That was just one example of how a nutrient insufficiency impacts the development and progression of a disease—every nutrient has multiple disease associations, and every ailment has multiple nutrient associations. The nickel-and-diming effect of nutrient insufficiencies gradually chips away at your health, increasing your risks for every disease and symptom under the sun, from type 2 diabetes to cancer, cardiovascular disease to Alzheimer's disease, headaches to PMS, asthma to osteoporosis, fatigue to increased susceptibility to infection. These important links between nutrient shortfalls and diseases and symptoms are summarized in appendix B. Of course, I'll discuss many of the most fascinating connections in part 2, and you can get even more into the nitty-gritty details at Nutrivore.com.

HEALTH IMPACTS BEYOND FOOD

Yes, we're talking about the essentiality of nutrients for supporting health and wellness, but I want to make sure we also acknowledge the importance of social determinants of health, health-related habits—like smoking, alcohol consumption, and drug abuse—social connection and support, stress levels, and lifestyle factors like activity and sleep. We can think of these factors as nourishment of the body beyond nutrients.

While this book is focused on how to improve your diet, it's important to understand that the foods we eat, while very consequential, are just one piece of the health puzzle.

Our behavior, including food and lifestyle choices, accounts for 40 to 50 percent of health outcomes. What contributes to the remainder? Roughly 30 percent of health outcomes are determined by genetics, 10 to 20 percent are determined by medical care, and 20 percent are determined by our social and physical environment.[14] The latter, accounting for one fifth of health outcomes, is also referred to as *social determinants of health.*

Social determinants of health have a major effect on people's health, well-being, and quality of life.[15] Examples of social determinants of health include safe housing, transportation, and neighborhoods; racism, discrimination, and violence; education, job opportunities, and income; access to nutritious foods and physical activity opportunities; polluted air and water; and language and literacy skills. Social determinants of health also contribute to health disparities and inequities. For example, people who don't have access to grocery stores with healthy foods are less likely to have good nutrition.[16] That raises their risk of health conditions like heart disease, type 2 diabetes, and obesity—and even lowers life expectancy relative to people who do have access to healthy foods. Yes, there's an integral connection between social determinants of health and other factors, including access and quality of medical care and our behavior.

Since social determinants of health affect access to healthy foods, I want to help by making healthy eating as easy and affordable as possible. In chapter 10, I will debunk food myths that stigmatize healthy foods, making you think you need to spend more money on groceries, or more time in the kitchen, in order to be healthy. Despite the scaremongering on the internet, foods like vegetable oil, white rice, canned beans and fish, conventional meat, and nonorganic vegetables are all healthy options. Furthermore, stress harms our health, and unnecessarily worrying about toxins in our foods or straining our food budget because we're afraid of certain foods does us a disservice. You'll learn more about sourcing healthy foods on a budget in chapter 11.

You'll also see the recurring theme in this book that progress is greater than perfection, and every better choice counts. I'll back up the health benefits we can glean from even small, affordable, and accessible changes—like grabbing a can of green beans at the gas station to add to dinner tonight, or choosing a side salad at the drive-through window in addition to your usual meal—with statistics from scientific studies. You do not need to eat a perfect diet to improve your health. In fact, I'd argue there's no such thing as a perfect diet. Instead, use the information in this book to guide the changes that make the most sense for you, given your circumstances, while recognizing that there's more to health than what's on, or not on, your plate.

YOU KEEP USING THAT TERM: ALL-CAUSE MORTALITY

"All-cause mortality" is a term used by epidemiologists to refer to death from any cause. It's used in studies to assess whether or not something benefits or harms our health on average. That something could be patterns of behavior (such as eating a specific food, exercising a specific amount, or smoking); social determinants of health (such as education, race/ethnicity, or zip code); environmental exposures (such as polluted air or drinking water); or biological factors (such as genetics, vitamin D status, or age). Sophisticated analyses are employed to account for confounding variables in these studies, and analyses typically account for things like age, sex, smoking status, socioeconomic status, race/ethnicity, education level, exercise, previous diagnoses, diet quality or levels of intake of certain foods, weight or BMI, and alcohol consumption.

When something increases or decreases all-cause mortality, even when all the confounding variables are controlled for, causality is not established, but rather a statistical link is created. These data must necessarily be followed up with mechanistic studies (cell culture or animal experiments that look at the causal biological pathways) and/or intervention studies (where you change something in one group of people and compare against a control group). Please know that I only discuss all-cause mortality data when mechanistic studies have established and explained causality.

Okay, so what do all-cause mortality data mean for us in real life? While there is a whole lot of variability, we can say that very roughly, decreasing all-cause mortality by 10 percent translates to an additional year of life on average.[17] So the more changes we make that reduce all-cause mortality, the longer we can live. A 2022 study estimated that adopting a healthier diet starting at age twenty—defined as eating more vegetables, fruits, legumes, fish, and whole grains, as well as a handful of nuts each day, while reducing ultraprocessed foods—could add nearly eleven years to the life span of females and thirteen years to the life span of males.[18] The same study showed that making these healthy diet changes at age sixty could still add eight additional years of life, and making these changes at age eighty could still add 3.4 years of life! It's never too late to benefit from healthy changes.

THE NUTRIVORE PHILOSOPHY

The alarming statistics discussed so far can be summarized in two main conclusions:

1. Almost nobody gets enough nutrients from the foods they eat.
2. Dietary nutrient shortfalls are worsening, if not driving, nearly every health problem.

While the scope of the problem is vast, it requires the simplest of solutions: Get all the nutrients our bodies need from the foods we eat.

That's it! Of course, even though the idea is basic, achieving this worthy goal is not easy to do, that is, unless you know how. The rest of this book is dedicated to teaching you exactly what it looks like to apply the Nutrivore philosophy to however you eat now.

The guiding principles of Nutrivore help us to choose foods such that the total of all the nutrients contained within those foods adds up throughout the day to meet or safely exceed our daily requirements for the full complement of essential and nonessential (but still very important) nutrients, while also staying within our caloric requirements. When we eat a diet replete in nutrients, we reduce our risk of future health problems while alleviating many of the symptoms we're currently facing.

The Nutrivore philosophy appreciates the inherent nutritional value of foods, but no food is off-limits. By extension, no singular food choice is a bad one, and Nutrivore fully embraces treats, cultural foods, and food traditions without derision. Nutrivore has a permissive dietary structure, rather than a restrictive one.

Have you ever told yourself you're not allowed to have a food because that food is bad for you? Or have you ever told yourself that you don't deserve a treat because you skipped a workout, ate something else earlier in the week that was off-plan, or just didn't like the number on the scale that morning? Studies show that dichotomous approaches to diet, i.e., diets defined by a yes-food list and no-food list (or variations of that concept), increase the risks both of developing eating disorders and regaining lost weight.[19]

Food prohibition tends to cause fixation and can trigger disinhibition. Disinhibition refers to when, after giving in to that one thing that was against your rules—that piece of cake or that day of being a couch potato—your health behaviors unravel, driving more and more unhealthy choices. Basically, disinhibition is the technical term for falling off the proverbial wagon.

In a 2007 study, kids were given a bowl of yellow and red M&M's

and told they could eat as many as they wanted.[20] In the first phase, one group of kids had no restrictions, whereas the other was told they weren't allowed to eat the red ones. In the second phase, both groups of kids were told they could eat as many M&M's as they wanted of either color. The kids who were at first prohibited from eating red M&M's had an increased desire for them. When the kids were finally allowed to eat whatever M&M's they wanted in the second phase, they ate a higher proportion of red ones compared to the kids who didn't have any restrictions. Perhaps not surprisingly, the kids who had food restrictions at home ate the most M&M's (and total calories) in the study, regardless of which group they were in.

This effect isn't limited to children. When we label a food as "bad" and tell ourselves we're not allowed to eat it, the net result is that we become fixated on that food. When we eventually succumb to our craving, our eating behaviors unravel, and the diet yo-yo begins its upwards momentum. This can also set the stage for disordered eating patterns.

Dismayingly, 77 percent of people who lose weight gain all the weight back (and often more) within five years.[21] And, while we've already discussed why weight loss is not a primary goal of Nutrivore, it's worth noting that the psychological and behavioral impacts of restricting disallowed foods, while certainly not the only reason, are a major contributor to yo-yo dieting. (Another major contributor to weight regain is the concurrent reduction in basal metabolic rate, meaning we burn fewer calories, and increase in the hunger hormone ghrelin, which drives up appetite, together making it harder and harder to stay in a caloric deficit.) If weight loss is a goal for you, understanding the psychological impact of food restriction and letting go of value judgments of foods (and yourself for eating them) is a prerequisite for healthy, maintainable weight loss.

While labeling foods as bad does us a disservice, on the flip side, self-compassion helps us stay on track rather than falling into disinhibited eating patterns. A 2021 study showed that among overweight and obese individuals, the ones who cut themselves some slack when they ate something off-plan were able to stick to their diets the best and persevere toward their weight-loss goals.[22] By applying self-compassion, it's so much easier to surround one less nutritious food choice with other healthier, more nutrient-dense food choices. And that's the Nutrivore way!

We measure success on Nutrivore by asking whether all the foods you eat altogether supply your body with the nutrients it needs. Furthermore, because we are able to store at least a modest amount of most nutrients, the goal isn't even meeting nutritional requirements for the whole diet on a daily basis but rather doing so on average. It's okay if you don't reach the recommended dietary allowance (RDA) for zinc one day, but it's a good idea to look for a way to incorporate more zinc-rich foods into your diet if you find yourself falling short most days. So we're looking at the collective nutritional contribution of all the foods we eat. Nutrivore is about the whole diet.

Why evaluate the quality of the whole diet rather than each individual food you eat, like most diets do?

First, there's no such thing as a nutritionally complete food or food group, meaning there's no single food that provides all the nutrients we need to thrive. As an example, what if you decided to eat only watercress because it's one of the most nutrient-dense foods in the world? Well, you'd get impressive amounts of vitamin C, vitamin K, and phytonutrients (especially carotenoids and glucosinolates, discussed in more depth in chapter 8), and if you ate enough of it (285 cups of watercress would get you to 2,000 calories), you could reach the RDA of most vitamins and minerals. But you'd still be lacking in vitamin D, vitamin B_{12}, choline, omega-3 fats, and some essential amino acids, especially methionine and tryptophan. You'd also miss out on the full diversity of polyphenols as well as some functional compounds that just aren't available in watercress, like taurine, carnitine, carnosine, creatine, ergothioneine, and thiosulfinates. Eventually, you'd develop megaloblastic anemia due to vitamin B_{12} deficiency (in contrast, pernicious anemia causes vitamin B_{12} deficiency), plus symptoms such as increased pain sensitivity and aggression due to tryptophan deficiency, and dementia from methionine deficiency. Yes, it's an extreme example, but it helps drive the point home that we necessarily must eat a variety of different foods that supply complementary nutrition in order to get the full range of nutrients that our bodies need.

Second, foods can fill important nutritional niches in a diet without being objectively nutrient dense. A great example of this is white rice, which is totally underwhelming from a nutrient density perspective, yet research has shown that white rice can indeed contribute to good health. This is thanks to its resistant starch content, which has significant prebiotic activity, meaning it feeds probiotic bacteria in our guts, greatly benefiting gut health and, by extension, overall health. In a 2011 study of more than eighty-three thousand Japanese adults, steamed rice consumption was associated with reduced risk of cardiovascular disease in men, even after adjusting for other diet and lifestyle factors.[23] The men who ate the most rice had a 30 percent reduced risk of coronary heart disease and heart failure, and an 18 percent reduced risk of cardiovascular disease, compared to the men who ate the least amount of rice.

Furthermore, not every food you eat needs to be the pinnacle of nutrient density in order for your whole diet to supply all the nutrition you need. There is room in a healthy diet for empty calories—let's call them quality-of-life foods. For example, let's say you enjoy a breakfast of a mushroom and spinach omelet, as well as yogurt and berries topped with some granola on the side; then you have chicken, lentil, and vegetable soup for lunch, an apple for a snack, and salmon with roasted potatoes and steamed veggies for dinner. Pat yourself on the back for such a nutrient-dense menu. Now what if you add a delicious slice of decadent chocolate cake for dessert? Does that sweet treat negate all the nutrients from the other foods you ate that day? Absolutely not! That slice of cake in no way takes away from all those healthy food choices throughout the day, plus you're most likely still within your caloric requirements, i.e., not overeating—take that pat on the back!

The more nutrient-dense foods you choose at each meal, the more room there is for quality-of-life foods while still reaching your nutrient goals and avoiding overeating. And you can maximize nutrient density with the weekly serving targets for each of the nutritionally distinct foundational Nutrivore foods highlighted in chapter 9. These serving targets are derived from studies that evaluate the health effects of various levels of consumption of different foods and food groups, and are set to the minimum amount to eat per week associated with most of the benefits. We'll get into the details in chapter 9, but for now, just know that the twelve Nutrivore foundational foods are:

vegetables in general
cruciferous vegetables (the cabbage family)
leafy vegetables
root vegetables
alliums (the onion family)
mushrooms

fruit in general
citrus fruits
berries

pulse legumes
nuts and seeds
seafood

Before you accidentally apply a typical diet mindset to this list of foundational foods, let me emphasize that this does not mean these are the only foods you eat, nor are these the only nutrient-dense or healthy food options, nor does this even mean that you *have to* eat these foods to be a Nutrivore. I am highlighting these food families because they each offer something special nutritionally that when combined most easily contribute to us meeting our nutritional needs from the foods we eat. These foods expedite reaching the goal of getting all the nutrients our bodies need from the foods we eat, so you can truly stop counting, weighing, measuring, or otherwise overthinking your food choices.

It's important to emphasize that a Nutrivore approach isn't about perfection. With there being no foods that are strictly off-limits (unless you have an allergy, intolerance, or strong aversion to it, of course), we can take a step back from diet dogma. We can ditch the guilt associated with eating an off-plan food because there are no off-plan foods on Nutrivore! To simplify the Nutrivore philosophy into a catchy tagline, it's nourishment, not judgment.

NUTRIVORE IS A DIET MODIFIER

Frankly, the last thing we need is another diet. Good thing for us, Nutrivore is not a diet itself but rather a food philosophy or diet modifier. By deepening your understanding of what nutrients do in the body and which foods supply them, you can apply Nutrivore principles atop other dietary structures, intuitive eating, or anti-diet, thereby increasing your consumption of vital nutrients that are essential for your health.

Despite the long-established recommended daily intake levels of essential nutrients and the increasing awareness of the importance of nonessential nutrients (like coenzyme Q10 and polyphenols), no mainstream or fad diet, or government dietary guidelines, have ever integrated the concept of completely meeting our nutritional needs from the foods we eat. But that doesn't mean that we *can't* integrate the Nutrivore philosophy into these diet plans.

In fact, there are myriad combinations of foods we can eat in a day that will supply the full complement of nutrients that our bodies need to thrive. You can customize your food choices to fit not only your preferred diet but also your food preferences, budget, and how much time you have to prepare foods. But doing so does require nutrient awareness, meaning some basic knowledge of what nutrients do in the body, what foods contain them, and how to combine nutritionally complementary foods in order to get the full range of nutrients your body needs. The great news is that once you have this basic knowledge, you can choose foods within your preferred dietary framework to easily improve the nutritional quality of your diet.

That's the goal of part 2 in this book, to teach you the base knowledge you need to give you the confidence in your food decisions moving forward, so you can successfully implement Nutrivore in your kitchen. I will teach you the importance of specific nutrients and what foods supply those nutrients, as well as which foods are most strongly associated with better health outcomes, all outside of any specific dietary framework. But don't think these chapters will be a snooze fest—I've tracked down dozens of superfascinating studies, incorporated amusing historical anecdotes, and highlighted the relevance of specific nutrients to your health challenges. I promise you won't feel like you're back in class but instead like your social media feed is so chock-full of useful tidbits that you keep scrolling for hours.

RISK IS A VOLUME KNOB, NOT A LIGHT SWITCH

If you're already starting to feel overwhelmed by a health to-do list, let me quickly remind you that you don't need to make every better choice, every day, starting immediately, and forever after.

Risk for disease is not an on-off switch, where if you do everything perfectly, you have no risk, and if you fall short of that high bar, you have high risk. Instead, think of risk for disease as a volume knob. Every good choice you make turns the volume down, lowering your risk for an undesirable health outcome. Some suboptimal choices will turn the volume up, increasing your risk, and many will simply have no effect—you might have missed out on a chance to turn the volume down, but that choice isn't hurting anything either. The goal here is to make more volume-lowering choices than volume-raising ones, overall bettering your chances of good lifelong health.

I will say it yet again: No one decision, nor one food eaten, nor one workout missed, nor one late night, is going to make or break your health. And there's a huge benefit to acknowledging that our health is affected by long-term patterns rather than any given choice on any given day: it allows us to avoid disinhibition, a fall off the proverbial wagon triggered by eating something that's against the rules. If instead we can remember that disease risk is a volume knob, and our next choice is another opportunity to lower the volume, it's easier to not let that one decision make us give up on trying. As we start stacking those good choices, we also start to develop them into healthy habits, which means that making those better choices becomes automatic and easy.

Yes, every better choice counts.

CHAPTER 3

The Nutrivore Score

The Nutrivore Score is a tool to identify the most nutrient-dense options within every food group and subgroup, to inform your day-to-day choices.

The term "nutrient density" refers to the concentration of nutrients (mainly vitamins and minerals, but also protein, fiber, phytonutrients, and other micronutrients) per calorie of food. High nutrient-density foods supply a wide range of nutrients (or alternatively, high levels of a specific, important nutrient) relative to the calories they contain. In fact, this is the entire premise of the Nutrivore Score system—a way to quantify the nutrient density of foods and make the nutritional evaluation of foods objective.

THE SCIENTIFIC BACKDROP FOR THE NUTRIVORE SCORE

The concept of a nutrient-dense food was first defined in the 1970s as any food that provided "significant amounts of essential nutrients" per serving. Because of a lack of formal criteria for determining whether or not a food met this definition, inconsistent and subjective standards were applied, largely built around broad food groups, and overly focused on fat and sugar content as problematic, rather than vitamins, minerals, and other important nutrients as beneficial. As a result, some foods were labeled as unhealthy, like nuts, olives, and avocadoes, purely because of their fat content—we now recognize these foods contain heart-healthy fats that reduce cardiovascular disease risk.

In addition, the terms "good source" and "excellent source" were coined, defined as providing 10 or 20 percent of the daily value respectively of a specific nutrient per serving. As a result, some nutritionally underwhelming foods were labeled as healthy based on being a good source of a single nutrient. For example, a sugary fruit punch can include the phrase "A good source of vitamin C" on its label if it contains 10 percent of our daily vitamin C per glass.

In the early 2000s, the definition of nutrient density was updated—instead of referring to nutrients per serving, nutrient density is now defined as a measure of nutrients per calorie.[1] This switch came from acknowledging that almost everyone had dietary shortfalls of essential nutrients, while consuming abundant, often overabundant, calories. We needed a way to help people consume more nutrients for each calorie, rather than more servings of foods.

Thus, nutrient profiling was born, the science of categorizing foods according to their nutritional composition.[2] In 2006, the European Commission proposed that nutrient profiles should be used in order to make nutrition and health claims. What followed was the development by scientists of a confusing array of relatively similar methods to quantify the nutritional value of foods, including (but not limited to) nutrient for calorie (NFC), calorie for nutrient (CFN), nutritious food index (NFI), naturally nutrient rich score (NNR), nutrient-rich foods (NRF) index, nutrient adequacy score (NAS), and nutrient density score (NDS).[3] But despite two decades of work, none of these nutrient-density scores have yet been adopted by any agency or institution. Why? They're just not ready for prime time.[4]

When you look at how foods stack up using these various nutrient-density scores, the results don't quite add up. When the NNR of 120 foods was compared to the average healthiness ratings from more than seven hundred registered dietitians, nutritionists, and other health professionals, there was only 62 percent agreement.[5] That means that for 38 percent of foods, the NNR showed that the food was healthy, whereas health professionals disagreed, or the other way around. Certainly, some of this difference can be explained by the unearned reputation of some foods swaying the scores given by the health professionals, but the bigger issue is that the NNR uses only fourteen nutrients in its calculation. When the quality of people's diets was evaluated using the NRF compared to the Healthy Eating Index, it did not align particularly well—the NRF only explained 44.5 percent of the variance in the Healthy Eating Index.[6] The most complex algorithmically of the nutrient profiling systems is the Food Compass, which incorporates fifty-four food attributes into its calculation, including assessing things like additives and processing. However, the Food Compass has been criticized because it weighs certain attributes more heavily, which skews the results toward plant foods in a way that doesn't reflect the current scientific literature. For example, Lucky Charms cereal scores twice as high as ground beef or cheddar cheese, and a boiled egg scores the same as pineapple canned in heavy syrup.[7]

So with a complete lack of consensus in the scientific community on the best way to measure nutrient density, I developed my own nutrient profiling method, the Nutrivore Score.

The Nutrivore Score is built on the scientific foundation already laid by studies in the field of nutrient profiling. The best way to make this calculation comprehensive and unbiased was easy for me to see, perhaps because I have no loyalty to government dietary guidelines, no food lobby breathing down my neck, no prejudgment on which foods should score high or low, and no feeling of any necessity to align a nutrient-density score with any specific diet.

WHAT GOES INTO THE NUTRIVORE SCORE CALCULATION

Now before you get worried, no, I'm not going to ask you to do any math! I have done all the calculations for you. Not only can you search the entire Nutrivore Score database at Nutrivore.com but I've also included Nutrivore Scores for all the most common whole foods and ingredients in appendix D (see page 299).

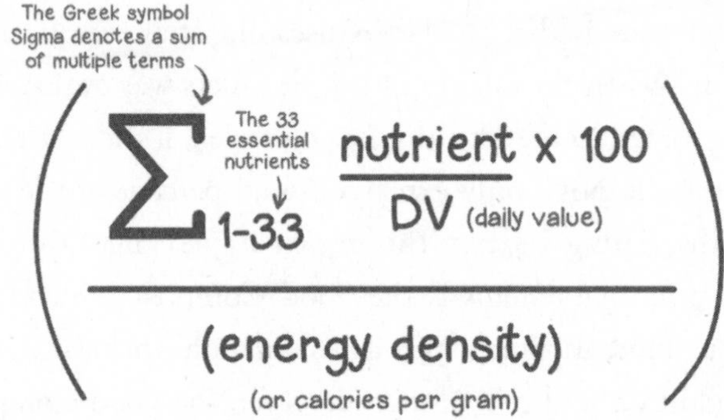

TL;DR: The Nutrivore Score is a measure of the total amount of nutrients per calorie of a food. The Nutrivore Score is calculated as the sum of each of thirty-three nutrients relative to its daily value present in the food, divided by the food's energy density. By dividing the amount of each nutrient by its daily value, we're factoring into the calculation how much of each nutrient our bodies require. And by dividing by the energy density—i.e., the calories per serving—we're converting the sum of percent daily values to a measure of total nutrients per calorie.

The nutrients used in the Nutrivore Score calculation are protein, fiber, calcium, copper, iron, magnesium, manganese, phosphorous, potassium, selenium, zinc, vitamin A, vitamin B_1 (thiamin), vitamin B_2 (riboflavin), vitamin B_3 (niacin), vitamin B_5 (pantothenic acid), vitamin B_6 (pyridoxine), vitamin B_7 (biotin), vitamin B_9 (folate), vitamin B_{12} (cobalamin), vitamin C, vitamin E, vitamin D, vitamin K, choline, monounsaturated fat, linoleic acid, alpha-linolenic acid (ALA), the long-chain omega-3 fatty acids eicosapentaenoic acid (EPA) and docosahexaenoic acid (DHA), carotenoids, phytosterols, and polyphenols.

The main dataset for the calculation is the USDA Food Central Database. Unfortunately, it's surprising how much nutrition information is missing from this database. So my team and I have filled as many gaps as possible from scientific papers and other databases like Phenol

Explorer and other national databases such as Fineli, the nutrition database maintained by the Finnish Institute for Health and Welfare. Where the level of several nutrients in a food remains unknown, the Nutrivore Score is marked with a footnote to denote that the score is likely underestimated for that food and should be thought of as a minimum.

The Nutrivore Score calculation also adds the highest value of available data for one bonus nutrient, relative to a threshold set using epidemiological studies for that nutrient, similar to a percent daily value. The bonus nutrient can be any of the following: glucosinolates, thiosulfinates, coenzyme Q10 (coQ10), conjugated linolenic acid (CLA), betaine, betalains, myo-inositol, ergothioneine, taurine, and medium-chain triglycerides. The reason only one bonus nutrient is included in the Nutrivore Score is because these are all nutrients for which there is limited data—too much incomplete data would mean less commonly studied foods are unnecessarily penalized.

INSIGHT FROM THE NUTRIVORE SCORE

The Nutrivore Score is an amazing lens through which to view food, and the results are a surprise a minute. Without this calculation, who would have guessed that strawberries are about twice as nutrient dense as blueberries? Or that cantaloupe has about double the nutrients per calorie of honeydew? Who knew that iceberg lettuce is slightly *more* nutrient dense than artichokes, celery, and sockeye salmon? Or that beef liver and kale have about the same nutrient density? Who could have predicted that fennel and whitefish are equally nutrient dense? Or that dark-meat turkey is more nutrient dense than light meat turkey? Or that the single most nutrient-dense food is . . . wait for it . . . canned clam liquid?

Some of these nonintuitive results come from comparing high-energy-density foods with low-energy-density foods.

Kale has a Nutrivore Score of 4,233, making it one of the most nutrient-dense foods on the planet. Per 2-cup serving, kale delivers 2.1 grams of fiber, 162 percent daily value vitamin K, 60 percent daily value biotin, 54 percent daily value vitamin C, 20 percent daily value manganese, 13 percent daily value vitamin A and vitamin B_2, 12 percent daily value alpha-linolenic acid (ALA), 10 percent daily value calcium, 4,580 micrograms of carotenoids, 159 milligrams of glucosinolates, and 178 milligrams of polyphenols—all for just nineteen calories. That makes kale a very valuable food!

There's only a 5 percent difference in Nutrivore Score between kale and beef liver. Beef liver has a Nutrivore Score of 4,021, so it also qualifies as one of the most nutrient-dense foods on the planet. Per 3.5-ounce serving, beef liver delivers 2,471 percent daily value vitamin B_{12}, 1,084 percent daily value copper, 552 percent daily value vitamin A, 333 percent daily value biotin, 212 percent daily value vitamin B_2, 143 percent daily value vitamin B_5, 82 percent daily value vitamin B_3, 73 percent daily value folate, 72 percent daily value selenium, 64 percent daily value vitamin B_6, 61 percent daily value choline, 36 percent daily value zinc, 31 percent daily value phosphorus, 27 percent daily value iron, 16 percent daily value vitamin B_1, and 13 percent daily value manganese, plus 20.4 grams of protein—and all for only 135 calories. Wow!

Kale and beef liver, while comparably nutrient-dense, do not contribute equal nutrients to our diets. When we look per serving, we see that kale delivers 50 percent daily value or more of three essential nutrients, whereas liver delivers more than half your recommended intake of eleven essential nutrients. These are both awesome food choices that contribute different nutrients to our diets, and ideally we'd incorporate both into our meal plans. We can say the same for the comparison of fennel to whitefish or sockeye salmon to iceberg lettuce.

Very-low-energy-density foods can have extremely high Nutrivore Scores if they offer good amounts of even a single nutrient. For example, coffee and tea, with average Nutrivore Scores of 6,832 and 3,721, respectively, offer very high amounts of polyphenols for just two calories per cup. On the flip side, very-high-energy-density foods must offer enormous amounts of multiple nutrients to boost their score even a little bit. For example, walnuts are jam-packed with healthy fats, biotin, vitamin E, copper, and manganese, but because they also deliver 183 calories per ounce, their Nutrivore Score comes out to a middling 303.

So the first lesson here is the importance of using the Nutrivore Score only to compare highly related foods. For example, cantaloupe, with its Nutrivore Score of 457, beats out honeydew, which has a Nutrivore Score of 228, thanks to much higher levels of vitamin A, vitamin C, carotenoids, and polyphenols. We can similarly use the score to identify the most nutrient-dense mushroom (enoki, with a Nutrivore Score of 4,434); leafy vegetable (watercress is the most nutrient dense you're likely to find at the store or farmers' market, with a Nutrivore Score of 6,929, but if you want to grow your own, garden cress is actually the highest, with a Nutrivore Score of 11,265); seafood (Eastern oysters are at the top, with a Nutrivore Score of 3,049); or apple (Granny Smith, with a Nutrivore Score of 204).

Other nonintuitive results from comparing Nutrivore Scores come from years of diet culture programming going against what the data actually says. Iceberg lettuce is not just "crunchy water" or the nutritional equivalent of cardboard—it's impressively nutritious thanks to its vitamin K, folate, manganese, and polyphenol content, while being a low-calorie food. Although light-meat turkey is leaner, you get more nutrition overall from dark-meat turkey, including double the amount of zinc and more than three times the amount of vitamin B_{12}. And while blueberries are definitely a fantastic choice with their impressive Nutrivore Score of 396 and lots of scientific studies supporting the health claims, strawberries, blackberries, and raspberries are all even more nutrient dense—their Nutrivore Scores are 762, 743, and 491, respectively, thanks to overall higher vitamin content—and equally as health promoting in scientific studies.

How does canned clam liquid earn its chart-topping Nutrivore Score of 14,744? A one-cup serving has only five calories, making it a very-low-energy-density food, but delivers an impressive 500 percent daily value vitamin B_{12}, 104 percent daily value copper, 22 percent daily value phosphorus, 18 percent daily value selenium, 8 percent daily value potassium, 6 percent daily value magnesium and choline, 5 percent daily value vitamin E, and 4 percent daily value vitamin B_2 and iron. Clam chowder, anyone?

The Nutrivore Score reinforces the value of whole foods, but also shows that minimally processed options like frozen vegetables and canned fish are almost as nutrient dense, and sometimes more so, than the raw, fresh version of these foods. For example, fresh broccoli has a Nutrivore Score of 2,833, whereas frozen unprepared broccoli has a Nutrivore Score of 2,925. Raw Brussels sprouts have a Nutrivore Score of 2,817, whereas frozen is nearly identical at 2,815. And canned pink salmon has a Nutrivore Score of 752, whereas raw fresh pink salmon fillet has a Nutrivore Score of 625. Yes, we can finally view these budget-friendly options as the nutritional equivalent of the more expensive fresh options, and stop feeling guilty about reaching for convenience.

A key tenet of the Nutrivore Score system is that all foods lie on a spectrum of nutrient density. There is no cusp above which a food is "good" and below which a food is "bad." While any food with a Nutrivore Score over 150 contributes more nutrients than calories to the diet, there are plenty of examples of foods with lower scores that are still incredibly valuable sources of nutrients. For example, cheese has an average Nutrivore Score of 140 but is also the most concentrated food source of calcium.

HOW TO USE THE NUTRIVORE SCORE

The best way to use the Nutrivore Score is to identify the most nutrient-dense option within the foods you like, have access to, and can afford.

For example, let's say you're planning on roasting chicken for dinner, and want to serve it with something starchy and some kind of steamed vegetable. Instead of a dinner roll (with a Nutrivore Score of 130), consider a baked sweet potato (Nutrivore Score of 497) or butternut squash (Nutrivore Score of 718). And instead of steaming green beans (Nutrivore Score of 605), swap them out for asparagus (Nutrivore Score of 1,385) or broccoli (Nutrivore Score of 2,833). Making spaghetti? Instead of regular pasta (Nutrivore Score of 145), consider whole wheat pasta (Nutrivore Score of 202); options made with edamame, chickpeas, or lentils (Nutrivore Scores up to 509); zoodles (aka zucchini noodles; Nutrivore Score of 1,477); or baked spaghetti squash (Nutrivore Score of 297). You also can't go wrong by adding a serving of berries to your breakfast, veggies and dip or hummus to your lunch, or a side salad to your dinner.

Anytime you can swap out a lower Nutrivore Score food or ingredient for a higher one, you're upping your overall nutrient intake. You can apply this to your choice of breakfast cereals, pizza toppings, snack foods, salad dressings, sandwich fixings, barbecue side dishes—everything you eat! A list of seven hundred common foods and their Nutrivore Scores can be found at the back of this book, and you can look up the Nutrivore Scores of thousands more foods at Nutrivore.com.

Another great strategy to up the nutrient density of your meals is to simply season liberally with herbs and spices, which has the added bonus of boosting flavor. For example, let's say you add one tablespoon of chopped garlic (about three cloves), which has a Nutrivore Score of 5,622, and a half cup of chopped fresh basil, which has a Nutrivore Score of 3,381, to an entire forty-ounce jar of store-bought marinara sauce to liven it up. That would boost the Nutrivore Score of your spaghetti sauce from 575 to 707! And many condiments are very nutrient dense. For example, hot sauce has a Nutrivore Score of 1,193, mustard has a Nutrivore Score of 718, fish sauce has a Nutrivore Score of 593, and soy sauce has a Nutrivore Score of 433.

There is a caveat when it comes to the Nutrivore Score. If you find yourself obsessing over nutrient-density gamification, or finagling high–Nutrivore Score swaps or additions in a way that detracts from your enjoyment of the foods you're eating, then I want you to disregard the Nutrivore Score completely. The Nutrivore Score is a superuseful tool, but not every tool works for every person, and thankfully for us, it isn't the only one in our nutrient-density toolbox.

If this seems a little overwhelming, don't worry, you will gain more clarity on how to refine food choices in part 3. I have created other resources to help you implement Nutrivore principles without sweating the Nutrivore Score, so if you would prefer, you can instead just use the Nutrivore Meal Map (see page 66) and Weekly Serving Matrix (see page 234). The Nutrivore Score was instrumental for the development of these resources, but you don't need to compare scores to use them. Instead, you can use the healthy eating patterns identified through the Nutrivore philosophy to guide food choices, all while embracing flexibility and flavor without guilt or seeking perfection.

THE TOP ONE HUNDRED NUTRIVORE SCORE FOODS

You can buy nutrient-dense foods at any grocery store and in almost any aisle.

Here are the one hundred most nutrient-dense whole foods that can be found at just about any grocery store year-round, ranked by Nutrivore Score. (I didn't include foods that you're likely only to find at specialty stores or would need to grow yourself, but these are included in appendix D if you're curious.) Shopping from this list is a great way to up the nutrient density of your whole diet. Remember, frozen and canned options are great!

The Nutrivore Scores in the table below are calculated using the nutrition data for the raw, fresh version of the food, unless stated otherwise. Some of the scores are an average of representative foods—such as averaging Swiss and rainbow chard for chard and averaging green, black, and oolong tea for tea—and are marked with an asterisk when that's the case.

Top 100 Nutrivore Score Foods

Food	Nutrivore Score
*Coffee	6,832
*Chard	6,386
Turnip greens	6,370
Radishes	5,863
Garlic	5,622
Parsley	5,491
Mustard greens	5,464
Spinach	4,548
Shiitake mushroom	4,343
Kale	4,233
*Tea	3,721
*Liver	3,692
Chives	3,531
Bok choy (aka pak choy, Chinese cabbage)	3,428
Basil	3,381
Collard greens	3,323
Curly endive (aka chicory greens)	3,086
Broccoli	2,833
Brussels sprouts	2,817
Red leaf lettuce	2,684
*Oysters	2,652
Cilantro (aka coriander leaves)	2,609
Oyster mushroom	2,550
Kohlrabi	2,497
*Kidney	2,543
Radicchio	2,471

Food	Nutrivore Score
Endive (aka Belgian endive, chicory spear)	2,390
Chinese broccoli (aka Chinese kale, gai lan)	2,365[1]
Cremini mushroom (aka brown mushroom, Italian brown mushroom, baby bella)	2,279
Green leaf lettuce	2,245
Romaine lettuce (aka cos lettuce)	2,128
Green onions	2,097
Arugula (aka rocket)	2,019
Cabbage, green	2,034
Beets	2,013
Turnip	1,954
Dillweed	1,940
Butterhead lettuce (aka Boston lettuce, Bibb lettuce)	1,934
White button mushroom	1,872
Summer squash	1,596
Cauliflower	1,585
Mussels	1,564
Laver (aka nori)	1,520
*Tomatoes	1,501
Portobello mushroom	1,483
Zucchini	1,477
Asparagus	1,385
Cabbage, red	1,369
*Peppers, sweet (aka bell peppers)	1,226
Leeks	1,128
*Crab	1,114
*Peppers, hot chili	1,111

Food	Nutrivore Score
Clams	1,046
Pumpkin	1,036
Cocoa, unsweetened	1,024
Herring	996
*Mint	962[2]
Mackerel	922
*Kimchi, sauerkraut	904
Alfalfa sprouts	902
Carrots	899
Squid	890
Okra	859
Lobster	839
Anchovies	805
Iceberg lettuce	773
Artichokes	771
Celery	767
Rutabaga (aka swede)	766
Strawberries	762
*Tuna	752
Flatfish (aka flounder, sole)	749
Blackberries	743
Shallots	740
*Salmon	731
Mung bean sprouts	711
Pickles, sour	702
Brazil nuts	694
*Trout	678
Butternut squash	670

Food	Nutrivore Score
Edible-podded peas	669
Fennel	663
Whitefish	663
Sardines (canned in oil)	654
Scallops	645
Papaya	636
Pears, Asian	621
Green beans (aka green snap beans)	605
Eggplant (aka aubergine)	563
Catfish, wild	559
Swordfish	557
Snapper	548
Persimmons, Japanese (aka kaki fruit)	537
Shrimp	535
Halibut	523
Plums	521
Flaxseed (aka linseed)	515
Raspberries	491
Lentils	489
*Kiwi	477

1 Nutrivore Score may be higher, since 10 to 25% of data is missing.

2 Nutrivore Score is likely higher, since 25 to 50% of data is missing.

* Average of representative foods

CHAPTER **4**

Easy Steps to Nutrivore

This chapter summarizes all the easy action steps to increase your nutrient intake, so you can start being a Nutrivore at your very next meal!

I'm a firm believer that knowledge is power. The more we understand why certain foods are nutritionally important, and the more we grasp how our specific health challenges are linked to nutrients, the more motivating it is to change how we eat. But you don't need a graduate degree in nutritional sciences to start choosing more nutrient-dense foods; you don't even need to finish reading this book (although I hope you will; there are some really fascinating studies to talk about and crazy interesting fun facts for me to dispense, not to mention a few choice puns). This chapter is for all you go-getters eager to start effecting change in your life, starting with your very next dinner plate.

I confess I have an ulterior motive for putting all these easy steps to Nutrivore toward the beginning of this book, before you get to read all the captivating stories I've written about individual nutrients. I want you to see just how straightforward a Nutrivore approach really is. With just a few small changes to your current diet, you can make huge improvements in your nutrient intake.

So what are these easy steps? Let's break it down.

CHOOSE MOSTLY WHOLE FOODS

To understand why whole foods are so fundamental to a healthy diet, all we need to do is define what they are. *Whole foods* are those in which the inherent nutrients are still intact. Mic drop! I mean, it's tough to argue against the value of whole foods when we're prioritizing nutrients. But let's go into a bit more detail anyway, not just to drive this point home but to reveal some of the interesting nuance here.

Whole foods may be completely unprocessed—such as raw carrots, apples, or berries. Or they may be minimally processed, which can include removal of inedible parts (like shelling or peeling), drying, crushing, cooking without adding ingredients (roasting, boiling, steaming, etc.), freezing, or pasteurization—such as roasted chicken, steamed broccoli, a peeled banana, or unsalted mixed nuts.

Processing is any treatment of a whole food that alters it from its natural state, including removing otherwise edible parts (like removing the bran and germ from brown rice to make white rice), or by adding ingredients (like salt, oil, and sugar). Examples of processed foods include white rice, all-purpose flour, fruits canned in syrup, or sardines canned in oil with added salt. This type of processing can remove some, although not all, of the inherent nutrients. Many processed foods (like canned vegetables and fish) are still nutrient-dense options.

Ultraprocessed foods are made mostly or entirely from ingredients extracted from foods through a series of industrial techniques and processes. The more processed or refined a food is, the more nutrients are degraded and ultimately stripped out of it, so one of the things these foods have in common, besides being super convenient and addictively delicious, is they tend to have very little to offer in terms of essential nutrients. Examples of ultraprocessed products include soft drinks, energy drinks, salty packaged snacks, candy, packaged bread and cookies, cake and cake mixes, margarine and other spreads, sweetened breakfast cereal, deli meats, American cheese, chicken or fish nuggets, hot dogs, instant soups, and regular pasta noodles.

It's worth noting that ultraprocessed foods can be made with organic, non-GMO ingredients and sold in health food stores, with deceptive labels that make you feel good about an alternative that doesn't have any more nutrition to offer than what you're swapping it out for—this is sometimes referred to as the "health halo" effect, or "greenwashing."

But if you're lamenting giving up one of your favorite foods, stick with me for a few more paragraphs. I promise the news isn't all bad.

Let's start with what happens when we eat a lot of ultraprocessed foods. Besides providing the dopamine rush that drives hunger, cravings, and food addiction, the more ultraprocessed foods we eat, the higher our risks of obesity, cancer, type 2 diabetes, cardiovascular disease, depression, and dementia.[1]

A 2019 prospective study of nearly twenty thousand Spanish university graduates (average age was thirty-seven at the beginning of the study) followed for fifteen years showed that after accounting for confounding variables, people who consumed four or more servings of ultraprocessed foods daily had a 62 percent increased risk of total mortality.[2] Plus, with every additional daily serving of ultraprocessed foods above that amount, risk of total mortality went up another 18 percent. A similar 2022 study out of the UK, which followed more than sixty thousand people over the age of forty for ten years, showed that people who got 43 percent or more of their calories from ultraprocessed foods had a 17 percent higher risk of cardiovascular disease and a 22 percent higher risk of total mortality than people getting 20.8 percent or less of their calories from ultraprocessed foods.[3] A 2021 meta-analysis calculated that for every 10 percent of our daily calories that comes from ultraprocessed foods, our risk of total mortality goes up by 15 percent.[4] Yikes!

Despite those scary statistics, this doesn't actually mean that ultraprocessed foods can't fit into a healthy diet. Just because something is harmful in large quantities doesn't mean that it's harmful in any quantity. The Spanish study above shows us that there isn't much effect on health if we stay below about two or three servings of ultraprocessed foods per day; the British study above measured that cusp of negative effect at about one fifth of our daily caloric intake. And there's definitely enough data to say that a couple of servings of ultraprocessed foods per day, especially in the context of an otherwise whole foods diet, is not going to have a meaningful effect on our health.

A 2022 meta-analysis showed that not all ultraprocessed foods are equally problematic.[5] While sugar-sweetened beverages, artificially sweetened beverages, and processed meat all increased risk of total morality, breakfast cereals were associated with lower mortality. The people who consumed the most breakfast cereals (including everything from oatmeal and All-Bran to Fruity Pebbles and Lucky Charms) had a 15 percent lower mortality risk than the people who consumed the least breakfast cereal; and those who mainly consumed whole grain breakfast cereals had a 23 percent lower mortality risk. (Those who only consumed sugary cereals had no change in mortality risk.) This may reflect the fortification of breakfast cereals, meaning they have more to offer nutritionally than, for example, a can of cola, in addition to the fiber content of whole grain breakfast cereals. Certainly, more research is needed to fully understand which ultraprocessed foods get an exemption from the list of foods that increase risk of health problems.

That's right, I'm saying that you don't need to completely give up ultraprocessed foods. Aren't you glad you stuck with me? I think a fair interpretation of the current scientific evidence is that if you're meeting your body's nutritional needs from the 80 percent of your diet that is whole and minimally processed foods, the 20 percent of your calories that comes from ultraprocessed foods is unlikely to cause any harm. Some people refer to this as the eighty-twenty rule. What would that look like? If you eat a two-thousand-calorie-per-day diet, that would translate to four hundred calories from your favorite packaged or fast food, about what you'd get in a quarter pounder with cheese, seven Oreo cookies (five and a half, if Double Stuf), one slice of pepperoni pizza, or a medium glazed doughnut plus a can of Coke.

Remember, risk is a volume knob, not an off switch. No one food will make or break your health. By choosing mostly nutrient-dense whole foods, you can still achieve your Nutrivore goals—and dial that volume knob way down—while including some quality-of-life foods, even if they are the emptiest of calories.

I have an important caveat, though. Approximately one fifth of people globally are addicted to ultraprocessed foods.[6] If continuing to incorporate a few ultraprocessed foods into your diet is driving disordered eating habits (like binging or purging) or food addiction (like if you're jonesing for your Twinkies when you try to cut back), then you may benefit from eliminating them completely; you might additionally benefit from working with an eating disorder specialist.

Choosing mostly whole foods is also the easiest way to moderate added sugars and sodium intake. Let's briefly talk about the compelling reasons to consume added sugars and sodium in moderation, independent of their presence in ultraprocessed foods.

Moderate Added Sugars and Sweeteners

Added sugars are defined as sugars and syrups that are added to foods during processing or preparation, including sugars and syrups added at the factory, during cooking, and at the table. Science shows that it's important to keep our added sugar intake below 10 percent of total calories.

A 2014 study showed that consuming 10 to 24.9 percent of calories from added sugars increased cardiovascular disease risk by 30 percent, and consuming 25 percent or more of calories from added sugar increased cardiovascular disease risk by 2.75 times![7] But note that staying below the 10 percent of calories from added sugars threshold doesn't have any clear detriment to our health, so there's absolutely room in a healthy diet for some sugar!

It's worth emphasizing that the 10 percent rule applies to *added* sugars, not carbohydrates in general or sugars that come from whole foods like fruit. When we consider all dietary sugars, including those inherent in whole foods like fruit, we see that limiting to 25 percent of calories is the way to go.[8] And if you're intentionally hypercaloric, perhaps in a bulking phase at the gym or looking to gain weight if you are underweight, it would be better to keep total sugar intake lower than 25 percent, although there isn't clear guidance on an exact cutoff in the scientific literature.

The science is mixed on whether replacing sugars with sweeteners facilitates weight loss or improves insulin sensitivity, with some studies showing benefit, some showing no effect, and some actually showing, counterintuitively, that sweeteners also contribute to insulin resistance. Nonnutritive sweeteners are sugar substitutes that include artificial sweeteners like aspartame as well as "natural" sweeteners like stevia and monk fruit extract. While they're marketed as a healthier option than sugars, the science doesn't really bear this out.

Whether there is an association between sweeteners and cardiovascular disease has not been as extensively studied as other foods or food additives. But a large 2022 study out of France that included over a hundred thousand participants followed for about ten years showed that total sweetener intake—including cyclamates, saccharin, thaumatin, neohesperidine dihydrochalcone, steviol glycosides (i.e., stevia), and salt of aspartame-acesulfame potassium—increased risk for cardiovascular disease, including heart disease and stroke.[9] High intake (mean was seventy-seven milligrams per day, the equivalent of about one and a half cans of diet soda) versus zero intake showed an overall 9 percent increased risk of cardiovascular disease. The statistical model accounted for age, sex, physical activity, smoking, education, family history of cardiovascular disease, energy intake without alcohol, alcohol consumption, sodium, saturated fatty acids, polyunsaturated fatty acids, fiber, sugar, fruit and vegetables, red and processed meat.

Interestingly, the same cohort was analyzed for associations between sweetener intake and cancer risk.[10] High intake of sweeteners increased total cancer risk by 13 percent compared to no intake, with the highest association being with aspartame and acesulfame potassium and breast cancer and obesity-associated cancers. Although not all studies have shown an association between sweeteners and cancer.[11] All in all, much more science looking at outcomes other than weight is required to fully understand the health effect of sweeteners.

While this sounds pretty damning for sweeteners, it's still better to consume them than to exceed 10 percent of total calories from added sugars. A 2022 study analyzing data from the Women's Health Initiative showed that consuming one or more artificially sweetened beverages daily increased the risk of cardiovascular disease by 14 percent, whereas drinking one or more sugar-sweetened beverages daily increased the risk of cardiovascular disease by 19 percent.[12] A 2021 study calculated that, for each sugar-sweetened beverage daily that is replaced with the equivalent amount of an artificially sweetened beverage, unsweetened coffee or tea, or plain water, all-cause mortality risk is decreased by 4 to 7 percent.[13]

Unfortunately, from a health perspective, it just doesn't look like sweeteners are that much better than sugar. But will a diet Coke here and there wreck your health? Absolutely not, nor will a regular Coke, a slice of cake, an ice cream cone, a brownie, a candy bar, a . . . Hmm, writing this is making me hungry. My point is that 1) sweeteners are not a cheat code for tasting sweet and getting off scot-free, and 2) added sugars and/or sweeteners in moderation can absolutely fit into a healthy diet.

Avoid Excessive Salt (Sodium) Intake

Excess sodium intake increases the risk of cardiovascular disease, osteoporosis, kidney stones, kidney disease, and stomach cancer, especially when potassium and calcium intake is concurrently low. Ideally, we'd consume between 1.5 and 2.3 grams of sodium per day.

How does this translate to salt? Table salt is roughly 40 percent sodium by weight and 60 percent chloride by weight. It works out that there are about 2.4 grams of sodium in one teaspoon of salt (which weighs about six grams). Unrefined sea salt has less sodium per teaspoon (thanks to some sodium being displaced by other minerals), but it varies. A good general guide is to limit to about one teaspoon of salt total throughout the day, including salt inherent in foods or added during processing, while cooking, and at the table. This is really easy to do if you prepare most of your meals at home.

Nearly three-quarters of the sodium most people eat comes from prepackaged foods, processed store-bought foods, and restaurant meals.[14] In fact, the five biggest contributors to the high sodium intake of the average American are bread and rolls, pizza, sandwiches, cold cuts and cured meats, and soup. By contrast, only 11 percent of dietary sodium comes from salt added at home, including during cooking and at the table. Most people who cook the majority of their meals at home don't need to worry about getting too much salt.

BIG BENEFITS FROM A DIVERSE DIET

Few things seem to make people angrier on the internet than giving them permission to eat foods. I'm sure you've seen it, the backlash on a social media post sharing the science proving that vegetable oils are actually healthy, or that we don't need to worry about the mercury in seafood or pesticide residues on fruit and vegetables. (Shocked? I'll talk about each of these in more depth in chapter 10.) But with the rise of ever more restrictive eating patterns and the pervasiveness of food myths, permission to expand your diet is the most important thing I can offer.

The number-one best thing we can do to improve diet quality is eat a wide variety of foods. But one of the biggest nutritional challenges of the typical Western diet is that while it may feel like you're eating a wide variety of foods, with so many being made from only a handful of ingredients (wheat, corn, soy, and dairy), the diet isn't actually diverse. We can increase variety and nutrient density by replacing these types of foods (breads, cereals, pasta, pizza, crackers, cookies, etc.) with a diversity of whole foods instead.

Dietary diversity is typically defined as the total number of different food items in a diet. One way to measure dietary diversity is *dietary species richness,* the number of different species represented in the diet during a one-year period. This is a technical way to classify foods for a measurement of dietary diversity, and you don't need to sweat the confusing details here, but you can think of this as a methodical way of measuring the number of different whole foods represented in the diet. Strawberries count as one species, blueberries count as one species, salmon counts as one species; but semolina and whole wheat pasta only count as one species since they're both made of the same singular ingredient, the species *Triticum turgidum*, commonly called durum wheat.

In a 2021 study that included nearly half a million people living in nine European countries and followed for twenty-two years, the people with the highest dietary species richness (eighty-one or more different species in the diet over the course of a year) had a 37 percent reduced risk of all-cause mortality compared to those with the lowest dietary species richness (forty-eight or fewer different species in the diet over the course of a year).[15] The authors calculated that for every additional ten species we consume annually, all-cause mortality decreases by 10 percent! And a 2022 meta-analysis found that high dietary diversity reduced all-cause mortality risk by 22 percent compared to low dietary diversity, as well as reducing cardiovascular disease mortality by 17 percent and cancer mortality by 10 percent.[16] Quite simply: The more different foods we eat, the healthier (on average) we'll be.

Why is dietary diversity so effective at improving health outcomes? Perhaps unsurprisingly, more diverse diets are higher quality and more nutrient dense.[17] In fact, dietary diversity scores can be used as a proxy for nutrition, with low scores equating to malnourishment and high scores equating to healthy diets.[18] Essentially, a diversity of different foods equates to a diversity of nutrients, increasing the likelihood of getting all the nutrients we need from our diets, i.e., Nutrivore!

All in all, these studies make a compelling case for eating as many different foods as possible. What's a good goal? While more studies are needed to determine the best target number of different foods per day or per week, a case can be made to aim for at least twelve different whole foods per day, and thirty-five different whole foods over the course of the week.

Every little bit counts, so a great goal is simply to mix it up in whatever way feels achievable to you right now. Maybe that's just adding a single new vegetable or fruit to your rotation or trying a new recipe once per week.

Tips for Diversifying Your Diet

Here are some easy ways to increase dietary diversity:

- **Embrace soups, stir-fries, and salads.** These are easy dishes to pack a bunch of different foods into, often containing eight to ten different foods or more. Check out the recipes for these in chapter 12.
- **Think of easy swaps.** If you normally make a dish with salmon, try it with trout instead. Swap your go-to cut of steak for a different cut, or meat from a different animal (like lamb chops). If you normally put blueberries on your yogurt, mix it up with some blackberries. If you normally put lettuce on your sandwich, try spinach or chard instead. Love mashed potatoes? Try mashing other root veggies instead.
- **Try different varieties of your staple foods.** Look for different varieties of apples, bananas, grapes, oranges, pears, kiwis, carrots, kale, lettuce, potatoes, sweet potatoes, snap beans, asparagus, cauliflower, broccoli, Brussels sprouts, cabbage, summer and winter squash, and so on. You can usually find even more varieties at a local farmers' market.
- **Add variety with garnishes.** Add fresh chopped herbs to your roasted veggies, toss a handful of nuts or sliced fruit into your salad, or serve a chutney or salsa with your steak or fish.
- **Eat seasonally.** In-season vegetables and fruit (like peaches and cherries in the summer, apples and squashes in early fall, pomegranates and persimmons in the late fall, citrus in winter, and berries in spring) are more likely to be fresher, cheaper, and locally grown, even from large grocery store chains.
- **One of each shopping.** When walking up and down the produce aisles at your local grocery store, instead of loading up on just a few different veggies for the week, grab one bunch/head/bag of as many

different veggies as you can. When cooking, pair veggies that have similar cooking times, like broccoli and cauliflower, spinach and rainbow chard, turnips and potatoes, asparagus and green beans.

- **Be adventurous!** If you see a fruit or vegetable you've never tried at the store, get some. Once you're home, you can search online for how to prepare and eat it. Try different meals at your favorite restaurants, and cook different recipes from your go-to cookbooks. Try some new cuisines, new flavors, new ingredients. You might just find some new favorites, too.

EAT THE RAINBOW OF FRUITS AND VEGGIES

One of the single most important things we can all do to improve the nutritive value of our diets and lower risk of health problems is eat the full color spectrum of vegetables and fruits, typically referred to as "eating the rainbow," and eat plenty of them.

It's impossible to overstate how important it is for our health to eat an abundance of vegetables and fruits. A 2019 review summarized a wealth of scientific studies showing that the more vegetables and fruit we eat, the lower our risk of cancer, cardiovascular disease, type 2 diabetes, obesity, chronic kidney disease, osteoporosis and bone fragility fractures (including hip fracture), cognitive impairment and dementia (including Alzheimer's disease), neurodegenerative diseases, asthma, allergies, chronic obstructive pulmonary disease, age-related macular degeneration, cataracts, glaucoma, depression, anxiety, ulcerative colitis and Crohn's disease, rheumatoid arthritis, inflammatory polyarthritis, nonalcoholic fatty liver disease, acne and seborrheic dermatitis, and lowers markers of inflammation.[19] In fact, the amount of vegetables and fruit we eat is a better predictor of our health outcomes than any other food in our diets; and eating eight hundred grams (equivalent to 1.75 pounds, or twenty-eight ounces) reduces all-cause mortality by a humongous 31 percent compared to eating less than forty grams daily.[20]

A prudent goal is to consume five or more servings of vegetables per day, along with two servings of fruit. Why? Most studies show that this amount and relative ratio provides the majority of the benefits we can glean from high fruit and vegetable intake. The dose response relationship between vegetable and fruit consumption and our overall health isn't linear, meaning that each serving we add to our diets doesn't affect our health equally. Instead, going from eating no vegetables to a single serving per day delivers a similar amount of health benefit as going from one serving per day to five—yes, eating five servings of veggies per day is about twice as good for you as eating one. This is particularly great news if you currently don't eat vegetables because any effort you put in to upping your veggie intake will return dividends in terms of your health. Consuming more than five servings of vegetables per day, while still beneficial, provides diminishing returns. For fruit, the optimal amount is around two to three servings daily—both less and more than this amount isn't as beneficial, although even up to four or five servings per day is still better than eating no fruit.

So, what is a serving for fruits and veggies? It's standardized to:

- one cup for most vegetables and fruit, measured raw
- two cups for leafy vegetables, measured raw
- one quarter cup for fatty fruits (like olives or avocado)

It's not as much as you think! These measurements have a helpful visual aspect to them. For example, one cup is about the size of a fist, and a tablespoon is a similar volume to the top half of a thumb. Plus, most vegetables and fruits shrink by about half when cooked. When you realize that a serving of steamed broccoli is only about half a fist's worth, it's nowhere near as intimidating. See page 241 for more visual approximations of serving sizes.

Given what we know about dietary diversity, choosing a wide variety is extremely important. This means that eating a serving of seven different vegetables and fruits per day delivers more benefits than eating seven servings of the same vegetable or fruit.

Here's where the idea of eating the rainbow comes in. The pigments that give different fruits and vegetables their characteristic colors are phytonutrients. Each one of these classes of phytonutrients has distinctive benefits, which is why choosing vegetables and fruits of different colors is important for ensuring that we consume a wide variety of these beneficial compounds. (See also pages 166–67.) A 2022 umbrella review that included 86 studies, 449 health outcomes, and data from more than 37 million participants concluded that 42 percent of health outcomes were improved by color-associated pigments. Those health outcomes that were improved by *multiple* pigments included body weight, lipid profile, inflammation, cardiovascular disease, type 2 diabetes, cancer, and total mortality.[21] In fact, this review shows that color-associated fruit and vegetable variety may confer additional benefits to population health beyond total fruit and vegetable intake. So aim for dietary representation of each of the five color families for fruits and veggies: 1) red; 2) orange and yellow; 3) green; 4) blue and purple; and 5) white and brown.

It's also worth noting that frozen, canned, and dried vegetables and fruit are all great options if those are more accessible, affordable, and/or convenient for you. I'll bust many myths about food quality, including the nutritional value of frozen and canned foods, in chapter 10.

The Best Incentive to Eat More Fruits and Veggies

When you hear a rationalization for making a healthier (but maybe harder) choice that is based on improving long-term health outcomes, it can sometimes be hard to feel the relevancy and urgency to today's choices. I'll wrap up this section with one last reason to eat more veggies and fruit: Doing so can make you happier!

A 2016 study showed that for each serving of fruit and vegetables you eat daily, you increase happiness, well-being, and life satisfaction, up to eight servings per day.[22] The researchers calculated that going from almost no fruit and veggies to eight servings per day would increase life satisfaction equivalent to moving from unemployment to employment. While the mental health benefits of eating lots of veggies doesn't happen overnight, it is a much faster time frame than other metrics of health like cardiovascular disease or cancer risk—benefits to overall well-being occurred within twenty-four months.

THE NUTRIVORE MEAL MAP

Whether you're cooking at home or eating out, the easiest way to eat a Nutrivore diet is to follow the Nutrivore Meal Map for most of your meals. The science behind these recommendations will be expanded on throughout this book, but there's no reason why you can't start using this simple guide right now. Mentally, divide your plate into four roughly equal quarters. Each quarter will supply a different collection of vital nutrients, and together they will add up to a balanced, nourishing meal.

Fill one quarter of your plate with a starchy food.

One to two servings of a starchy food (defined as one cup raw for starchy vegetables and fruit like plantains, or one ounce raw for pulse legumes and whole grains, all of which translate to about half a cup cooked) at each meal is sufficient to meet carbohydrate needs for most people and contribute substantial dietary fiber to the diet (one serving of sweet potato has four grams of fiber and one serving of lentils has seven grams of fiber). The benefits of starch and fiber are discussed in more depth in chapter 5.

Fill one quarter of your plate with a protein food.

One to two servings of a protein food (defined as three ounces for cooked meat and seafood; two large eggs; one cup of bone broth, milk, or yogurt; one and a half ounces of cheese; a quarter cup for tofu, and half a cup for cooked pulse legumes like lentils) at each meal is sufficient to meet protein needs for most people, and provided you're consuming a variety of protein foods, ensure adequate intake of all nine essential amino acids. When you select a whole food plant protein—for example, the classic combination of rice and beans (together, a complete protein)—merge the quarter of your plate filled with protein foods with the quarter of your plate filled with starchy foods. Processed plant proteins like tofu, tempeh, seitan, plant-based meats, and protein powders count only toward the protein quarter and not toward the starch quarter of your plate. Protein and amino acids are discussed in more depth in chapter 5.

Fill the remaining half of your plate with a variety of vegetables and fruit.

Covering half of your plate with vegetables and fruit (and three quarters of your plate if your starchy food is a root vegetable or winter squash) at each meal is a simple way to easily achieve the goal of five or more servings of vegetables and two servings of fruit daily. Ideally, choose two or more different ones (for example, a quarter of your plate covered in broccoli and a quarter filled with beets) at each meal, hitting all five color families (red, orange and yellow, green, blue and purple, and white and brown) throughout the day, and with as much variety in the veggie family during the week as possible.

Cook and dress your food with healthy fats—such as olive oil, avocado oil, soybean oil, canola oil, corn oil, or sunflower oil. (See chapter 10 for more discussion on vegetable oils.) Alternatively or additionally, incorporate whole food sources of healthy fats into your meal—think fish and shellfish, olives, avocados, nuts and seeds. It's totally fine to use butter or other animal fats (like bacon drippings) for flavor when cooking calls for it, but know that studies show that swapping out butter and other highly saturated cooking fats for vegetable oils reduces risk of all-cause mortality as well as mortality from specific causes, including cardiovascular disease, diabetes, cancer, respiratory disease, and Alzheimer's disease.[23] It's not a huge effect compared to most of the other dietary tweaks we're talking about in this book, so using these healthier oils whenever it makes culinary sense to do so is a good way to go. The most important dietary fats are discussed in more depth in chapter 5.

Season as you enjoy with spices and herbs, and know that you're upping the health benefits of your meal when you do! Thanks to their super phytonutrient content, herbs and spices have been shown to have powerful antioxidant activity, exhibit cancer-preventive effects, reduce inflammation, and reduce cardiovascular disease risk. The benefits of herbs and spices are discussed in chapter 8.

And finally, drink mostly water.

Choosing mostly water—including flavored or infused waters, sparkling water, club soda, spring or mineral water, and regular ole tap water—helps to keep us hydrated. But some other beverages are health promoting when consumed in moderation, too. The many health benefits of tea and coffee are discussed in chapter 8. Juice, while it has the reputation of being a glass full of sugar, is also beneficial in moderation. A 2019 study showed that five ounces (150 milliliters) of fruit juice per day is optimal and lowered risk of all-cause mortality by about 10 percent—higher or lower than that amount wasn't as beneficial.[24] In comparison, there's no intake level above zero where soda improves health outcomes. A 2021 meta-analysis showed that dairy consumption—including drinking milk—was associated with a 10 percent lower risk of stroke, a 4 percent lower risk of coronary heart disease, and a 9 percent reduced risk of hypertension (high blood pressure).[25] Fermented beverages like kombucha, kefir, and kvass are a good source of probiotics, which are discussed on pages 93–94. And when choosing fruit punch, soda, sports drinks, energy drinks, or sweetened coffee and tea, make sure to keep added sugar consumption below 10 percent of total calories.

While we're on the topic of beverages, and not to be a complete Debbie Downer, we now know that no amount of alcohol is beneficial. A 2023 systematic review of more than forty years of research found that many of the early studies showing benefits of moderate alcohol consumption (the famous J-shaped curve) were flawed.[26] A 2022 study found that any amount of alcohol increased risk for high blood pressure and coronary heart disease.[27] Alcohol dramatically (as much as five times) increased risk of head and neck cancers (oral cavity, pharynx, and larynx), esophageal cancer, stomach cancer, liver cancer, gallbladder cancer, breast cancer, and colorectal cancer.[28] And a 2018 systematic analysis concluded that the safe amount of alcohol to imbibe to minimize harm across health outcomes is zero drinks per week.[29] It's okay to have an occasional drink, it's just not going to improve your health like we were told in the 1990s. Instead, the risk of all-cause mortality increased by

5 percent in females who consumed twenty-five grams of alcohol daily (less than two drinks) and males who consumed forty-four grams of alcohol daily (just over three drinks). A drink is defined as containing fourteen grams of alcohol, which usually translates to twelve ounces of beer, five ounces of wine, or one and a half ounces of distilled spirits.

Using the Nutrivore Meal Map as a visual guide to construct most of your meals will help you eat a balanced, nutrient-dense diet without additional effort. Incorporate a further focus on choosing mostly whole foods, embracing a wide diversity of different foods, and eating the rainbow of fruits and vegetables, and you've got most of your nutritional bases covered! As we enter part 2 of this book and examine the relationships between specific nutrients and your health complaints, think of this information as ways to refine your food choices and take each plate to the next level nutritionwise.

Nutrivore Snacks

Snacks are another opportunity to choose nutrient-dense foods.

There are compelling reasons to treat snacks like minimeals and include some protein, fiber, and healthy fats. A 2014 study of healthy women concluded that compared to high-fat or high-carb snacks, eating high-protein snacks, even if lower in calories, improved appetite control, satiety, and reduced food intake at subsequent meals.[30] A 2011 study in type 2 diabetics showed that high-protein snacks resulted in fat mass loss, despite no change in total energy intake.[31] And a 2006 study in healthy women showed that a high-protein, high-fiber snack not only reduced energy intake at the next meal but reduced glucose and insulin responses over the whole day.[32]

If you don't have time for a minimeal-type snack, a piece of fruit is also a healthy option. In fact, a 2021 study showed that eating fruit for a snack lowered risk of all-cause mortality by 22 percent and cancer mortality by 45 percent compared to other snack patterns.[33] On the other hand, a starchy snack increased risk of all-cause mortality and cardiovascular disease by about 50 percent! So a muffin or bag of chips isn't as good a choice as an apple.

NUTRIVORE MEAL MAP

50%
Vegetables & Fruit

2-5 SERVINGS

E.G., leafy veggies, root veggies, cruciferous veggies, mushrooms, alliums, citrus, and berries

*Season and garnish with herbs and spices

25%
Starchy Foods

1-2 SERVINGS

E.G., pulse legumes, whole grains, and starchy vegetables

DRINK MOSTLY WATER

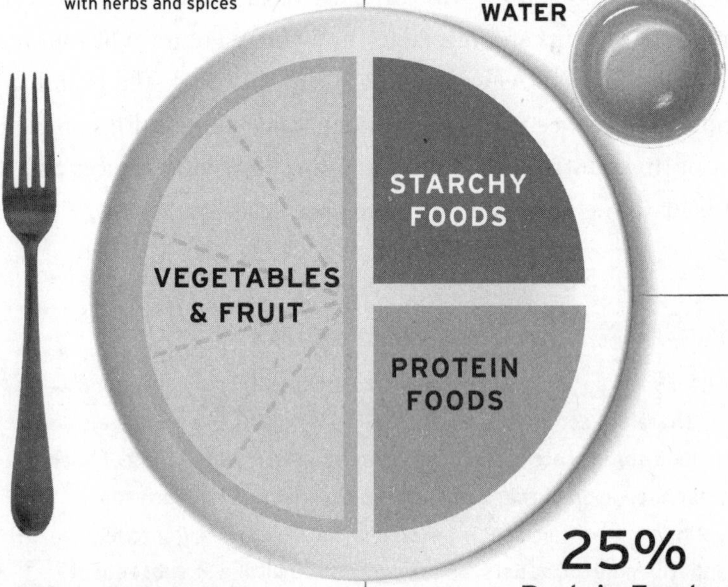

STARCHY FOODS

VEGETABLES & FRUIT

PROTEIN FOODS

25%
Protein Foods

1-2 SERVINGS

* E.G., meat, seafood, broth, eggs, dairy, and plant proteins

* If choosing whole-food plant proteins like lentils or edamame, merge with the starch quarter of your plate

* Choose mostly whole foods and vary the foods you eat day to day

Eat the Rainbow

AIM FOR AT LEAST ONE SERVING OF PLANT FOODS FROM EACH OF THE COLOR FAMILIES DAILY

* Red
* Orange + yellow
* Green
* Blue + purple
* White + brown

CHOOSE HEALTHY FATS

to cook and dress your foods and for meal components

E.G., nuts and seeds, fish, avocados, olives, olive oil, vegetable oils

Part 2

NUTRIENTS AND YOUR HEALTH

I have two teenage daughters, and I marvel at the well-rounded general education that they're getting in public school: language arts, social studies, history, mathematics, science, music, and arts. Among the scientific fields they learn about are physics, chemistry, biology, geology, astronomy, computer sciences, and environmental sciences. They even can opt to learn some multidisciplinary sciences as well—my oldest is currently taking organic chemistry. It's so much more than I had the opportunity to learn when I was young. But there's a big, important topic that's missing from their education, and even from the electives from which they can choose: nutritional sciences.

Imagine if by the time we graduated high school we all had the same type of broad knowledge base of nutrition as we do of grammar or algebra. Imagine how much easier it would be to navigate the grocery store and to critically evaluate diet claims online if rooted so deep in your brain that you know it as well as your multiplication tables (even if fuzzy and you feel like you need to double-check with a calculator) was a practical collection of facts about nutrients, a general idea of their biological roles and relations to health and disease, and lists (even if incomplete) of the types of foods that contain them. Imagine if we all were nutrient aware. It would inure us from predatory marketing, foster healthier lifelong eating habits, and banish the yo-yo diet from our lives.

I hope that someday nutritional sciences will make it into the required high school curriculum. In the meantime, I will use these next four chapters to teach you this essential knowledge foundation so you can move forward in your day-to-day decision making, empowered by information—i.e., we will build nutrient awareness. But don't worry, you won't feel like you're back in class, or if you do, it will feel like those special days with your favorite substitute teacher who had such flare and pizzazz that you couldn't help but be enraptured by the lesson.

While I will endeavor to leave you with a newfound appreciation for nutrients along with practical knowledge of how to choose foods to get enough of them, I will not be sharing every single thing that every nutrient does. Instead, I will home in on one particular health effect of interest for each of a relatively small selection of nutrients, with chapters organized by nutrient type—think of it as a highlights reel. Rather than just the greatest hits, though, over the next four chapters I will cover the majority of ailments and symptoms you might be facing—from PMS to osteoporosis, from headaches to high cholesterol, and from brain fog to diabetes. Every reader will find nutritional solutions to their own health challenges and goals.

Think of this section of the book as a series of short stories; you can read them all in order for the most fulfilling experience, or pick and choose the ones you're most interested in.

For each nutrient I'll share in what foods it can commonly be found and any related benefits of foods that are particularly valuable sources of it. In this way, we'll also build brick by brick the collection of Nutrivore foundational foods, as well as highlight nutritionally interchangeable foods that are also health promoting—these foods are awesome day-to-day choices even if they don't offer anything particularly unique nutritionally. Don't worry, it won't be all liver and kale! Sure, you'll be a veggie fiend by the end of this book when you fully understand the myriad ways they benefit us, but we'll also cover some fun (and, yes, healthful) foods like coffee, chocolate, and steak.

Why am I sharing historical anecdotes while teaching modern nutritional sciences? As you'll see, these stories illustrate not just the ingenuity, and sometimes serendipity, that went into the scientific discovery of nutrients but also how often assumptions about nutrients (that later turned out to be wrong) have intertwined with diet advice, leading us astray. For several centuries, influential scientists, doctors, and politicians have been able to disseminate their unfounded beliefs about foods far and wide—yes, misinformation spread long before social media—and many of the diet myths that are still pervasive today have roots in erroneous conclusions and opinions about optimal diet that became common knowledge before the hypotheses being proven false.

For example, Sarah Tyson Rorer is often considered the first American dietitian thanks to her work with doctors to develop special diets for the infirm and malnourished.[1] Self-educated in chemistry and medicine, she founded the Philadelphia School of Cookery in 1884, authored many cookbooks, and worked for decades as a columnist for and editor of magazines, including *Ladies' Home Journal* and *Good Housekeeping*. A century before the earliest Instagram influencers, Rorer is still best understood in those terms, or as the Martha Stewart of her day. She gave lectures at Madison Square Garden, had a weekly radio show, was a sought-after endorser of then-new products like Pyrex and Shredded Wheat, and was even honored at the Chicago Woman's World Fair in 1925.

With her massive platform, Rorer hubristically shared her beliefs on healthy eating and hygiene, railing against overcooked vegetables (she had a point with that one); raw bananas (she believed they should only be eaten cooked); potatoes, strawberries, and citrus fruits (each of which she called poison); and breakfast. Before the first vitamin was even discovered, before we understood metabolism or knew about insulin, what Rorer said about which foods were healthy became gospel in households across America thanks to her reach and renown. And while Rorer lost her fortune during the Great Depression, and certainly is no longer a household name, many of the nutrition myths she espoused still have legs today.

The problem isn't that nutritional sciences is still an evolving field but rather how often dietary recommendations and public health policy decisions have preceded the necessary scientific underpinnings. Remember, this isn't about guilt or blame but rather about creating a clean slate in our brains for so much new, invaluable information. And, with that, let's dig in (pun intended)!

CHAPTER 5

Mighty Macronutrients: Protein, Carbs, and Fat

Nutritional science is a very young field of research, with its earliest beginnings dating from 1785 when chemists turned their attention to understanding the chemical composition of plants and animals.[1] The discovery that nitrogen was a constituent of both wheat and rotting beef was the first hint that we are what we eat, at least in the sense of raw materials. By comparison, Eratosthenes estimated Earth's circumference around 240 BCE; the printing press was invented in 1440; Sir Isaac Newton published his theory of gravity in 1687; and even the invention of the steam locomotive in 1712 preceded the earliest beginnings of nutritional sciences by more than seventy years. And it wasn't until 1839 that the nitrogenous substances in both plants and animals were identified as protein. The last of the twenty amino acids our bodies use to form proteins wasn't discovered until 1935. When you realize how recently most nutritional sciences discoveries were made, it's easy to see why so many misnomers persist in both folk remedies and common knowledge.

Yes, the first essential nutrient to be discovered was protein, originally referred to as nitrogenous substances or "animal matter" even when referring to plant proteins. Carbohydrates, fats, and the idea of combustion energy to create body heat (which would eventually be called calories, culminating in Wilbur Atwater's definitions thereof in 1887) all followed soon after.[2] Numerous scientists conducted experiments over the ensuing decades that iteratively improved our understanding of digestion and macronutrients. But despite the fact that scientists were gaining an understanding of oxidation of carbohydrates and fats for energy (a full century before Hans Adolf Krebs figured out cellular respiration, no less), many of them still believed that protein was all we really needed.[3]

In 1842, German organic chemist Justus von Liebig published a widely read book entitled *Animal Chemistry or Organic Chemistry in its Application to Physiology and Pathology* in which he argued that protein was the only true nutrient, supplying both "the machinery of the body and the fuel for its work." His rationale was that because he didn't find any fat or carbohydrates in muscle tissues, the only possible source of energy for muscle contraction was the explosive breakdown of protein molecules, producing urea as a by-product. He explained away the oxidation of fats and carbohydrates as mopping up oxidants produced by respiration. He was completely wrong about all of it.

As still happens today when a charismatic character is espousing some nutrition concept that sounds logical on the surface, many people adopted Liebig's idea that protein was the only required nutrient.[4] For example, during a scurvy outbreak in a Scottish prison in 1846, the treating physician, a Liebig groupie, concluded the inmates were not receiving enough protein despite the fact that 1) their average daily protein intake was 134 grams, and 2) lemon juice (which contains no protein) had been a proven treatment for scurvy for nearly a century by this time, thanks to James Lind and his famous controlled clinical trial of sailors in 1753.

Most of Liebig's ideas about nutrition, which he believed ardently and conveyed widely, were later shown to be false.[5] Of course, Liebig continued to be protein's biggest hype man—he's the inventor of Oxo beef stock cubes and tinned corned beef[6]—and his ideas heavily influenced the earliest USDA dietary guidelines, the 1894 Farmers' Bulletin written by Atwater (yes, the calorie guy, who was also the USDA's first chief of nutrition investigations). The bulletin, which sought to explain the nutritional merits of foods relative to their cost, heavily promoted the value of meat and dairy products and actually disparaged vegetables for lacking protein and fat and because they did not "gratify the palate."[7] To be fair, vitamins and most minerals hadn't been discovered yet, and scientists at the time did not yet know just how much about nutrition they didn't know.

The origin of the phrase "you are what you eat" comes from these early days of nutritional sciences and protein fanaticism. Often considered the father of the low-carb diet, politician Jean Anthelme Brillat-Savarin staunchly recommended avoiding starch, grains, sugar, and flour in his gastronomy book *Physiologie du Goût* (*The Physiology of Taste*) published in 1825.[8] Although a better direct translation of his words is "Tell me what you eat and I will tell you what you are," Brillat-Savarin thought that the foods you ate marked you as a certain type of person. If you ate the same types of foods he did, you were a good person in the moral sense. Current fad diets continue to moralize foods in a similar way.

It's shocking to realize that low-carb, high-protein diets can trace their origins to a time when scientists still didn't understand the biological fate of carbohydrates, fats, and proteins when we consume them, how they're used differently in the body, nor even what they're made of and the physiological roles of their constituents.[9] And nearly two centuries later, the erroneous beliefs of a few influential figures continue to permeate modern diet culture, with subsequent diet gurus doubling down on faulty nutrition principles. These ideas have been around for so long—some of them since the days of balancing too much black bile with beef to treat depression (yes, that was a real thing before the germ theory of disease)—you're forgiven for thinking that these were proven concepts rather than the reality. Fortunately for us, since these early days of nutritional sciences research, our knowledge has increased exponentially, and we can now correct the record on macronutrients.

Here's what you need to know about protein, carbohydrates, and fats, and more important, how their constituents affect our health.

MACRONUTRIENTS 101

Protein, carbohydrates, and fat are the three essential macronutrients, that is, the nutrients we need in large quantities. They all can be used for energy, to fuel the chemical reactions of life, but more important, their building blocks—amino acids, saccharides, and fatty acids, respectively—serve diverse structural and functional roles in our biology.

We're going to examine some broadly relevant benefits to our health of consuming specific types of proteins, carbohydrates, and fats. But to do so, we need first to set the stage with a quick primer on what makes up each macronutrient and why they are essential.

Proteins and Amino Acids

Proteins are the molecules that perform most of the various functions of life. In addition to being major structural components of cells and tissues, proteins have incredibly diverse roles that range from driving chemical reactions (e.g., enzymes) to signaling (e.g., hormones) to transporting and storing nutrients. Proteins are synthesized within cells through a two-phase process (transcription and translation), during which their basic building blocks, amino acids, get linked to form long chains, spanning anywhere from twenty to more than two thousand amino acids in length.

Of the twenty amino acids used to build the proteins in our bodies, only nine are considered nutritionally indispensable, meaning that we absolutely have to get them from food—our bodies can't make them. These nine essential amino acids are isoleucine, histidine, leucine, lysine, methionine, phenylalanine, threonine, tryptophan, and valine. Six additional amino acids are considered conditionally indispensable, meaning that while other amino acids can be converted into these amino acids, the process is so inefficient that most of the time we still need to get them from food. These six conditionally indispensable amino acids are arginine, cysteine, glycine, glutamine, proline, and tyrosine. The remaining five amino acids are considered nutritionally dispensable, meaning that our bodies can make them in sufficient quantities provided there's enough protein in our diets. These nutritionally dispensable amino acids are alanine, aspartic acid, asparagine, glutamic acid, and serine. There are hundreds of additional amino acids that have important biological roles, but our bodies don't use them to make proteins. We'll talk about one example, ergothioneine, in this chapter.

The term "complete protein" refers to a food that supplies sufficient quantities of all nine nutritionally indispensable amino acids. This includes all animal foods (meat, seafood, eggs, and dairy) but only a few plant foods. Complete plant proteins include soy (like edamame, tofu, natto, and tempeh), buckwheat, quinoa, hemp, chia seed, and amaranth. Note however that while technically we only need to get the nine essential amino acids through diet, it is far preferable from a health standpoint to get all the amino acids from foods. That way, we don't have to rely on sometimes inefficient conversion processes for the amino acids our bodies need to make all the various proteins in our cells and tissues. Nevertheless, amino acid deficiencies are incredibly rare in people consuming sufficient protein.

Carbohydrates: Sugar, Starch, and Fiber

Carbohydrates are a class of organic molecules with the basic structural components being sugar molecules, or *saccharides*, most commonly glucose. Their main roles in supporting health are as an energy source, as fermentable substrate for the gut microbiome (i.e., food for our gut bacteria), and as molecular components important for cellular health and immune function. One way to classify carbohydrates is based on how they're digested and absorbed when we eat them, i.e., as sugars, starches, and fiber.

Sugars, also called simple carbohydrates, are made of one or two saccharides—like sucrose (made of one glucose and one fructose), lactose (made of one glucose and one galactose), glucose, and fructose—and are easily digested and enter the bloodstream rapidly, providing quick energy. Glucose is the preferred fuel source for our cells, powering the full range of physiological processes, from nerve transduction to muscle contraction to respiration. When we talk about blood sugar, we're referring to the presence of glucose in the bloodstream. While other saccharides like fructose and galactose can also be used for energy, they must first undergo conversion into glucose or intermediary energy molecules, a process primarily carried out in the liver.

Starches are complex carbohydrates made up mostly of glucose molecules. They are usually digested more slowly than sugars, so have a more gradual effect on blood sugar levels, offering sustained energy.

While sugars and starches get a bad rap for spiking blood sugar levels and insulin secretion, the development of insulin resistance and type 2 diabetes are much more complex than how they are often represented as being the direct result of simply eating too much sugar and white bread. We don't need to be afraid of sugars and starches; in fact, eating too few of them can be detrimental to thyroid function, skeletal muscle health, bone density, mental health and cognition, and immune function.

Fiber is a type of complex carbohydrate that our body can't digest and instead is a food source for the beneficial bacteria and other microbes that inhabit our digestive tract. Fiber also regulates peristalsis of the intestines (the rhythmic motion of muscles around the intestines that pushes food through the digestive tract), stimulates the suppression of the hunger hormone ghrelin (so we feel more full), lowers cholesterol, and slows the absorption of simple sugars into the bloodstream to regulate blood sugar levels and avoid the excess production of insulin. We'll talk about fiber and the gut microbiome in more depth later in this chapter.

It's of course always best to choose whole food sources of carbohydrates—like fruits, vegetables, legumes, and whole grains—because they contain a mix of carbohydrates, including fiber, that slows down digestion and blunts the blood sugar response. Blood sugar regulation is further improved by ingesting carbohydrate-containing foods as part of a complete meal that also includes protein and fats.

Fats and Fatty Acids

Fats are a type of lipid, which is broadly defined as a molecule that is insoluble in water but that dissolves in organic solvents like ether and chloroform. Lipids encompass fats and oils, fatty acids, phospholipids, and sterols like cholesterol.

Lipids perform three primary biological functions within the body:

1. They serve as structural components of cell membranes.
2. They are an energy-storage molecule and some can be directly used for energy.
3. They function as important signaling molecules (how our cells communicate with each other), including being integral to the structure of steroid hormones (like testosterone, estrogen, cortisol, and vitamin D).

The effect of dietary fat on our health is dependent on both the type of fat and how much of it we're eating.

Fats and oils are more technically called *triglycerides* (or triacylglycerol), which are composed of three fatty acids linked together (esterified) by a glycerol molecule. Fatty acids are the building blocks of fats. They are used not only for energy but for many basic structures in the human body, such as the outer membrane of every single cell. Fatty acids can be broadly characterized by chemical traits such as by molecule length (short-chain, medium-chain, and long-chain fatty acids) and by the number of double bonds between carbon atoms (saturated, monounsaturated, or polyunsaturated). If you've heard of omega-3 and omega-6 fats, these are polyunsaturated fatty acids that are further categorized based on the location of the first double bond. We don't need to get into the weeds on these various chemical traits—all you need to know is that they affect the shape and size of the fatty acid, which determines its biological functions. There are many different fatty acids, each with different effects on and roles in human health.

There are two essential fatty acids: alpha-linolenic acid (ALA; the shortest omega-3 polyunsaturated fatty acid) and linoleic acid (LA; the shortest omega-6 polyunsaturated fatty acid). The term "essential" is misleading here. The fatty acids with the most profound roles in the human body are arachidonic acid (AA), an omega-6 polyunsaturated fatty acid, and eicosapentaenoic acid (EPA) and docosahexaenoic acid (DHA), both omega-3 polyunsaturated fatty acids. Our bodies can convert any omega-6 polyunsaturated fatty acid to any other omega-6 polyunsaturated fatty acid, and similarly can convert any omega-3 polyunsaturated fatty acid to any other omega-3 polyunsaturated fatty acid—which means that we can make EPA and DHA from ALA and AA from LA. But that conversion can be extremely inefficient, so it's important to get these from food. While ALA and LA are abundant in plant foods, AA, EPA, and DHA are found in seafood, meat, and poultry.

The Real Stars Are Macro Building Blocks

The most important thing to know about macronutrients is that they are not monolithic; not all proteins, carbohydrates, and fats have the same effect on our health. In fact, the various amino acids, saccharides, and fatty acids that make up macronutrients have hundreds, if not thousands, of important roles in human biology beyond energy. So while it's typical to think of macronutrients simply in terms of energy and weight loss, the real magic is how specific macronutrients and their building blocks interact with our health at the cellular and molecular level. It's the small things these big things are made of that really matter.

It would take several volumes to describe the details of all of these effects (and several vats of coffee to keep you awake long enough to read them), so for the rest of this chapter I'll instead focus on a few select examinations of especially relevant health effects of specific macronutrient constituents. Through these examples, we'll build an appreciation for macronutrients beyond the typical low-carb, low-fat, and high-protein diets to more fully understand how shifting our focus from macronutrient manipulation to macronutrient building blocks as important nutrients can benefit our health in innumerable ways.

JOINT PAIN? TRY EATING MORE COLLAGEN

The wearing down of joint cartilage in osteoarthritis causes inflexibility, pain, and stiffness of predominantly weight-bearing joints such as the knees, hips, and spine. Osteoarthritis is the most common form of arthritis and accounts for about 25 percent of primary care physician visits among the elderly. There's accumulating evidence that a specific protein, called collagen, can prevent and even reverse cartilage degradation in osteoarthritic patients.[10]

Collagen accounts for 30 percent of the protein in our bodies. The word "collagen" is derived from the Greek "*kólla*," which means glue. Collagen functionally acts both as a glue—holding our cells, tissues, and organs together—and as a structural scaffold, including being a main building block of bone, cartilage, ligaments, tendons, and skin. There are twenty-nine currently identified types of collagen, all rich in the amino acid glycine and each with different biological roles in human health.

Normal aging, chronic inflammation, chronic stress, nutritional deficiencies, UV radiation, and smoking can all decrease collagen production as well as degrade collagen structure. This leads not only to wrinkles but to osteopenia and osteoporosis, osteoarthritis, cardiovascular disease, and decreased organ function, including heart, lungs, and kidneys. A variety of studies have shown that increasing collagen intake can mediate these effects, and indeed, collagen supplementation has been shown to improve conditions related to bone, joint, tendon, skin, muscle, and cardiovascular health!

A 2011 study of people with mild to moderate knee osteoarthritis showed that ten grams of collagen hydrolysate daily over twenty-four weeks significantly improved a measure of cartilage quality (called the dGEMRIC score, measured by MRI), while those receiving a placebo saw a continued deterioration of cartilage.[11] A similar 2009 study showed improvements to joint comfort and reduced pain.[12] Collagen supplements improve joint health in other contexts as well. A 2008 study in athletes with activity-related joint pain showed that ten grams daily of collagen hydrolysate for twenty-four weeks substantially reduced joint pain (including at rest, standing, walking, carrying objects, and lifting).[13]

Of course, you don't have to rely on supplements to get your collagen. It's a myth that collagen supplements are more digestible than the collagen we get from foods.[14]

While bone broth (or stock, if you include aromatics like celery, onion, and carrot) isn't the magical elixir it's often portrayed to be online, it is an especially collagen-rich food to include in our diet. This flavorful liquid is made by boiling the bones (and joints and ligaments, etc.) of just about any vertebrate you can think of (typically poultry, beef, bison, lamb, pork, or fish) in water for anywhere from an hour or so to several days. A 2019 study showed that long-simmered homemade bone broths—especially using the most collagen-rich tissues like beef marrow bones, chicken feet, or fish heads—can deliver up to twenty grams of collagen protein in one cup of broth, although the amount of collagen in broth varies greatly depending on preparation method and types of bones used.[15]

That reminds me of a joke. I went to the store for some broth, but they were all out of stock! Hyuck!

Other collagen-rich foods include gelatin (or aspic), offal, and any meat that you eat off the bone or that includes skin. Fish and shellfish are also great sources of collagen.

THE "LONGEVITY VITAMIN" ISN'T ACTUALLY A VITAMIN, IT'S ERGOTHIONEINE

Want to live a long and healthy life? I do, too! While nonessential, one nutrient worth focusing on is a little-known amino acid called *ergothioneine*. Ergothioneine is a nonproteinogenic amino acid, meaning an amino acid that isn't one of the twenty our bodies use to make proteins, with powerful antioxidant and anti-inflammatory properties. Ergothioneine is known to mitigate diseases associated with aging, including cardiovascular disease, cancer, liver disease, cataracts, and Alzheimer's disease.[16] It has been shown to enhance memory, reduce risk of depression, reduce neuroinflammation, and improve sleep.[17] There's even evidence for a role in fetal development, female fertility, and reducing risk of preeclampsia.

Ergothioneine is sometimes called the "longevity vitamin" (even though it's not technically a vitamin), since studies show that it reduces all-cause mortality and is associated with longer life span. For example, a 2020 study that followed thirty-two hundred health-conscious people for more than twenty years evaluated the association of 112 different metabolites in their blood with cardiovascular disease and all-cause mortality. The one that made a difference out of all 112 was ergothioneine; the higher the blood levels of ergothioneine, the lower the risk of cardiovascular disease and death.[18] Another 2020 study in elderly hospital patients that evaluated 131 metabolites in their blood showed that those with low ergothioneine levels were much more likely to be frail and have impaired cognition.[19] And while further research is needed, yet another 2020 study showed that lower dietary intake of ergothioneine in America compared to four European countries correlated strongly with shorter average life span.[20]

Mushrooms are the dominant food source of ergothioneine, which is particularly high in medicinal mushrooms and some culinary varieties like shiitake, maitake, and oyster. For example, oyster mushrooms contain double the ergothioneine per kilogram of button mushrooms. Ergothioneine can be found in a few other foods, including tempeh, kidney beans, asparagus, and chicken liver.

Ergothioneine Content of Foods

Food	Serving Size (measured raw)	Nutrivore Score	Ergothioneine (milligrams per serving)
Shiitake mushrooms	1 cup	4,343	24.4
Enoki mushrooms	1 cup	4,434	19.4
Maitake mushrooms	1 cup	3,551	12.2
Oyster mushrooms	1 cup	2,550	11.3
Tempeh	1/4 cup	438	3.4
White mushrooms (button)	1 cup	1,872	3.3
Morel mushrooms	1 cup	2,271	3.2
Brown mushrooms (cremini)	1 cup	2,279	3.2

Food	Serving Size (measured raw)	Nutrivore Score	Ergothioneine (milligrams per serving)
Asparagus	1 cup	1,385	1.5
Portobello mushrooms	1 cup	1,483	1.4
Chanterelle mushrooms	1 cup	1,555	1.1
Chicken liver	3.5 ounces	2,502	1.1
Red kidney beans	1 ounce	413	0.2

GUT HEALTH CONCERNS? FANTASTIC FIBER AND FERMENTS

If you've ever been forced to stay home so you could be close to a toilet, or lain awake at night unable to sleep due to abdominal pain or cramping, then you know just how much gastrointestinal symptoms can erode your quality of life. And for a huge swath of the population, these are common experiences, owing to conditions such as diverticular disease, inflammatory bowel disease, and irritable bowel syndrome. While getting enough dietary fiber is linked to reduced risk of just about everything that could go wrong with your health, this type of carbohydrate is particularly important for preventing these gastrointestinal conditions.

Fiber is the quintessential example of a nutrient that isn't labeled as essential but that is absolutely fundamental for our health. What separates fiber from other carbohydrates is that the ways the constituent saccharides link are not compatible with our digestive enzymes; our bodies just aren't capable of breaking apart those types of molecular bonds. Instead, fiber passes through the digestive tract mainly intact. And once it reaches the colon, the magic begins: Fiber serves as a substrate (food) for a wide range of bacteria, including some of the most important and beneficial species we can harbor.

In fact, many of the health benefits attributed to fruits, vegetables, nuts, legumes, and whole grains are due to the way the fiber in these foods affects the gut microbiome. It's worth going on a bit of a tangent to talk about the gut microbiome, because it helps to illustrate why getting enough fiber is so fundamental to our health.

Fiber and the Gut Microbiome

The term "gut microbiome" refers to the massive collection of microorganisms that inhabit our gastrointestinal tract and the beneficial metabolic by-products they produce.[21] And "massive" is far from hyperbole: An estimated thirty to a hundred trillion bacteria (along with other microorganisms including fungi, viruses, and archaea) comprise the microbiome, collectively weighing around 4.5 pounds and containing more than 150 times more genes than our own human genome! These microbes include a mixture of commensal (neutrally existing), symbiotic (mutually beneficial, also called probiotic), and some pathogenic (harmful to us) organisms. Every person's gut contains approximately four hundred to fifteen hundred different species of the possible thirty-five thousand different microorganisms that are well adapted to survive in the human gastrointestinal tract, although about 99 percent of the microorganisms in your gut come from thirty to forty species of bacteria.

Our gut microbes perform many different essential functions that help us to stay healthy. These include digestion, vitamin production, detoxification, regulation of cholesterol metabolism, providing resistance to pathogens, immune regulation, neurotransmitter regulation, regulation of gene expression, and more. In fact, every human cell is affected by the activities of our gut microbes. A healthy gut microbial community—one with a high diversity of microbe species including representation of all the keystone probiotic species and with pathogen populations kept in check—is essential for our health. And the converse is also true. An aberrant gut microbiome—one with low microbial diversity, missing important probiotic species, and/or with too-high growth of pathogens—has been linked to conditions as wide-ranging as cancer, obesity, diabetes, cardiovascular disease, anxiety, depression, neurodegenerative diseases, autism, autoimmune disease, ulcers, inflammatory bowel disease, irritable bowel syndrome, liver disease, gout, PCOS, osteoporosis, systemic infections, allergies, asthma, and more.[22]

The composition and metabolic activity of the community of microbes in our guts is influenced greatly by the foods we eat, most notably the amount and types of fiber.[23] There are many types of fiber—like the glucans in oats, the cellulose in celery, the pectin in apples, the lignin in strawberries, and the chitin in mushrooms—each supporting the growth of a different collection of beneficial microbes. Some bacteria are very picky eaters and will only survive if you feed them their favorite food.[24] In fact, very small differences in fiber structure can make a huge difference in which bacteria are supported, which is why fiber supplements, while they can help regulate bowel movements, have limited utility from a gut microbiome perspective.[25] A good rule of thumb is to aim to eat a serving of at least thirty different plant foods per week.[26]

IBS, IBD, and Diverticular Disease

Inadequate fiber consumption increases risk of diverticular disease, inflammatory bowel disease, and irritable bowel syndrome via alterations to the gut microbiome that increase inflammation and via direct effects of fiber on intestinal motility and gastrointestinal function. So let's circle back to the links between the fiber content, or lack thereof, of our diets and the development and management of these gastrointestinal conditions.

Diverticular disease (including diverticulosis and diverticulitis) prevalence increases with age, affecting about 10 percent of people under the age of forty and at least half of adults over the age of sixty.[27] Diverticular disease is considered to be a complication of chronic low fiber consumption, although there are additional risk factors such as low vitamin D levels, smoking, and sedentary lifestyle.[28] It used to be that a diagnosis of diverticulitis or diverticulosis came with a lifetime ban on insoluble fiber-rich foods like corn, popcorn, nuts, and seeds, and often low-residue diets (very low fiber) were recommended.[29] This has changed in recent years in response to research showing the exact opposite, that high-fiber foods reduce the risk of diverticular disease complications.[30]

Inflammatory bowel disease (IBD) collectively refers to Crohn's disease and ulcerative colitis, which are high-morbidity autoimmune conditions characterized by chronic inflammation of the gastrointestinal tract, and which affect 1.3 percent of Americans.[31] Eating a high-fiber diet is well known to reduce risk of IBD. For example, a 2011 systematic review identified fiber, vegetables, and fruit as protective against inflammatory bowel diseases, with fiber and fruit being more protective against Crohn's disease and vegetables being more protective against ulcerative colitis.[32] And a 2013 prospective study showed that high-fiber diets (about twenty-four grams of fiber daily) reduced risk of developing Crohn's disease by 40 percent compared to low-fiber diets (less than twelve grams daily). It is currently unclear whether increasing dietary fiber intake is helpful once IBD has developed, but studies also show that it doesn't increase disease activity, and a few small studies indicate that high fiber intake may help prolong remission in ulcerative colitis.[33]

Irritable bowel syndrome (IBS) is a diagnosis of exclusion, and refers to gastrointestinal symptoms—such as constipation, diarrhea, cramping, abdominal pain, bloating, and gas—without a clear cause such as IBD, celiac disease, diverticular disease, or stomach ulcer. It's estimated that 11 percent of people globally are affected by IBS.[34] IBS is believed to be primarily caused by low dietary fiber causing an unhealthy gut microbiome, although fiber supplements have shown limited utility in symptom management, likely because probiotics are additionally required to improve gut microbiome composition.[35] Probiotics supplements containing *Bacillus coagulans* have the best track record for IBS, but *Lactobacillus plantarum* and *Lactobacillus acidophilus* have also been shown to be very beneficial.[36] While there's still some uncertainty on the best types of fiber and best probiotic combinations for different manifestations of IBS, it seems as though both are required for effective treatment.[37]

Fiber Goalz and the Best Food Sources

The RDA of fiber is fourteen grams per one thousand calories. So, if you eat a two-thousand-calorie-per-day diet, aim for at least twenty-eight grams of fiber. Fiber is one of those "the more, the better" nutrients. For example, a 2015 meta-analysis calculated that for every ten grams of daily fiber you consume, risk of all-cause mortality decreases by 10 percent.[38]

All whole plant foods—whole grains, legumes, vegetables, fruits, nuts, and seeds—contribute fiber to our diets. While pulse legumes and certain fruits and veggies stand out as being particularly fiber rich, the most important thing you can do to up your fiber intake is to simply fill three quarters of your plate with whole plant foods, à la Nutrivore Meal Map (see page 70).

Fiber content is retained quite well through preparation and cooking, so as long as you're eating the whole plant food, you can enjoy your fruits and veggies raw, roasted, boiled, steamed, grilled, fried, microwaved, pureed in smoothies, or snuck into baked goods. Ditto for whole grains and pulse legumes, with the exception that these should not be eaten raw. You get more fiber per serving when you leave the peel or skin on fruits and veggies, when it's edible. Juicing fruits and veggies removes most of the fiber, which is discarded with the pulp, so it's best to stick with whole options most of the time.

High-Fiber Foods

Here is a selection of some high-fiber foods that make it easy to hit your fiber goals.

Food	Serving Size	Fiber Content per Serving
Kumquats	1 cup	14.6 grams
Chia seeds	1 ounce (about 3 tablespoons)	9.8 grams
Artichoke (globe or French)	1 cup	9.1 grams
Guava	1 cup	8.9 grams
Green peas	1 cup	8.3 grams
Split peas, boiled	1/2 cup	8.2 grams
Raspberries	1 cup	8.0 grams

Food	Serving Size	Fiber Content
Lentils, boiled	1/2 cup	7.8 grams
Blackberries	1 cup	7.6 grams
Black beans, boiled	1/2 cup	7.5 grams
Kidney beans, boiled	1/2 cup	6.6 grams
Chickpeas, boiled	1/2 cup	6.3 grams

Increasing Fiber Intake? Go Slow!

If you're looking to up your fiber intake, it's best to do so gradually. This is because a sudden increase in fiber intake can cause a variety of unpleasant symptoms, such as gas, bloating, constipation, and diarrhea—your gut microbiome needs time to adjust to your dietary changes.

It's recommended to step up your fiber intake weekly, giving your digestive tract a full week to acclimate to each incremental increase, until you hit your target fiber intake levels—the recommended amount to increase each week is five grams per day.[39] If you're starting out at ten grams of fiber daily, go up to fifteen grams for all of next week, the week after go up to twenty grams for the whole week, and the week after that, go up to twenty-five grams for the whole week. If a five-gram incremental increase causes gastrointestinal symptoms, it's okay to take smaller steps and give more time between each increase.

It's also helpful to make sure your fiber is coming from a variety of sources (not from supplements or fiber-fortified meal replacement products like protein bars) and that you're incorporating some probiotic fermented foods, like sauerkraut, yogurt, kefir, and kombucha.

When in doubt, consult your doctor.

Fermented Foods for Gut Health

Probiotics are often recommended to fix an out-of-whack gut microbiome, but rather than reach for supplements, consider fermented foods. They reduce risk of cancer, cardiovascular disease, osteoporosis, type 2 diabetes, obesity, allergies, and gastrointestinal disorders. This is thanks to their probiotics (when raw and unpasteurized), beneficial bioactive compounds created as a result of the fermentation (also called *postbiotics*, like short-chain fatty acids), and the nutrients inherent in the food that was fermented.[40]

A 2021 study showed that eating fermented foods more reliably improved gut microbiome composition and reduced inflammation, compared to a high-fiber diet.[41] Specifically, eating an average of six servings of fermented foods daily—one serving defined as six ounces for kombucha, yogurt, kefir, buttermilk, and kvass; a quarter cup for kimchi, sauerkraut, and other fermented veggies; and two ounces for vegetable brine drink (the liquid leftover after fermenting vegetables)—increased gut microbiome diversity and reduced inflammation across the whole cohort. In contrast, gut microbiome composition was more stable after increasing fiber intake to an average of forty-three grams daily, and the effects on inflammation were mixed—for some study participants it went down, but for others it went up. The authors of this landmark study make a great case for doing both, upping fiber intake *and* eating more fermented foods.

There isn't a specific daily recommended intake for probiotics, and the amount and bacteria strains present in fermented foods vary widely, so there's no definitive guidance on how much fermented foods to consume. But a 2013 study showed that as little as fifteen grams of kimchi daily (about 1.5 tablespoons) for one week reduced LDL and total cholesterol, triglycerides, and fasting blood glucose levels in healthy young adults.[42] So every little bit counts! A great goal is to eat some fermented foods every day.

What can we load our plates with? Let's start with some of these: fermented vegetables (sauerkraut, kimchi, pickles), fermented fruits (chutneys, pickled jackfruit), fermented condiments (relishes, pickled ginger), kombucha, kefir, yogurt, kvass, natto, miso, tempeh, and vinegars—all teeming with beneficial microbes!

OLÉ, OLÉ, OLÉ, OLEIC ACID TO LOWER CHOLESTEROL

Approximately 117 million Americans live with some kind of cardiovascular disease, and cardiovascular disease is responsible for about 875,000 deaths each year in the United States alone (and more than 19 million deaths globally each year).[43] It is the single biggest killer and the single biggest health care cost. Risk factors for cardiovascular disease include high cholesterol, high blood pressure, type 2 diabetes, smoking and secondhand smoke exposure, unhealthy diet, and physical inactivity. Let's zoom in on cholesterol and why a specific fatty acid called *oleic acid*, the dominant fat in olive oil, is so good at lowering it.

Even though many people associate cholesterol with heart disease, it's a nutrient that plays an essential biological role. It is the molecular backbone of steroid hormones—including vitamin D, estrogen, testosterone, progesterone, and cortisol—and bile acids, which help us to digest fats. Plus, cholesterol is a structural component of cellular membranes that helps to maintain membrane fluidity. What is often referred to as serum or blood cholesterol isn't actually cholesterol itself but rather lipid transport molecules called lipoproteins. There are four classes of lipoproteins that circulate in our blood: chylomicrons, very low density lipoproteins (VLDL), low-density lipoproteins (LDL), and high-density lipoproteins (HDL), the latter of which can transport thousands of lipids in a single lipoprotein particle. The two major lipids that are transported by these lipoproteins are triglycerides and cholesterol. As such, it isn't high cholesterol per se that is associated with cardiovascular disease but rather high levels of VLDL and LDL (or "bad cholesterol") along with high levels of free triglycerides (triglycerides that aren't transported by a lipoprotein) in the blood. High levels of high-density lipoproteins (HDL, or "good cholesterol") are protective against heart disease.

The fear of dietary cholesterol started in the 1950s and peaked in the 1970s due to an assumption made by prominent scientists like Ancel Keys that dietary cholesterol increased blood cholesterol and that this directly caused cardiovascular disease.[44] But it's been known since the 1990s that for most people, dietary cholesterol does not translate to elevated LDL and VLDL.

In response to extensive scientific research, the recommended daily limit of three hundred milligrams of cholesterol was removed in the 2015–2020 edition of the USDA Dietary Guidelines for Americans. Even though dietary cholesterol doesn't affect serum cholesterol for most people, bad news on a serum lipid panel—high total cholesterol, high LDL "bad" cholesterol, high triglycerides, and low HDL "good" cholesterol—will still have your doctor emphasizing the need for major dietary shifts, like recommending a Mediterranean-style diet, the generic term for a diet pattern that emphasizes fruits and vegetables, whole grains, seafood, nuts, legumes, and (ding, ding, ding, ding) olive oil.

Countless research studies have demonstrated that olive oil can help to prevent cardiovascular disease by protecting the integrity of your vascular system (think healthy blood vessels) and lowering your dangerous LDL cholesterol (a marker of inflammation, too).[45] For example, a 2014 prospective study showed that participants who consumed the most olive oil had a 35 percent reduced risk of cardiovascular disease, and a 39 percent reduced risk if they mainly consumed extra virgin olive oil, compared to the lowest intake of olive oil.[46] The authors calculated that for every ten grams per day of extra virgin olive oil you add to your diet (one tablespoon is fourteen grams), your risk of cardiovascular disease decreases by 10 percent and your risk of mortality from cardiovascular disease decreases by 7 percent. In fact, a 2019 meta-analysis showed that olive oil was the best plant oil for reducing LDL cholesterol, total cholesterol, and triglycerides, and it additionally increased HDL cholesterol.[47] And a 2022 study showed that just seven grams—about half of a tablespoon—of olive oil daily reduced all-cause mortality by 19 percent compared to rarely consuming olive oil.[48] What's in olive oil that is responsible for these heart health benefits? It's a long-chain monounsaturated fat called *oleic acid*, which reduces cardiovascular disease risk factors like high blood pressure, cholesterol, triglycerides, inflammation, and oxidative stress, and reduces actual cardiovascular disease incidence and events.[49]

Switching to oleic acid–rich fats like olive oil is more beneficial from a cardiovascular disease risk perspective than reducing total fat intake. A 1999 randomized controlled double-blind clinical trial evaluated several diets where 34 percent of total calories came from fat, and 20 percent or more of total calories were from monounsaturated fats (mainly oleic acid).[50] Compared to either a reduced fat diet or the control average American diet, the high monounsaturated fat diets reduced total cholesterol by 10 percent and LDL cholesterol by 14 percent. A 2021 meta-analysis calculated that for each additional 5 percent of total calories coming from monounsaturated fats, risk of all-cause mortality decreased by 3 percent.[51] A 2008 study showed that 80 percent of the reduction in blood pressure caused by increasing olive oil consumption could be attributed to the effects of oleic acid.[52]

While olive oil usually gets all the oleic acid love, you also get these heart-healthy fats from whole olives, avocados, high-oleic sunflower oil (which is made from sunflower seeds specially selected to have more oleic acid), palm olein (the separated liquid fraction of palm oil that is higher in oleic acid), and some nuts, notably macadamia nuts and cashews.

FISH FOR THOUGHT: HOW EPA AND DHA IMPROVE COGNITION AND BRAIN HEALTH

Do you often misplace your keys only to find them later in your pocket? Do you ever leave the stove burner on only to remember when your burned meal sets off the smoke detector? Do you regularly blank on a word or someone's name midconversation? These can be early signs of Alzheimer's disease or other forms of dementia—which affects about one in ten US adults over the age of sixty-five—so it's worthwhile mentioning to your doctor next time you see them.[53] But they can also be signs of what we colloquially refer to as brain fog, the mild cognitive impairment that can be associated with stress, not getting enough sleep, and many chronic health conditions, and which affects 22 percent of people sixty-five years and older. Whether your concern is dementia, or simply enhancing attention, focus, and memory, increasing intake of two fatty acids in particular, EPA and DHA, can help.

Eicosapentaenoic acid (EPA) and docosahexaenoic acid (DHA) are the long-chain omega-3 fatty acids found in seafood that are most famous for their cardiovascular and immune health benefits. But they also improve brain health in a variety of ways, including supporting neuron function, reducing neuroinflammation, increasing neurogenesis (the formation of new neurons), enhancing cerebral blood flow, reducing amyloid aggregation (implicated in dementia), and playing roles in neurotransmission (the transfer of information between neurons via chemical signaling).[54] It's no surprise therefore that low omega-3 levels have been associated with a number of mood disorders and neurological conditions, including depression, bipolar disorder, attention deficit and hyperactivity disorder (ADHD), autism spectrum disorder, dementia (including Alzheimer's disease), and schizophrenia.[55]

DHA has some specific additional roles in nervous system health. In fact, it serves as a major component of neuronal plasma membranes, and makes up about 40 percent of the polyunsaturated fatty acid content of the brain.[56] Along with being incorporated into postsynaptic cells (neuron cells that receive signals), DHA increases the release of the neurotransmitter acetylcholine, which plays a role in brain plasticity and memory.

EPA and DHA have been shown to improve working memory and processing accuracy in healthy adults, young and old alike, and to reduce the rate of cognitive decline in the elderly. For example, a 2012 study in young adults showed improvements to working memory after six months of taking a supplement containing a combined 1,680 milligrams of EPA and DHA.[57] A 2015 meta-analysis showed that just one gram daily was enough to improve working memory in healthy adults.[58] And a 2022 study showed that Alzheimer's disease patients with lower serum levels of DHA had more rapid cognitive decline than those with higher levels.[59] This study also showed that levels of omega-3 fats in the blood are directly related to dietary intake.

Rich sources of DHA and EPA are fish, particularly fatty cold-water fish (like salmon, herring, mackerel, and sardines) as well as some algaes and cod liver oil. Shellfish such as crab, oysters, and squid also contain some long-chain omega-3s. There are trace amounts (about 1.2 milligrams per two-cup serving) in the leafy green vegetable purslane, but the type of omega-3 found in plant foods is more typically ALA. If you don't eat seafood, fish oil, krill oil, or algal oil, supplements can be used to increase your intake of these important healthy fats.

Eating more seafood is one of the best things you can do to prevent cognitive decline and dementia as you age. One 2018 analysis found that eating four or more servings of fish per week (compared to less than one weekly serving) was associated with a significantly slower decline in global cognition and memory in the elderly, the cognitive equivalent to being four years younger.[60] Similarly, a 2016 meta-analysis found that each additional serving of fish per week was associated with a 5 percent reduction in dementia risk and a 7 percent reduction in Alzheimer's risk.[61] And a 2022 meta-analysis showed that just two servings of fish per week reduced Alzheimer's disease risk by a whopping 30 percent and all-cause dementia by 10 percent.[62]

Eating more fish can improve cognition in kids, too! A 2020 randomized trial of healthy eight- and nine-year-old children found that the addition of three hundred grams of oily fish per week (just shy of three servings) led to significant improvements in cognitive function (particularly cognitive flexibility and attention) while also reducing social and emotional behavioral issues.[63]

HYDRATION MOTIVATION: PREVENTING KIDNEY STONES

Kidney stones affect approximately 10.6 percent of males and 7.1 percent of females in the United States.[64] Although there are different types of kidney stones, calcium oxalate kidney stones are the most common, accounting for about 80 percent of cases. Certain dietary factors increase risk—high meat intake, high salt intake, low calcium intake, and low intake of fruits and vegetables, all things we're going to fix with Nutrivore—but the biggest risk factor is inadequate hydration.[65]

Water is an essential nutrient; staying hydrated is essential for kidney health and helps optimize digestion, neurological function, circulation, body temperature regulation, and muscle contraction. The latest research suggests that adult males should consume about thirteen cups (101 ounces, or three liters) of fluid per day, and adult females should consume about nine cups (seventy-four ounces, or 2.2 liters)—but this includes all beverages (yes, even tea and coffee), as well as the water content of the food we eat.[66] We get about 20 percent of our daily water from food, particularly fruits, vegetables, and soups.

How does hydrating ourselves better prevent kidney stones? When we have too-high concentrations of oxalates in the urine, a condition called hyperoxaluria, calcium oxalate crystals can form in the kidneys and develop into stones. Increasing fluid intake reduces the risk of kidney stones by increasing urine volume and diluting oxalate levels, in turn helping prevent stones from forming. In fact, ingesting enough fluids to keep urine flow greater than one milliliter per kilogram of body weight per hour nearly eliminates the risk of oxalate oversaturation in the urine, and can dramatically reduce kidney stone formation. There's some indication that drinking up to 50 percent more than the standard recommendations is important for people with recurring kidney stones.

While we're talking about hydration, go ahead and skip the alkaline water—not only are the various claims unfounded but too-high pH water can negatively affect the gut microbiome.[67]

BALANCED MACRONUTRIENTS: WHAT DOES THAT EVEN MEAN?

There's one more important topic related to macronutrients: the benefits of consuming them in relative balance, meaning neither high nor low of any macronutrient. The Food and Nutrition Board of the Institute of Medicine has set accepted macronutrient distribution ranges (AMDR) for protein, fat, and carbohydrates:

- 10 to 35 percent calories from protein
- 20 to 35 percent calories from fat
- 45 to 65 percent calories from carbohydrate (but no more than 25 percent from sugars)

This is what is referred to as *balanced macronutrients*, the happy medium range for protein, fat, and carbohydrates that a wealth of scientific studies prove best supports overall health. In fact, a rigorous 2020 systematic review showed that diets outside of the AMDR for protein, fat, and/or carbohydrates increase risk for all-cause mortality.[68]

A *balanced diet* refers to eating a wide range of foods in the right proportions to deliver balanced macronutrients. Importantly, there's a lot of wiggle room within these AMDR ranges, which means there's a lot of flexibility in adopting a balanced diet. For example, if you eat a 2,000-calorie-per-day diet, your macronutrients would be balanced if you consume anywhere between 50 and 150 grams of protein, 44 to 78 grams of fat, and 190 to 270 grams of carbohydrates with at least 28 grams of fiber.

Contrary to purported claims, rigorous and well-controlled metabolic ward studies have confirmed that low-carb and ketogenic diets don't turn us into "fat-burning machines" with increased energy expenditure and preferential fat mass loss—if anything, they do the opposite.[69] Plus, very low carbohydrate diets are associated with a variety of unwanted side effects, such as fatigue, headaches, gastrointestinal symptoms, increased risk of infection, menstrual irregularities, kidney stones, and heart problems. Far from this being a transitory "low-carb flu," these potentially serious side effects are a reflection of how many amazing things insulin does in the human body beyond simply shuttling glucose into cells. And while there is no recommended dietary allowance (RDA) for carbohydrates, there is one for fiber: fourteen grams per thousand calories. It is very challenging to consume sufficient fiber on a low-carbohydrate diet.

Too-high carbohydrate intake is a problem if it means insufficient fat and protein intake, or if those carbohydrates are coming largely from sugar. In addition to staying below 10 percent of calories from added sugar, as discussed in chapter 4, it's important to moderate sugar from whole foods like fruit as well. A 2013 systematic review showed that when 25 to 30 percent of our calories come from sugar, even when we're not consuming excess calories, cardiovascular disease risk factors increase.[70] This research is behind the AMDR for carbohydrates including a limit on calories from sugars of 25 percent of total calories.

Our Gut Bacteria Also Love Starchy Foods

Another reason to avoid going too low carb is that it's not great for our gut microbiomes. Resistant starch is abundant in foods like potatoes, rice, plantains, lentils, and oats—so cutting down on these types of foods to reduce carbohydrate intake can have negative consequences for those gut bacteria that prefer resistant starch to other fiber types.

A 2019 study of children following a ketogenic diet to help manage therapy-resistant epilepsy showed that three months of a very low carb diet caused significant reductions in important probiotic *Bifidobacterium* species.[71] A 2019 study of adults following a low-carb Paleo diet showed reduced levels of probiotic *Bifidobacterium* and *Roseburia* species.[72] Why is this a big deal? Reduced levels of *Bifidobacterium* are associated with inflammatory bowel disease, irritable bowel syndrome, allergies, asthma, atopic dermatitis (aka eczema), obesity, metabolic syndrome, type 1 and type 2 diabetes, autoimmune disease, colorectal cancer, depression, and Alzheimer's disease.[73] Reduced levels of *Roseburia* are associated with inflammatory bowel disease, irritable bowel syndrome, obesity, type 2 diabetes, cardiovascular disease, neurological diseases, autoimmune disease, asthma, and allergies.[74]

Excessive fat intake is associated with increased risk of obesity, type 2 diabetes, cardiovascular disease, dementia, certain cancers, and even certain autoimmune diseases.[75] Of course, it's not as simple as "go low fat," which comes with its own health risks like obesity, type 2 diabetes, cardiovascular disease, depression and anxiety, certain cancers, and certain autoimmune diseases.[76] (Yes, those lists are nearly identical! Mind blown, right?) It turns out that a huge variety of factors are at play here, like the overall quality of the diet, whether the diet includes excess calories, and whether the person is overweight.

The amount of fat in the diet seems to be overall more important than the types of fat, provided we're getting enough of those fatty acids that are extremely beneficial to our health, like oleic acid, DHA, and EPA, as we've already discussed. Yes, this may even be true with regards to saturated fat, although this question is currently being hotly debated by scientists, akin to the debate over cholesterol that happened in the 1990s and early 2000s.[77]

The argument in favor of ditching the current limits on saturated fat intake in dietary guidelines is based on meta-analyses of prospective studies that show no association between how much saturated fat people eat and what are called "hard end points," like all-cause mortality, cardiovascular disease mortality, total coronary heart disease, ischemic stroke, and type 2 diabetes.[78] And, the argument in favor of continuing to recommend limiting saturated fat to 10 percent of total calories is based on clinical trials where participants reduce their saturated fat intake (for example, by replacing butter with vegetable oils) showing a reduction in cardiovascular disease incidence (although not cardiovascular disease mortality nor all-cause mortality).[79]

One explanation for these opposing results put forward by scientists is that what really matters is the dietary patterns in which saturated fats are consumed, pointing to studies showing that whole food sources of saturated fat—like cheese, red meat, and chocolate—have a neutral or slightly beneficial effect on cardiovascular disease risk, whereas saturated fats used for cooking or added to ultraprocessed foods increase risk.[80] While the jury is still out on this question, it's prudent to rein in saturated fat intake. Fortunately for us, adopting Nutrivore principles—including sticking with balanced macros, eating a wide diversity of whole foods, and prioritizing heart-healthy fats like those in olive oil and seafood—will typically result in saturated fat intake easily below the 10 percent threshold. But when in doubt, talk to your doctor.

A flexible metabolism is one that can easily switch between carbohydrates and fats, depending on what's available. Although protein is not a preferred source of energy, it can be used if needed—this is why people lose muscle mass in addition to fat stores when they are too severely calorically restricted, fasting, or starving. In fact, protein is the only macronutrient to have an RDA in addition to the AMDR.

The RDA of protein is 0.8 grams per kilogram of body weight (0.36 grams per pound body weight). That amounts to fifty-six grams of protein per day for a 150-pound person. However, it's important to emphasize that many studies have evaluated diets containing three to four times more protein than this minimum and proven benefits to weight management, body composition, hormone regulation, and cardiovascular health.[81] These studies suggest that an optimal protein intake for most people is probably in the range of 1.2 to 1.8 grams of protein per kilogram of body weight (82 to 122 grams daily protein for that same 150-pound person), and that people who are very active may see the best results at even higher intake (up to as high as 2.4 grams of protein per kilogram of body weight, 164 grams of daily protein for that same 150-pound person).

While the primary goal of Nutrivore is lifelong health, not losing weight, it's also worth noting that a plethora of studies show that higher protein consumption can help to preserve lean mass during a caloric deficit, facilitating fat loss, should that be a goal for you.[82] A 2010 study compared the effect of moderate protein intake (1.0 gram of protein per kilogram of body weight per day) to high protein intake (2.3 grams of protein per kilogram of body weight per day) on lean body mass in athletes over a four-week-long caloric deficit.[83] While the moderate protein group lost more weight (3.0 kilograms), more than half of that was muscle mass (1.6 kilograms). In comparison, the high protein group lost about the same amount of fat, and only 0.3 kilograms of muscle mass. A similar 2013 study that included normal weight and overweight participants who were physically active found that higher protein intake (1.6 or 2.4 grams of protein per kilogram of body weight) preserved muscle mass during a month of eating 30 percent fewer calories and exercising more to burn 10 percent more calories, compared to following the RDA.[84] Again, while the number on the scale dropped more for the lower protein intake group, the participants consuming higher protein lost more fat mass (1.8 kilograms compared to 1.3 kilograms, for 1.6 grams protein per kilogram of body weight compared to 0.8) and much less muscle mass (0.9 kilograms compared to 2.2 kilograms). This study interestingly showed that there's a maximum benefit—there

More Protein as You Age Is a Good Idea

Sarcopenia—gradual loss of muscle mass, strength, and function associated with aging—can greatly affect your quality of life as you age by reducing your ability to perform daily tasks. Up to 13 percent of people aged sixty to seventy years, and up to 50 percent of people over the age of eighty, are affected by sarcopenic symptoms such as fatigue, weakness, loss of coordination, difficulty balancing, and slower speed of walking and standing.[85] Importantly, menopause seems to accelerate sarcopenia—a 2021 study showed that females lost 10 percent of their muscle mass during the perimenopausal period.[86]

Physical activity and consuming adequate protein are the two best things you can do to prevent sarcopenia.[87] A 2015 study showed that upping protein intake by just 20 percent reduced risk of frailty in sixty- to ninety-year-old women by 32 percent, thanks to preserving muscle mass.[88] And a 2008 study in men and women aged seventy to seventy-nine showed that consuming at least 1.2 grams of protein per kilogram of body weight reduced muscle mass loss by 40 percent compared to consuming 0.8 grams of protein per kilogram of body weight during the three-year follow-up period.[89]

wasn't a difference between 1.6 and 2.4 grams per kilogram of body weight, so there doesn't seem to be a good rationale to go much above 1.6 grams per kilogram of body weight for nonathletes. It's worth noting that at higher body weight concurrent with lower caloric intake, there may be a discrepancy between protein intake goals using these formulas and the AMDR—if this is the case for you, please consult your doctor.

So how do you get enough protein? Let's look at the protein content of some common food options:

Protein Content of Common Foods

Food	Serving Size (measured raw)	Nutrivore Score	Protein Per Serving
Grass-fed beef loin strip steak	3.5 ounces	371	23.1 grams
Shrimp	4 ounces	535	23.1 grams
Wild Atlantic salmon	4 ounces	868	22.8 grams
Chicken breast, skinless	3.5 ounces	309	22.5 grams
Eggs	2 large	355	12.6 grams
Tofu	1/4 cup	339	10.0 grams
Sharp cheddar cheese	1.5 ounces	121	10.2 grams
Quinoa	1 ounce	227	4.0 grams

A three- to four-ounce serving of meat or seafood, or two servings of a plant protein like tofu or lentils, at each of three meals per day would satisfy the lower end of the recommended protein consumption for an average person, with about double that satisfying the higher end of protein requirements for people looking to lose weight or support athletic performance. Provided you're getting enough total protein from a variety of different foods (animal foods and/or complete plant protein foods), you don't need to worry about amino acid deficiencies—these are typically only seen in the context of malnourishment and starvation.

While you certainly can apply Nutrivore principles to a macronutrient manipulation–based diet if you desire, the default on Nutrivore is balanced macronutrients for all the reasons outlined here. The Nutrivore Meal Map (see page 70) and the Nutrivore Weekly Serving Matrix (see page 234) have balanced macronutrients principles baked in, so if you're using these tools, even casually or haphazardly, you're extremely likely to be eating a diet within the AMDR ranges for protein, carbohydrates, and fat.

CHAPTER 6

Magnificent Minerals

Nutritionally, a mineral is defined as a chemical element (that is, a member of the periodic table) required as an essential nutrient. In our food, minerals may be present in inorganic salts (like table salt, aka sodium chloride) or as part of carbon-containing organic compounds (like the magnesium in chlorophyll, the pigment that makes plants green).

The discovery of minerals as essential nutrients followed closely on the heels of the "chemical revolution," a scientifically exuberant era in the late eighteenth and early nineteenth centuries, when chemists isolated many chemical elements for the first time in addition to developing chemical analysis methodologies.[1] The first mineral to be identified as an essential nutrient was iodine, which is necessary for thyroid health since it's a structural component of thyroid hormones.[2] This is an interesting story; let me set the stage.

Before iodine's discovery, goiter due to iodine deficiency was so widespread that it is depicted in paintings dating from the Byzantine Empire. Beyond the signature swelling in the neck caused by enlargement of the thyroid gland, symptoms of goiter include hoarseness, dizziness, coughing, trouble swallowing, and even difficulty breathing. In England during the mid-1700s, the treatment du jour for goiter was an elixir called the "Coventry Remedy," whose closely guarded secret ingredient was burned sea sponge, an ancient medicine whose earliest recorded use dates from Chinese physicians in 1600 BCE. But in

1779, the Coventry Remedy formula was published, making its active ingredient widely known—insert a Shock Horror sound effect: *dun-dun-dunnnnn!*

Meanwhile, iodine as a chemical element was first discovered completely by chance in 1811, when a French chemist named Barnard Courtois was extracting potassium and sodium from the ashes of seaweed, trying to find an alternative way to create gunpowder. When he accidentally added too much sulfuric acid to the seaweed ash, a cloud of purple vapor erupted, condensed onto the copper vats in the room, and formed blue-black crystals of solid iodine. Fun fact: That unusual vapor color inspired iodine's name, which comes from the Greek word *iodes*, meaning violet.

The person who put two and two together was a Swiss physician named Jean François Coindet, who showed in 1820 that iodine was indeed the active constituent of burned sea sponge for treating goiter. Coindet created a tincture of iodine crystals dissolved in distilled alcohol and administered it to people with long-standing goiters. Amazingly, their goiters started shrinking within eight days, and many were completely gone in as little as six weeks. No prior remedy for goiter had ever come close to this impressive efficacy. And a century after Coindet's pioneering work, in 1924 iodized table salt, the first fortified food, was introduced in the United States, reducing risk of goiter by 74 percent.[3]

Iodine is a relatively simple mineral from a biological perspective, since 80 percent of all the iodine in the adult human body is found in the thyroid gland. Other essential minerals have much more complex roles, most of which weren't discovered until the twentieth century, and some of which are still not fully understood.

We now divide essential minerals into macrominerals, which are those we need in excess of a hundred milligrams per day to avoid symptoms of deficiency, and trace minerals, which are those we need in much smaller amounts, one to one hundred milligrams per day, to avoid symptoms of deficiency. Macrominerals include sodium, chloride, potassium, phosphorus, magnesium, and calcium. Trace minerals include copper, chromium, iodine, iron, molybdenum, manganese, selenium, and zinc.

Just as we did in chapter 5, let's zoom in on some specifics, highlighting particular and broadly relevant health effects of some of the most fascinating essential minerals.

Seaweed vs. Sea Salt for Iodine

If you consume iodized table salt, or foods made with iodized table salt like fast food or packaged salty snacks, you don't need to worry whether you're getting enough iodine. But if you switch to unrefined sea salt—Himalayan pink salt, Celtic sea salt, or French cel gris—you're trading that iodine (and some of the sodium) for a wider diversity of trace minerals. For example, a 2020 study measured the amounts of twenty-five trace minerals in Himalayan pink salt, finding that most samples contained calcium, magnesium, potassium, iron, copper, chromium, manganese, molybdenum, phosphorus, selenium, zinc, barium, boron, cobalt, silicon, sulfur, and vanadium (in order from highest to lowest amounts, on average).[4]

If you do switch to noniodized salt to benefit from all those trace minerals, it's important to make sure you're still getting enough iodine. While fish, shellfish, eggs, and dairy are all good sources, your best food source of iodine is sea vegetables like nori, wakame, arame, kombu, and kelp. Some sea vegetables can have very high iodine content (especially kelp and kombu), so it's worth making sure you don't exceed the tolerable upper limit of iodine by overdoing sea vegetables.[5]

And sea vegetables are definitely a plus when it comes to our health. A 2020 study showed that eating seaweed almost every day reduced risk of cardiovascular disease by 21 percent in men and 20 percent in women, compared to never eating seaweed.[6] A 2021 study showed that eating about one serving of sea vegetables per day (a serving is five grams for dried sea vegetables and three grams for sheets like nori wraps, one of which weighs about three grams) reduced risk of all-cause mortality by 6 percent.[7]

PMS AS A CONSEQUENCE OF CALCIUM INSUFFICIENCY

There are so many clichés about premenstrual syndrome, aka PMS, but the reality is that upward of 90 percent of people who menstruate report symptoms such as bloating, constipation, cramps, headaches, cravings, fatigue, anxiety, and moodiness the week or two before their period starts.[8] If you ever have felt like this monthly ebb and flow (pun intended) is something to suffer in silence while popping nonsteroidal anti-inflammatory drugs (NSAIDs), then your mind is about to be blown by the knowledge that PMS symptoms can be alleviated by upping nutrient intake, especially calcium.

Calcium is a major structural component of bones and teeth, and serves as an electrolyte—a type of electricity-conducting mineral needed for regulating nerve impulses, muscle contraction (including the beating of our hearts), blood pH, and fluid balance. Getting enough calcium is vital for protecting against osteoporosis and bone fractures, especially in conjunction with vitamin D and magnesium. But calcium can also help reduce your risk of kidney stones, protect against pregnancy-related high blood pressure, lower your risk of colorectal cancer (and improve survival following diagnosis), help you maintain a healthy body weight, and, yes, even reduce PMS symptoms!

Calcium improves PMS thanks to its antagonistic relationship with estrogen and how their interplay ultimately affects serotonin. No, calcium isn't nagging estrogen to do its homework and stop wearing goth makeup. This means that as estrogen levels gradually increase—first just before ovulation, and second during the midluteal phase (a few days to a week after ovulation)—that directly causes calcium levels to decrease, especially inside cells. The parathyroid gland senses this decrease in calcium, so it produces more parathyroid hormone, which helps to move calcium from the outside of cells to the inside. The problem occurs when there just isn't enough calcium for parathyroid hormone to normalize levels, and the combination of too much parathyroid hormone and too little calcium causes a series of biochemical changes ultimately resulting in abnormalities in neurotransmitter synthesis and release, especially serotonin.[9] Then, as estrogen levels start to drop the week or so before your period starts, so, too, does your serotonin.

You may recognize serotonin as the neurotransmitter important for mood regulation, and whose deficiency is associated with both depression and anxiety. But as a hormone neurotransmitter, serotonin does so much more than boost our mood! Serotonin also influences learning and memory, body temperature regulation, sleep, sexual behavior, addiction, appetite, and pain perception. Serotonin even helps to regulate intestinal peristalsis (that's the coordinated muscle contractions that help push food through our digestive tracts), which is why serotonin also plays a role in nausea, vomiting, constipation, and diarrhea. Yep, between those functions, all the symptoms we associate with PMS are covered!

Calcium supplementation has been shown to make PMS symptoms less severe, and people with high dietary calcium intakes (1,200 to 1,300 milligrams daily) have a 30 percent lower risk of experiencing PMS compared to people with low calcium intakes (around five hundred milligrams daily).[10] In a 1998 clinical trial, premenopausal women were randomly assigned either a 1,200-milligram calcium carbonate supplement daily or a placebo, and within three cycles, the women taking calcium saw their PMS symptom severity cut in half.[11] Calcium benefited all four symptom factors—negative affect, water retention, food cravings, and pain—and improved fifteen of the seventeen symptoms tracked by this study.

Low dietary calcium, especially in combination with low vitamin D, also increases the risk of severe period cramps and other discomforts during menstruation such as leg pain, nausea, vomiting, diarrhea, fatigue, weakness, fainting, and headaches.[12] So a more calcium-replete diet can help in this regard, too.

While dairy products aren't particularly nutrient dense, you just can't beat them from a calcium concentration perspective. One ounce of cheddar cheese has an impressive two hundred milligrams of calcium, or about one sixth of the daily value. One cup of skim milk has three hundred milligrams of calcium, or one quarter of the daily value. And a cup of low-fat yogurt has about 450 milligrams, over a third of the daily value!

And, as you would expect, studies show dairy consumption, especially skim and low-fat milk and yogurt, reduces PMS. In a 2005 study, women who consumed four or more servings of dairy products daily had a 32 percent lower risk of experiencing PMS, and women who consumed four or more cups of skim or low-fat milk specifically daily had a 46 percent lower risk of experiencing PMS, compared to one or fewer servings weekly.[13]

Can't do dairy? Other great sources of calcium include bone-in canned fish, green cruciferous vegetables (like kale, collard greens, and turnip greens), seaweed, and molasses.

Got Molasses?

Wait, molasses is a good source of calcium? Yes! Plus, it's by far the most nutrient-dense sugar option with its Nutrivore Score of 367. For comparison, maple syrup's Nutrivore Score is 103, honey's is 20, and granulated sugar's is 1. Molasses is so nutrient dense that it contains 40 percent more calcium per calorie than cheddar cheese and nearly three times more iron per calorie than grass-fed strip steak. A single tablespoon delivers 50 percent daily value manganese, 45 percent daily value biotin, 17 percent daily value potassium, 15 percent daily value each of iron, magnesium, and vitamin B5, and 11 percent daily value each of calcium and copper, for just fifty-eight calories. Have you ever heard the aphorism "good news travels like molasses"? Well, hopefully this good news about molasses will spread much faster!

HEAD POUNDING? THINK MAGNESIUM

Every day, an unbelievable 15.8 percent of the global population has a headache.[14] If you're one of the 14 percent of people who get migraines (I'm in that not particularly elite club with you) or the 26 percent of people who get tension headaches, or even worse, the one in twenty-two people who endure a headache more than half of the days each month, then understanding the link with magnesium insufficiency will be of particular interest to you.

Magnesium is an essential mineral needed by every cell in the body. In addition to being an electrolyte, magnesium serves as a cofactor for hundreds of different enzymes, giving it a role in more than three hundred metabolic reactions, including pathways for cell signaling, energy production, protein synthesis, nucleic acid synthesis, and ion transport. Magnesium also has important structural functions in cells and bone tissue. Consuming enough magnesium may help protect against a variety of chronic diseases, including cardiovascular disease, type 2 diabetes, and osteoporosis.

In the brain, magnesium plays several important roles that likely underlie the connection between low magnesium levels and headaches, such as improving cerebral blood flow, reducing inflammation, and supporting neuron communication.[15] The strongest link, however, is that magnesium deficiency is associated with something called *cortical spreading depression*, sometimes informally referred to as a "brain tsunami," which is believed to cause migraine auras and pain.[16]

Studies show mixed results when evaluating magnesium as a treatment for headaches, meaning that popping some magnesium supplements at the first sign of that migraine aura might work for some people but not for others.[17] But the good news is that taking a magnesium supplement regularly, or better yet, making sure your diet supplies sufficient magnesium, can reduce the frequency and severity of headaches. For example, in a 1996 double-blind, placebo-controlled study, migraine sufferers who took a six-hundred-milligram magnesium supplement (in the form of trimagnesium dicitrate) daily for four weeks experienced an impressive 41.6 percent decrease in migraine frequency and took about half the amount of pain medication per migraine attack.[18] This reminds me of a joke. What did the scientist say when she ran out of magnesium? 0Mg!

Magnesium-rich foods include all green vegetables, seeds (especially pumpkin seeds, almonds, and cashews), fish, legumes, and cocoa.

HIGH BLOOD PRESSURE? POTASSIUM IS YOUR NEW BEST FRIEND

Nearly half of American adults, and three quarters of adults over the age of sixty, have high blood pressure, over 130/80.[19] High blood pressure is sometimes referred to as the "silent killer" because it usually has no symptoms; meanwhile the damage to your body can quietly build up over years. And high blood pressure is a risk factor not only for cardiovascular disease (including heart disease, heart attack, heart failure, and stroke) but for hypertensive retinopathy, chronic renal failure, and even type 2 diabetes. While too much sodium usually gets the blame, too little potassium may be the real culprit.

High blood pressure is a problem because too much force on our artery walls causes them to adapt by becoming stiffer and thicker, a process called *arteriosclerosis*. The resulting narrower blood vessel diameter in turn increases blood pressure, causing a vicious cycle that sets the stage for an even scarier effect on blood vessels, *atherosclerosis*.[20] A sticky, fatty deposit, called *plaque*, starts building up on the inside of artery walls, which further narrows and hardens them. Arterial plaque is made up mainly of LDL cholesterol, calcium, inflammatory cells, cellular debris, and a clotting agent called fibrin. If an artery becomes blocked by plaque, this is referred to as a *thrombosis*—think deep vein thrombosis, coronary heart disease, and heart attack. If a piece of plaque breaks off and then blocks an artery downstream, this is referred to as an *embolism*—think ischemic stroke, pulmonary embolism, and heart attack. Yes, heart attacks can be caused by either thrombosis or embolism. (It's worth noting that there's a bit of a chicken-and-egg effect here. Factors other than blood pressure can cause arteriosclerosis and atherosclerosis, so hardening of the arteries can be both a cause and a consequence of high blood pressure.)

Why are low-sodium diets the go-to recommendation for lowering blood pressure? One of sodium's most important roles in the human body is regulating blood pressure and blood volume.[21] But when we consume too much sodium, defined by the World Health Organization as more than five grams of sodium per day, we retain water, so less urine gets produced, blood volume increases, and blood pressure rises. And a 2013 meta-analysis showed that reducing salt intake, from an average of 9.4 grams of sodium per day down to 5 grams, reduced blood pressure by a small but meaningful amount—systolic blood pressure reduced by an average of 4.2 millimeters of mercury (mmHg), and diastolic blood pressure reduced by an average of 2.1 mmHg. Remember these numbers because we'll come back to them.[22]

Potassium works in opposition to sodium—potassium is the main positively charged ion within cells, while sodium is the main positively charged ion outside of cells. The concentration difference between these two minerals is called the *membrane potential*, and it creates a gradient with an electrical charge that directs the flow of ions, ultimately allowing for the control of muscle contraction, heart function, and the transmission of nerve impulses. As a result of its role in membrane potential, potassium levels influence a wide variety of biochemical processes in the body, including blood pressure, but also vascular tone, hormone secretion, gastrointestinal motility, acid-base homeostasis, glucose metabolism, insulin metabolism, renal concentrating ability, electrolyte balance, fluid balance, and the action of mineralocorticoids (steroid hormones that help maintain the body's salt balance).[23] Yeah, potassium has quite the résumé!

Controlled trials of potassium supplements (usually in the form of potassium chloride, at doses of 2,340 to 2,535 milligrams daily) have found that increasing people's potassium intake leads to significant reductions in blood pressure, regardless of salt intake. A 2015 meta-analysis found that, among people with hypertension, potassium supplementation reduced their systolic blood pressure by 6.8 mmHg and diastolic blood pressure by 4.6 mmHg without changing sodium intake.[24] And if you're astutely thinking back to how much reducing sodium lowered blood pressure, then you've already noticed that upping potassium has an even greater benefit. It's also worth noting that the blood pressure–lowering effect of added potassium is greatest among people whose baseline potassium intake is under 3,510 milligrams per day—the adequate intake level is 4,700 milligrams per day—evidence that it's the ratio of sodium to potassium that matters most.

Similarly, some of the trials showing a benefit of sodium reduction on blood pressure (such as those using the famous dietary approaches to stop hypertension, or DASH diet) found that sodium reduction had an effect in the context of a standard Westernized diet, but not among participants eating a higher-potassium diet rich in vegetables, fruits, lean protein, and whole grains.[25] Even at a single meal, adding potassium to a high-sodium meal is able to attenuate the sodium-induced endothelial dysfunction typically seen.[26]

The takeaway? Ideally, you would consume more potassium than sodium to regulate blood pressure as well as support cardiovascular health in general, skeletal health, and kidney health, in addition to not going full Salt Bae. Of course, let's acknowledge the importance of lifestyle factors for regulating blood pressure like not smoking, being active, managing stress, and getting enough sleep.

Root vegetables include some of our best sources of potassium, most notably sweet potatoes, regular potatoes, cassava, plantains, and winter squash. But wait, even potatoes? Yep—but with the caveat that a 2021 study showed that eating baked and boiled potatoes reduces blood pressure, but eating French fries does not.[27]

Other great sources of potassium include heart of palm (the top food source with 54 percent daily value potassium per one-cup serving, raw and fresh), raisins, dried apricots, bamboo shoots, and molasses. Fun fact: Bananas, while having a reputation for being a great source of potassium, have only 11 percent daily value per serving (one cup, or about one extra-large banana). Isn't that bananas? (Hyuck!)

CHROMIUM DEFICIENCY COULD UNDERLIE TYPE 2 DIABETES

The prevailing message from both diet culture and the health care industry is that type 2 diabetes is a disease of excess affecting overweight and obese people. A diagnosis means that we must have consumed too many goodies loaded with sugar and white flour, and it is therefore our own glutinous fault if we develop this condition. As my father-in-law would say if there were little ears in the room, poppycock! While type 2 diabetes affects our body's ability to process simple carbohydrates, the oversimplified ideas that eating too many carbohydrates is the singular culprit and that it only affects fat people are laughable.

In reality, type 2 diabetes is caused by a complex interaction between genetics, epigenetics, and the environment (the latter of which includes diet and lifestyle factors) that together reduce the production of insulin and/or the sensitivity of our cells to the actions of insulin, leading to chronically elevated blood sugar levels. Furthermore, 21.8 percent of type 2 diabetics are considered an ideal weight (not that far off from the 30 percent or so of the American population with a normal BMI).[28]

While poor diet quality, typified by frequent consumption of ultra-processed foods, certainly increases the risk of developing type 2 diabetes, so, too, does smoking, high alcohol consumption, a sedentary lifestyle, too little sleep, too much stress, and having the wrong kinds of bacteria growing in our guts.[29] Deficiencies of vitamins and minerals involved in glucose metabolism and insulin signaling (which include vitamin D, as discussed on pages 24–27, vitamin B_1, vitamin C, biotin, and chromium) may be a prerequisite for the development of insulin resistance, making getting enough of these nutrients relevant not just for type 2 diabetics but for prediabetes, gestational diabetes, nonalcoholic fatty liver disease, polycystic ovary syndrome (PCOS), and even obstructive sleep apnea.

Chromium is particularly interesting here because, unlike most minerals and vitamins, the amount of chromium in different foods hasn't been thoroughly documented, which makes it impossible to accurately assess dietary intake and the prevalence of insufficiency. It's no longer even considered essential, even though studies dating from the 1960s have linked inadequate chromium intake with type 2 diabetes risk thanks to chromium's role in enhancing insulin signaling.[30]

A variety of controlled trials—with participants ranging from healthy adults to malnourished children to type 2 diabetics—have shown that chromium supplementation can boost the efficiency of insulin, improve blood lipid profiles, and in some cases, improve impaired glucose tolerance.[31] A 1997 controlled trial of 180 diabetics found that supplementing with a thousand micrograms of chromium per day for four months reduced fasting blood sugar levels by up to 19 percent compared to supplementing with a placebo; chromium supplementation was also associated with reduced insulin concentrations and lower glycated hemoglobin A1c.[32]

Unfortunately, we still need more research to be able to definitively state how much chromium is required for which specific benefit. So instead of reaching for high-dose supplementation, your best bet is shooting for the adequate intake level for chromium, thirty-five micrograms per day for males and twenty-five micrograms per day for females up to the age of fifty (forty-five micrograms while breast-feeding, and thirty micrograms while pregnant).

Chromium is found in small amounts in every food group, but is most abundant in organ meat, green vegetables, mushrooms, nuts, molasses, and chocolate.

Did I Hear Someone Say Chocolate?

One of the best sources of chromium is dark chocolate, and yes, studies show chocolate can reduce risk of developing type 2 diabetes and be a beneficial food for diabetics! Yay!

In fact, a 2017 meta-analysis found that people with the highest intake of chocolate (all chocolate, even the cheap stuff) had an 18 percent lower risk of developing type 2 diabetes compared to people with the lowest intake of chocolate. The greatest risk reduction occurred at two one-ounce servings per week (25 percent lower risk), with no additional protective effects occurring above six servings per week.[33] And a 2015 randomized controlled trial of sixty adults with type 2 diabetes and high blood pressure found that eating twenty-five grams of dark chocolate (versus white chocolate), which is just shy of one ounce, every day for eight weeks led to lower fasting blood sugar, hemoglobin A1c, and a marker of inflammation (high-sensitivity C-reactive protein), whereas the white chocolate group saw no changes in those parameters.[34] Of course, chocolate has other nutrients that are contributing to these benefits, too, most notably polyphenols, especially rich in higher-quality dark chocolate.

I love being the bearer of good news!

SELENIUM FOR THYROID HEALTH

Hypothyroidism, meaning your thyroid gland doesn't make enough thyroid hormone, is estimated to affect a whopping 11.7 percent of the American population.[35] Worse, many people don't even know they have a thyroid problem; a 2022 review estimated that 5 to 7 percent of the population in the United States and Europe have undiagnosed hypothyroidism.[36] And, getting enough selenium could make a big difference.

Let's quickly review what the thyroid does. The thyroid is an endocrine gland, meaning it produces hormones, located in your neck. Two main thyroid hormones (thyroxine, or T4, and triiodothyronine, or T3) regulate a variety of processes in the body: they help regulate metabolism; they act on small intestine cells to increase carbohydrate absorption; they act upon adipocytes (fat cells) to induce fatty acid release; and they play major roles in growth, development, and reproductive function. For example, approximately half of females with Hashimoto's thyroiditis or Graves' disease experience infertility.[37] And thyroid hormone deficiency can reduce energy expenditure (how many calories we burn in a day) by up to 50 percent, which is why unexplained weight gain is a common symptom of hypothyroidism.[38] So, yeah, having a healthy thyroid is super important.

Where does selenium fit in? Over two dozen selenoenzymes—enzymes with one or more selenium atoms as part of their molecular structure—play key roles in reproduction, thyroid hormone metabolism, antioxidant defense (including preventing and reversing oxidative damage in the brain), DNA synthesis, and immunity. As a result, selenium plays a protective role against cancer, heart disease, asthma, inflammatory bowel disease, neurodegenerative disease, and thyroid disease. Three selenoenzymes (called *iodothyronine deiodinases*, say that five times fast!) regulate thyroid hormone activation and deactivation—in fact, our thyroid glands contain more selenium per gram of tissue than any organ in our entire bodies![39]

Observational studies show an inverse relationship between selenium levels in the blood and risk of goiter and thyroid volume, particularly among women with iodine deficiency.[40] Plus, low selenium intake has been shown to be a risk factor for Hashimoto's thyroiditis and

Graves' disease.[41] Several randomized trials have reported a beneficial effect of selenium supplementation in patients with Hashimoto's thyroiditis (including a reduction in circulating antibodies and improved well-being) and Graves' disease (including enhanced quality of life, improvements in eye health, and a slower progression of symptoms).[42]

Fish and shellfish are some of our more reliable sources of selenium, often containing more than 50 percent of the daily value per four-ounce serving. Other good sources are organ meats, meat and poultry, cheeses, and mushrooms. But by far the most concentrated food source of selenium is Brazil nuts. A single Brazil nut provides 175 percent of the recommended daily intake of selenium. In fact, in a 2015 study, researchers gave one Brazil nut per day for three months to hemodialysis patients, who tend to have poor thyroid hormone conversion (T4 to T3) due to selenium deficiency caused as a treatment side effect. Even though a daily Brazil nut was insufficient to restore their T3 levels to normal, there was a significant improvement—their T3 levels nearly doubled![43]

Selenium Toxicity from Too Many Brazil Nuts?

While selenium toxicity from eating too many Brazil nuts has not been reported in the scientific literature (even among people eating traditional diets in the Tapajós River region of the Brazilian Amazon, which are very high in selenium), it's prudent not to go nuts on Brazil nuts.[44] Selenium toxicity is expected with usual daily intakes of nine hundred micrograms or more of selenium, and it would take only about ten Brazil nuts every day to get you there. Eating ten Brazil nuts every once in a while isn't likely to cause a problem, but to be on the safe side, if you eat Brazil nuts every day, limit it to three or four. Fun fact: One sign of selenium toxicity is garlic breath without the garlic, so that's one to watch for!

MORE ZINC COULD MEAN FEWER INFECTIONS

Feel like you're always getting sick, or that you're constantly battling inflammation? You might not be getting enough zinc.

Even though zinc is the second most abundant metal in the human body (after iron), it wasn't until 1963 that scientists discovered that zinc is essential for all forms of life. Since the discovery of its nutritional importance, research has revealed copious roles for zinc. It serves as a cofactor for an astounding three hundred–plus enzymes and more than a thousand transcription factors (proteins that control the first step of protein formation from the genetic map in our DNA, which is transcribing DNA into messenger RNA).[45] Among zinc's many functions, it is critical for a healthy immune system because it is needed for the development of cells mediating both the innate and the adaptive immune responses (including neutrophils, natural killer cells, macrophages, B-lymphocytes, and T-lymphocytes).[46]

Across studies, zinc supplementation has been shown to help reduce the duration of colds, with meta-analyses showing that using lozenges containing seventy-five to eighty milligrams total throughout the day of zinc acetate or zinc gluconate can help significantly reduce the length of illness (however, above eighty milligrams daily doesn't appear to have much added benefit).[47] A 2015 meta-analysis showed that when properly dosed and started early enough in the cold cycle, zinc supplementation was able to shorten the duration of nasal discharge by 34 percent, congestion by 37 percent, coughing by 46 percent, throat hoarseness by 43 percent, sore throat by 18 percent, scratchy throat by 33 percent, muscle ache by 54 percent, and sneezing by 22 percent.[48] And another meta-analysis found that on average, taking zinc reduced the length of the cold by 2.7 days (down from an average of seven days).[49]

These impressive benefits appear to be due to zinc's ability to prevent cold viruses (typically rhinovirus) from binding and multiplying in the mucous membranes of the throat and nose, as well as reducing nasal inflammation. Prophylactic zinc supplements lower respiratory infections in children;[50] and dietary zinc is a major predictor of infectious disease severity.[51] Getting sick less often is a great motivator for making sure you're getting enough zinc in your diet on a daily basis.

Of course, zinc's immune health benefits don't stop at the common cold. Besides zinc protecting against other infections (including pneumonia, tuberculosis, and malaria), there's also research showing it has a role in protecting against age-related immune decline, improving Covid-19 survival and health outcomes, preventing the recurrence of canker sores, speeding up wound healing, and reducing the risk of opportunistic infections and immune failure in HIV/AIDS patients.[52] Plus, getting enough zinc reduces risk of Alzheimer's disease, depression, heart disease, cancer, and autoimmunity. What an ama-zinc nutrient! (Hyuck!)

Oysters are our singular best dietary source of zinc along with tons of other nutrition—in fact, oysters are one of the most nutrient-dense foods we can choose; Pacific oysters have a Nutrivore Score of 2,255. Per four-ounce serving, which only contains 93 calories, Pacific oysters deliver a whopping 174 percent daily value zinc, plus 767 percent daily value vitamin B_{12}, 201 percent daily value copper, 161 percent daily value selenium, 157 percent daily value biotin, 48 percent daily value iodine, 33 percent daily value iron, 32 percent daily value manganese, 21 percent daily value vitamin B_2, 15 percent daily value phosphorus, 14 percent daily value vitamin B_3, 12 percent daily value vitamin B_5, 10 percent daily value each of vitamin C and vitamin A, and 791 milligrams of EPA and DHA. Other varieties of oysters and other mollusks, like clams and mussels, have similarly impressive nutrient profiles, including being amazing sources of zinc. Unfortunately, there aren't any studies showing that eating oysters specifically reduces our risk of getting the common cold, nor duration or severity of symptoms. Aw, shucks. (Get it?)

Other good sources of zinc include red meat, fish, eggs, legumes, and nuts. But due to the phytate content of zinc-rich plant foods, its bioavailability is much higher in animal products.

CAREFUL NOT TO GO OVERBOARD

In the quest for good health, it's eye-opening to realize that specific nutrients can be used strategically to alleviate various health concerns, so I want to add a note of caution here about not going overboard. The adage "everything in moderation" holds particular weight when it comes to nutrients. That's because there's an optimal range for the amount of each nutrient in which our body has enough to function well but not so much that other problems arise. The low end of this nutrient Goldilocks zone is defined by the recommended dietary allowance (RDA), and the top end is defined by the tolerable upper limit (TUL).

The TUL is the maximum daily amount of a nutrient that's safe to consume over the long term, based on scientific evidence and careful risk assessment. Going a little over the TUL once in a while usually isn't a big deal, but regularly exceeding this amount may increase the risk of adverse health effects such as chronic toxicity. Chronic toxicity occurs when someone consumes too much of something on a daily or near-daily basis for a long period of time, typically weeks to months. The symptoms and specific adverse effects differ depending on what's being consumed in excess. For example, the symptoms of chronic hypervitaminosis A (too much vitamin A) are dry or itchy skin, hair loss, bone and joint pain, fatigue, blurred vision, and loss of appetite. Iron overload, also called hemochromatosis, can cause liver disease, heart disease, type 2 diabetes, hormone abnormalities, and increased skin pigmentation (typically a gray or bronzy hue).

Remember the serendipitous discovery I shared at the beginning of this chapter that iodine is an essential mineral? In the 1820s, Coindet's successful treatment of goiter with iodine tinctures led to unrestrained enthusiasm for iodine as a purported therapeutic agent for many conditions. Yes, even prior to the age of the internet, unproven miracle cures went viral. But unlike celery juice, too much iodine is toxic, and the popularity of iodine therapy among Coindet-stans led to overuse and symptoms of iodine toxicity like heart palpitations, tremors, and rapid weight loss; as a result, iodine therapy fell into disrepute. As iodine therapy went the way of MySpace (albeit two hundred years earlier), other researchers, intrigued by Coindet's discovery, expanded our understanding of the role of iodine in thyroid health, eventually establishing both the RDA and TUL for iodine.

Yes, it is possible to get too much of a good thing when it comes to minerals and many vitamins.

Chronic toxicity is seen most commonly in the context of supplements—for example, if you were to take both a vitamin A supplement (perhaps to improve vision) and a multivitamin that contains a lot of vitamin A. But there are a few foods—like Brazil nuts, kelp, and liver—that are such great sources of certain nutrients that we actually do need to be careful about how much of them we consume and how often. If you aren't sure whether you're taking too much of a vitamin or mineral supplement, or getting too much from food, ask your doctor.

MARVELOUS MINERALS CHEAT SHEET

I hope you're sold on the value of getting all the minerals our bodies need from the foods we eat. But we didn't get a chance to talk about all of the essential minerals, nor the full range of benefits of the few we discussed—that could be a whole book just by itself (and one that could treat insomnia). So here's a handy-dandy cheat sheet of all the ways essential minerals benefit our health.

Essential Minerals: How Much, What, and Why

	Best Food Sources	Links to Health
Calcium RDA: 1,000 mg TUL: 2,500 mg	dairy products green vegetables bone-in canned fish seaweed molasses	essential for healthy bones, joints, and teeth reduces colorectal and kidney cancer risk reduces kidney stone and disease risk improves PMS and menopause symptoms reduces blood pressure reduces obesity risk

	Best Food Sources	Links to Health
Chloride RDA: 2,300 mg	salt salmon prawns seaweed celery	needed for digestion potentiates effect of high sodium intake most research focuses on problems from too much chloride
Copper RDA: 900 mcg TUL: 10,000 mcg	shellfish nuts and seeds organ meat legumes chocolate	reduces cardiovascular disease risk important for immune health supports bone health supports reproductive health may reduce cancer risk, but more research is needed
Iodine RDA: 220 mcg TUL: 1,100 mcg	fish shellfish seaweed eggs dairy products	essential for thyroid function may reduce breast and gastric cancer risk, but more research is needed
Iron RDA: 8 mg (m) 18 mg (f) TUL: 45 mg	red meat organ meat mollusks dark green vegetables	important for immune function can improve restless leg syndrome and insomnia
Magnesium RDA: 400 mg (m 19–30 years) 420 mg (m 31+ years) 310 mg (f 19–30 years) 320 mg (f 31+ years) TUL: 350 mg (from supplements only)	green leafy vegetables nuts and seeds fish legumes avocados	reduces risk of cardiovascular disease reduces risk of type 2 diabetes important for bone health reduces risk of asthma important for immune function reduces headache frequency and severity
Manganese AI: 2.3 mg (m) 1.8 mg (f) TUL: 11 mg	fish shellfish nuts and seeds dark green leafy veggies legumes	important for bone and joint health important for immune health reduces risk of type 2 diabetes may reduce seizures, but more research is needed
Molybdenum RDA: 45 mcg TUL: 2,000 mcg	legumes organ meat pork lamb eggs	reduces risk of esophageal cancer prevents tooth decay important for vascular health important for insulin signaling

	Best Food Sources	Links to Health
Phosphorus RDA: 700 mg TUL: 4,000 mg	dairy products fish shellfish poultry legumes	most research focuses on problems from too much phosphorus
Potassium AI: 4,700 mg	hearts of palm green vegetables melons potatoes sweet potatoes	reduces risk of cardiovascular disease reduces risk of kidney stones and disease important for bone health
Selenium RDA: 55 mcg TUL: 400 mcg	Brazil nuts fish shellfish organ meat mushrooms	reduces risk of cancer reduces risk of cardiovascular disease important for immune function important for thyroid health protects against mercury toxicity
Sodium AI: 1,500 mg TUL: 2,300 mg	salt shellfish seaweed celery spinach	most research focuses on problems from too much sodium
Zinc RDA: 11 mg (m) 8 mg (f) TUL: 40 mg	mollusks organ meat eggs legumes nuts and seeds	important for immune function reduces risk of neurodegenerative disease reduces risk of cardiovascular disease important for eye health reduces risk of type 2 diabetes may also reduce risk of depression, but more research is needed

RDA: recommended dietary allowance

AI: adequate intake

TUL: tolerable upper limit

m: male

f: female

*Only recommended dietary allowances for adults aged nineteen to fifty are shown. Except where otherwise noted, (m): recommendations for adult males; (f): recommendations for adult females. Visit Nutrivore.com for other age groups as well as recommendations for pregnant and lactating people.

CHAPTER 7

Vital Vitamins

The discovery of vitamins is one of the most important scientific achievements in history, greatly advancing our understanding of health and disease. Vitamins are organic compounds required for metabolic processes that don't provide energy or serve as building blocks, and that we have to get from the foods we eat. Vitamins can be broadly divided into two classes:

- *Water-soluble vitamins*, including all the B vitamins and vitamin C, dissolve in water.
- *Fat-soluble vitamins*, including vitamins A, D, E, and K, dissolve in fats and oils.

This property affects the way in which vitamins are absorbed, stored, and used in the body. We have limited capacity to store water-soluble vitamins, so low intake can cause deficiency in as little as a few weeks, whereas significant quantities of fat-soluble vitamins are stored in the liver and adipose tissues, so it can take months to years of low intake before signs of deficiency are evident. Water-soluble vitamins tend to act as coenzymes (a nonprotein compound that is necessary for the functioning of an enzyme), and fat-soluble vitamins tend to act as transcriptional regulators (turning genes on or off).

While there was no one singular moment of vitamin discovery—no equivalent of Archimedes jumping out of the bath and yelling *eureka* while running naked down the street—the story behind the earliest suspicions of the existence of vitamins, which dates from the first half of the nineteenth century, is a morbid tale worth telling. Trigger warning: The animal experiments performed in those days would never pass muster with an institutional review board today; feel free to skip ahead if this is something you'd rather not read about.

Until the late 1800s, it was believed that there were only four classes of essential nutrients—protein, fat, carbohydrates, and minerals—and that different fats and proteins were completely interchangeable in the diet. For example, scientists at the time thought that butter and olive oil had equal nutritional value, and that gelatin was nutritionally equivalent to meat. In fact, the discovery in the early 1800s that gelatin could be extracted from leftover bones was initially viewed as the solution to hunger—it was thought that one pound of bones could yield the same nutrition as six pounds of meat.[1] (In case you're wondering, it can't.)

In post–French Revolution Paris, it was a precarious time of rampant poverty and easily incited riots. The unrest surged in 1816, also known as "the year without a summer," when unusually cold, rainy weather blanketed Europe in a three-year-long volcanic winter caused by the eruption of Mount Tambora. The resulting crop failures caused bread prices to triple in rural France, resulting in famine and driving the poor to move into the city—the population of Paris nearly doubled in the following three decades, many living in squalor. At this time, one in every five infants was abandoned, typically left anonymously at government-run orphanages and hospices. But the impoverished had advocates, including a philanthropic organization called La Société Philanthropique, which, in an effort to feed the hungry, began supplying a gelatin-rich broth to the poor and infirm. Unfortunately, the broth's horrible taste and lack of observable benefits resulted in its edibility being questioned.

Then came physiologist François Magendie, who pioneered experimental physiology, the methodological basis for all nutritional sciences research as it is performed today.[2] Magendie had recently earned renown due to a series of long-term nutritional studies in dogs that he had performed in 1816. Magendie had been studying the importance of nitrogen (the ubiquitous molecular component of protein) in proper nutrition. He first fed dogs a diet of pure sugar and distilled water—the malnourished dogs developed corneal ulcers and early death, something that was also seen in the profusion of poorly fed, abandoned infants in Paris during this time.[3] Magendie then fed dogs a diet of gum arabic with either olive oil or butter; while the dogs still died of malnutrition, those whose diet included butter did not develop corneal ulcers—the first evidence of the effects of vitamin A.

In 1821, Magendie was tasked with understanding whether gelatin was a nutritionally suitable food, a research endeavor that took two decades.[4] Magendie fed dogs a diet of pure gelatin, comparing it to a diet of meat that had first been boiled in water; but neither diet met the dogs' nutritional needs. Surprised by this result, Magendie suggested something radical but that explained both his current results and those from his 1816 nutritional experiments: that some essential material was leached out of meat during boiling, and was present in butter but not sugar or olive oil. The question of what exactly this mysterious substance was (spoiler: it was vitamin A) wasn't revisited by scientists for another seventy-five years.

While Magendie was the first to suggest its existence, vitamin A wasn't officially isolated until 1937, 120 years after his trailblazing experiments. Just six years later, in 1943, the National Wartime Nutrition Guide published the Basic 7, a precursor to the modern USDA Dietary Guidelines for Americans, where butter got to be its whole own food group thanks to its vitamin A content. Yet another example of dietary guidelines predating the knowledge base to underpin it.

In fact, research continued well through the 1990s in an attempt to fully understand vitamin A's effects on immunity and childhood survival. You may know vitamin A (in the form of retinol) for its famous skin health benefits when applied topically, including reducing acne; reducing fine lines, wrinkles, and other visible signs of aging; and improving skin conditions such as atopic dermatitis (eczema). But vitamin A is also essential for a number of physiological functions—particularly vision (remember those corneal ulcers?), reproduction, thyroid health, immune function, and cellular communication.

Initially, vitamin research focused on diseases of deficiency, but in the last century, we've learned a metric ton about the many important and unique roles each vitamin plays in supporting human health more broadly. And while I'd love to tell you all about every role of each of them, I realize that would definitely break my promise that these informational midbook chapters won't be a snooze fest. So instead, let's continue with our theme of highlighting the most fascinating and broadly relevant connections between common health complaints and the vitamins that can alleviate or prevent them.

I Can't Believe It's Not Butter—It's Liver!

While butter may have risen to fame due to its vitamin A content (and probably also its delicious flavor had something to do with it), there are actually many far better food sources of vitamin A. Great sources of vitamin A include fish, shellfish, and egg. Although not particularly efficiently, your body can also convert some types of carotenoids, found in yellow, orange, and red fruits and vegetables into vitamin A.

The best food source of vitamin A is liver. While a one-tablespoon serving of butter contains about 12 percent daily value of vitamin A, lamb liver has 821 percent daily value, beef liver has 552 percent daily value, and chicken liver has 366 percent daily value vitamin A per hundred-gram (3.5-ounce) serving. Liver is one of the most nutrient-dense foods on the planet—it's packed with B vitamins and essential minerals like copper, selenium, iron, zinc, and manganese. Liver is a great food choice for packing in the nutrients in a single serving, helping us to meet our nutrient requirements within fewer calories and thereby earning more wiggle room for quality-of-life foods the rest of the day. (For example, see page 44 for a list of all the impressive nutrients you get in a serving of beef liver!) Although if you hunt or fish, note that the livers of certain animals contain so much vitamin A that they're toxic to eat, including from bear, seal, walrus, moose, and many species of fish such as red snapper, grouper, monkfish, cod, and tuna.

VITAMIN B6 FOR MENOPAUSE INSOMNIA AND DEPRESSION

Menopause can come with some very unwanted side effects. In addition to the stereotypical hot flashes and night sweats, females can experience a litany of other symptoms, including insomnia and depression. Approximately sixty million Americans, and upward of a billion people globally, are menopausal, yet awareness of how common these latter experiences are is low, due to the taboo nature of these symptoms. A whopping 42 percent of menopausal and perimenopausal females experience depression, with risk of depression being nearly double compared to premenopausal people.[5] Risk of insomnia also about doubles in menopause, affecting more than a quarter of postmenopausal people and upward of 44 percent of those who also experience severe hot flashes.[6] What can help? Vitamin B6!

More than a hundred different enzymes require vitamin B6 in order to carry out their various functions, including metabolism, hemoglobin synthesis, and neurotransmitter production. The link to mental health and sleep disturbances? Vitamin B6 is essential for the production of four neurotransmitters linked to mental health and sleep quality: serotonin, dopamine, GABA, and melatonin. Low levels of serotonin, dopamine, and GABA are each associated with poor mental health, and low levels of serotonin, GABA, and melatonin are each associated with poor sleep.

Inadequate vitamin B6 has been implicated in sleep disturbances. For example, a 2022 study showed that people with the highest levels of vitamin B6 were most likely to get eight hours of sleep per night. In contrast, those with the lowest levels were 29 percent more likely to get between five and seven hours of sleep per night, and 42 percent more likely to get less than five hours of sleep per night.[7] And in a 2021 study, supplementing with high-dose vitamin B6 (one hundred milligrams) daily resulted in participants getting about forty minutes of extra sleep per night.[8] In addition, various clinical trials combining melatonin and vitamin B6 (along with other B-complex vitamins, minerals, and/or sedating plant extracts) have shown that vitamin B6 potentiates the sleep-supporting effects of melatonin supplementation.[9]

A 2020 study evaluated how intake levels of forty-three nutrients affected risk of depressive symptoms, including insomnia, in menopausal and elderly women, and the only one found to have a significant effect was vitamin B6.[10] For every 0.084 milligrams per day (per two thousand calories) increase in vitamin B6 intake, risk of depressive symptoms decreased by a whopping 20 percent. The recommended dietary allowance for females over the age of fifty is 1.7 milligrams. This mental health benefit isn't specific to older females either. In a 2022 study, college students with self-reported anxiety or depression received a high-dose vitamin B6 supplement (one hundred milligrams) or a placebo for a month.[11] Those receiving vitamin B6 scored lower on a screening for anxiety-related disorders, both compared to their baseline and to the placebo group. Of course, vitamin B6 should be thought of as an adjunct to, rather than a substitute for, treatments for depression and anxiety, so make sure to talk to your doctor.

As for the other symptoms associated with perimenopause and menopause, estrogen hormone replacement therapy for menopause can reduce the frequency of hot flashes by 75 percent,[12] as well as help to preserve bone mineral density, reduce risk of sarcopenia (loss of muscle mass), and improve sexual health and esthetic concerns.[13] Provided estrogen hormone replacement therapy is started before the age of sixty and/or near the start of menopause, it also cuts cardiovascular disease risk in half and all-cause mortality risk by about one third.[14] However, estrogen therapy has limited benefit to menopause insomnia and does not appear to improve depressive symptoms, so it's a good thing vitamin B6 does.[15]

A hundred-gram (3.5-ounce) serving (weighed raw) of white meat chicken delivers an impressive 48 percent of the daily value of vitamin B6, but all cuts of poultry are also fantastic sources, from turkey to pheasant, giblets to ground, bone-in or boneless, skin optional. Other good sources of vitamin B_6 include fish, organ meat, red meat, and sunflower seeds.

VITAMIN B_9 FOR A HEALTHY PREGNANCY

If you are a female of reproductive age, making sure you're getting enough vitamin B_9, also known as folate or folic acid, is super important. You likely have heard this one before, but maybe didn't know the deets until now.

Folate is famous for its ability to prevent birth defects when taken by the mother during pregnancy, including cardiovascular malformations, orofacial clefts like cleft lip and cleft palate, and neural tube defects—congenital abnormalities that occur from the failure of neural tube (which becomes the spinal cord, spine, brain, and skull during development) closure during the first month of pregnancy (and which include encephalocele, anencephaly, and spina bifida).[16] This is why folic acid supplements are highly recommended during early pregnancy, or even before conception, and why vitamin B_9 is always included in prenatal multivitamins.[17] A 2003 study calculated that the incidence of neural tube defects was reduced by 77 percent in women who consumed at least 1,200 micrograms dietary folate equivalents per day.[18]

Unlike other B vitamins, which can have hundreds of functions in the body, the biochemical use of folate coenzymes is solely to mediate the transfer of "one-carbon units," also known as "methyl groups"—which means shuttling a molecule containing a single carbon atom and typically three hydrogen (CH_3) between carriers. But that's far from a small job: It means that folate serves a major role in metabolizing nucleic acid precursors (including DNA and RNA), breaking down amino acids, and assisting in methylation reactions.[19] Thanks to this one important function, folate is also important for other elements of reproductive health, too, including spermatogenesis (the origin and development of sperm cells) and the quality, maturation, implantation, placentation, and eventually fetal growth of oocytes (a cell within the ovaries that becomes an ovum, or egg). And, beyond the reproductive system, folate also supports cardiovascular health,[20] potentially protects against certain cancers,[21] and reduces the risk of cognitive and neurological disorders later in life.[22]

What's the difference between the natural forms of folate and its synthetic form found in supplements and fortified foods, folic acid? Food-derived folates must go through a two-step process to be absorbed in the gut, while the folic acid found in supplements and fortified foods is absorbed much more readily (it's estimated that folic acid is absorbed at a rate of 85 to 100 percent, in contrast to 50 to 60 percent for folate from food).[23] However, folic acid is unusable by the body until converted into its active form (called *5-methyltetrahydrofolate* or *L-methylfolate*), which is a four-step process. Natural folates, by contrast, occur in many chemical forms, including the active form, so while some food folate will need to go through the same series of four chemical reactions as folic acid before it's active in the body, some can be converted in fewer steps, and some do not require conversion at all. Thus, getting natural folate from foods, rather than vitamin supplements, is still a win. Of course, if you are pregnant or may become pregnant, folic acid is the gold standard supplement for preventing birth defects.

Pulse legumes include some of our best food sources of folate. For example, a serving of lentils, which is half a cup cooked (about the equivalent of one ounce raw) delivers 47 percent daily value of folate; chickpeas deliver 56 percent daily value, and pinto beans deliver 51 percent daily value. The only food that can give pulses a run for their folate money is liver. Pulse legumes are incredibly supportive of overall health, thanks to their high fiber content and often impressive nutrient density—the average Nutrivore Score of pulses is 358, the highest among starchy foods.

Other good food sources of folate include organ meats, green leafy vegetables (like spinach and lettuce), beets, artichokes, and seaweeds. Many processed grain products like cornmeal and breakfast cereals are also fortified with folic acid.

FATIGUED, FORGETFUL, OR FOGGY? YOU MIGHT NEED MORE VITAMIN B_{12}

Prior to the Covid-19 pandemic, general fatigue affected upward of 45 percent of Americans.[24] Add to that an estimated 17 percent of people who still have fatigue six months after Covid-19 infection, and the true burden of fatigue, while unknown, is astronomical.[25] Certainly, some fatigue can be explained by inadequate sleep—only about one third of Americans consistently get eight hours per night—and certain medical conditions like hypothyroidism. However, a shortage of iron, vitamin D, or B vitamins are also very common culprits. Let's focus on vitamin B_{12}.

Subclinical vitamin B_{12} deficiency—meaning your levels are lower than normal but not low enough to cause megaloblastic anemia (which is so, so, so much worse than iron-deficiency anemia, and can even cause irreversible neurological symptoms)—is associated with vague symptoms such as fatigue and mild cognitive deficits like forgetfulness and brain fog.[26] Subclinical vitamin B_{12} deficiency is more common in vegetarians and vegans, and risk also increases with age.[27] It's diagnosed with a simple blood test, and can typically be treated by increasing vitamin B_{12} intake (either via food or supplement), although depending on your levels and whether or not absorption issues are additionally identified, vitamin B_{12} injections may be indicated. But even for people with normal vitamin B_{12} levels, a little extra can help with fatigue. In a 1996 study, elderly adults received vitamin B_{12} injections twice weekly for eight weeks and scored significantly higher on a measurement of vitality.[28]

Like other B vitamins, vitamin B_{12} is important for metabolism, but it's also vital for maintaining brain and nervous system health due to its role in preserving the myelin sheath that surrounds neurons, as well as in synthesizing neurotransmitters.

Some researchers have postulated that low vitamin B_{12} could be driving cognitive decline in the elderly, increasing dementia diagnoses and eroding quality of life.[29] Accordingly, higher intake of vitamin B_{12}

and other B vitamins is associated with reduced risk of cognitive impairment in older adults. This seems to be a case where an ounce of prevention equals a pound of cure—while many studies have shown a strong association between low vitamin B_{12} and dementia, supplementation with vitamin B_{12} in older adults with cognitive decline seems to have limited benefits.[30]

In children and adolescents, too, insufficient vitamin B_{12} intake is associated with lower cognitive performance, including reduced short-term memory and attention, and lower performance in school.[31] There's also a link between low vitamin B_{12} and both attention deficit and hyperactivity disorder (ADHD) and autism spectrum disorder.[32] In children with ADHD, the lower their vitamin B_{12} levels, the worse their hyperactivity, impulsivity, and/or oppositionality symptoms.[33]

There are some promising ongoing clinical trials to evaluate the benefits of vitamin B_{12} supplementation for addressing postacute sequelae of Covid-19, aka long Covid.[34] There's a tremendous amount of overlap between the symptoms of vitamin B_{12} deficiency and those of long Covid.[35] In addition to the symptoms associated with iron-deficiency anemia—fatigue, pale mucus membranes and palms, weakness, and shortness of breath—megaloblastic anemia additionally causes a host of neurologic symptoms, such as numbness and tingling in the feet and hands, loss of taste and smell, difficulty walking, absent reflexes, disorientation, memory loss, nerve damage, and dementia, as well as gastrointestinal symptoms like appetite loss (and subsequent weight loss), sore tongue, diarrhea, loss of bladder control, and constipation. Perhaps as you read this, the results of these clinical trials are already available, but in the meantime, I know we all wait with bated breath for good news.

The best sources of vitamin B_{12} are organ meat, fish (especially sardines, salmon, tuna, and cod), shellfish, and red meat. Vitamin B_{12} is notoriously lacking in vegetarian and vegan diets, but some fermented soy products like tempeh and natto also contain vitamin B_{12}.

Noticing an Organ Meat Trend?

Are you starting to notice that organ meat like liver, kidney, and heart are frequently on the lists of good food sources of important nutrients? That's because organ meat delivers more nutrition per calorie and per serving than just about any other protein foods—mollusks like oysters, mussels, and clams are also impressively nutrient dense.

Liver and kidney tend to be very high in vitamin A, all of the B vitamins, choline, copper, iron, selenium, zinc, and coenzyme Q10. (Coenzyme Q10 is a vitamin-like compound with incredible benefits for human health, including helping to treat or prevent cardiovascular disease, type 2 diabetes, neurological diseases, gum disease, infertility, migraine headaches, and some cancers.) Even though heart isn't quite as vitamin and mineral rich as liver and kidney, it's the single best food source of coenzyme Q10, containing about four times more than liver or kidney.

While there's no rule saying you *have to* eat organ meat to be a Nutrivore, these are exactly the type of impressively nutritious foods that earn more room for quality-of-life foods.

FEELING STRESSED? MORE VITAMIN C CAN HELP

Quick: What's the square root of 729?

If you have math anxiety like 93 percent of adults, you might feel a jolt of panic just thinking about answering that question.[36] And, that's exactly what study participants were asked to do in a 2001 study that showed that loading up on vitamin C is super helpful for our mental health.[37] The study participants who took three one-thousand-milligram vitamin C supplements per day for just two weeks before being asked to perform mental arithmetic and public speaking had substantially better regulated stress responses—including lower cortisol (the master stress hormone) release, blood pressure, and subjective feelings of stress—compared to the unlucky participants who received a placebo.

Getting enough vitamin C reduces the risk of cardiovascular disease—including stroke and heart disease, as well as improving serum cholesterol and triglyceride levels—some forms of cancer, type 2 diabetes, cataracts, age-related macular degeneration, and gout. Studies confirm that higher intake of vitamin C brightens the skin and reduces the signs of aging, including sun damage, fine lines, and wrinkles, plus vitamin C can also speed up wound and burn healing.[38] Yes, vitamin C is quite the multitasker! Of course, vitamin C's most famous role is for immune function. While it's a myth that taking vitamin C reduces your risk of getting sick, it can reduce the length and severity of upper respiratory infections like the common cold.[39]

But that's not all it can do. Confirmed by subsequent research, there's a two-way street between vitamin C and our feelings of stress and anxiety—when you're stressed, you use up vitamin C more quickly, and low vitamin C levels magnify the stress response.[40] How does this work? Vitamin C is necessary for the generation of neurotransmitters like dopamine and serotonin, and of stress hormones including cortisol and catecholamines like adrenaline and noradrenaline. Plus, vitamin C potentiates the body's response to catecholamines via binding directly to adrenergic receptors, increasing their sensitivity, meaning that our bodies need vitamin C in order to respond normally to adrenaline and noradrenaline. Not getting enough vitamin C increases cortisol levels, decreases serotonin, increases blood pressure, and increases the subjective response to acute psychological stress. And a variety of studies show that vitamin C supplementation is associated with a decreased cortisol response after a psychological or physical stressor, reduced anxiety, and improved mood and cognition.

High dietary intake of vitamin C is known to reduce risk of stress-related disorders like depression and anxiety—it even supports what's called mental vitality, measured not just as an absence of stress-related disorders but also by increased focus, attention, and cognitive abilities.[41]

The reason citrus fruits are such valuable sources of vitamin C is not just because they contain a lot (which they do) but because they also are rich in flavonoids (like rutin, quercetin, hesperidin, and naringin) that increase the bioavailability of vitamin C by about 35 percent.[42] So as you would expect, eating citrus fruits is linked to the same health benefits associated with high vitamin C intake, including mental health benefits. For example, a 2016 study showed that older women who eat two or more servings of citrus fruit or juice daily have an 18 percent reduced risk of depression compared to those who consume less than one serving weekly.[43] And a 2011 study showed that eating a serving of whole citrus fruit most days reduces cardiovascular disease risk by 43 percent in men and 49 percent in women.[44] Yes, an orange per day about halves your risk of stroke and heart disease, so why do apples get all the aphorismic love?

Other great sources of vitamin C include berries, peppers, tropical fruit, and cruciferous vegetables.

VITAMIN E FOR SEASONAL ALLERGIES

The runny nose, itchy eyes, congestion, sneezing, and sinus pressure that you associate with hay fever, more technically called allergic rhinitis, are all due to the body's release of a single immune defense molecule, histamine. A 2022 study measured the prevalence of allergies bad enough to cause these miserable cold-like symptoms at up to 7.8 percent of the population.[45] And one nutrient with the capacity to alleviate these symptoms is vitamin E.

Vitamin E can improve allergy and asthma symptoms by inhibiting histamine release from activated mast cells.[46] And indeed, not only do people with allergic rhinitis tend to have lower levels of vitamin E but the severity of allergic symptoms increases the lower vitamin E levels are.[47] A variety of clinical trials have shown that vitamin E supplementation can improve both allergic asthma and exercise-induced asthma,[48] as well as atopic dermatitis.[49] And in a 2004 clinical trial, people with seasonal allergic rhinitis took an eight-hundred-milligram vitamin E supplement, or a placebo, through pollen season, which reduced their nasal symptoms.[50] It's worth noting here that high-dose vitamin E supplements can be harmful for some people; it's important to discuss with your doctor before taking vitamin E supplements, especially if you have a history of cardiovascular disease or diabetes.

Vitamin E is best known for its role as a fat-soluble antioxidant that can help reduce risk of cardiovascular disease, cancer, and neurodegenerative disease. So much more research is needed to fully understand its potential to alleviate allergies and allergic diseases like asthma and atopic dermatitis. In the meantime, it's best to think of vitamin E as an adjunct to traditional antihistamines or other treatments for allergies, rather than a replacement.[51] Yet in either case, there's ample rationale to make sure you're getting more vitamin E from your diet.

Vitamin E is found most abundantly in nuts and seeds. In fact, pumpkin seeds and sunflower seeds are the top two food sources of vitamin E, with 71 percent daily value and 69 percent daily value per one-ounce serving, respectively, and pecans and almonds deliver 50 percent daily value per one-ounce serving. Vitamin E is also found in other oily plant foods like avocados and olives (as well as their oils), vegetable oils, fatty fish, and organ meats.

VITAMIN K, OSTEOPOROSIS, AND BONE FRACTURE RISK

When you think of strong bones, you probably think of calcium and dairy products thanks to decades of Got Milk? ads. But in reality, a number of additional nutrients are required for skeletal health, including but not limited to boron, copper, iron, magnesium, manganese, phosphorus, potassium, zinc, vitamin A, vitamin B_6, vitamin B_{12}, vitamin C, vitamin D, and vitamin K. Phew! Let's focus on vitamin K, since it's one of the most common dietary shortfalls in Western countries, and not getting enough strongly increases risk for osteoporosis and bone fracture, which is a particular concern for postmenopausal females and older adults in general.[52] An estimated 50 percent of women and 20 percent of men over the age of fifty will experience an osteoporosis-related bone fracture, with hip fracture being particularly devastating due to high rates of disability and health care costs.[53]

Vitamin K plays a central role in calcium metabolism, basically controlling where in the body calcium ends up. Several bone-related proteins require a vitamin K–dependent chemical reaction called *gamma-carboxylation* (which transforms the amino acid glutamic acid into gamma-carboxyglutamic acid, a unique amino acid that binds to calcium) in order to carry out their functions.[54] (This same chemical reaction is required for normal blood clotting, which is why symptoms of low vitamin K levels include easy bruising, nosebleeds, bleeding gums, blood in the urine or stool, or heavy menstrual bleeding.)

A variety of studies have shown that vitamin K–rich diets reduce the risk of breaking a bone. For example, a 2022 study showed that older women with the highest dietary intake of vitamin K had a 41 percent reduced risk of a bone fracture than women with the lowest vitamin K intake, showing that consuming at least a hundred micrograms of vitamin K daily is extremely protective against any bone fracture.[55] And a 2000 study in elderly people showed a 65 percent decrease in hip fracture risk in those consuming the most vitamin K daily compared to the lowest intake levels of vitamin K.[56]

While getting enough vitamin K from the diet is incredibly important for healthy bones, when it comes to vitamin K supplementation to reverse osteopenia (reduced bone mineral density that's not bad enough yet to earn an osteoporosis diagnosis), forms of vitamin K_2 have the better track record. A 2013 study looking at supplementation of 180 micrograms of vitamin K_2 (specifically, menaquinone-7, aka MK-7) in postmenopausal women showed reduced loss of bone mineral density and improved bone strength over a three-year period.[57] And a 2022 meta-analysis concluded that vitamin K_2 supplementation could improve bone health and reduce fracture risk in postmenopausal females.[58] In the case of osteopenia and osteoporosis, getting vitamin D levels in the healthy range and eating enough calcium-rich foods is also extremely important.

Note that if you're taking some types of anticoagulant medications, vitamin K can cancel out the effects of these drugs, so it's best to seek medical advice from your doctor before increasing your habitual vitamin K intake.

Nutritionally, leafy vegetables, or greens, are our best food sources of vitamin K_1 (which is involved in photosynthesis, and therefore is particularly high in plant leaves). In fact, many leafy vegetables, especially dark green ones, contain more than the RDA of vitamin K in a single serving! Kale contains 162 percent daily value, spinach contains 241 percent daily value, chard contains 498 percent daily value, and dandelion greens contain 714 percent daily value per two-cup serving, measured raw.

Additional good sources of vitamin K include other green vegetables, like broccoli, Brussels sprouts, asparagus, and green beans. Vitamin K_2 is found in natto (a fermented soybean product), organ meats (especially liver), egg yolks, some hard cheeses, and dark chicken meat.

VALUABLE VITAMINS CHEAT SHEET

I hope you see why getting all the vitamins our bodies need from the foods we eat is so vital to our health. But of course, we didn't get a chance to talk about all of the essential vitamins, nor any of the vitamin-like compounds, nor the full range of benefits of the few vitamins we focused on—we'd be here for the next ten years if we did! So here's a helpful cheat sheet of all the ways essential vitamins benefit our health.

Essential Vitamins: How Much, What, and Why

	Best Food Sources	Links to Health
Vitamin A RDA: 900 mcg RE (m) 700 mcg RE (f) TUL: 3,000 mcg RE	liver and kidneys eggs seafood carrots sweet potato	essential for immune function important for male and female fertility essential for fetal development essential for eye health helps maintain thyroid health improves skin health and reduces visible signs of aging
Vitamin B_1 (thiamin) RDA: 1.2 mg (m) 1.1 mg (f)	pork liver soybeans seeds wild game	reduces risk of Alzheimer's disease reduces risk of cataracts reduces risk of type 2 diabetes improves survival during sepsis
Vitamin B_2 (riboflavin) RDA: 1.3 mg (m) 1.1 mg (f)	organ meat eggs milk and yogurt squid and octopus soybeans	reduces cardiovascular disease risk reduces frequency and severity of migraine headaches reduces risk of some forms of cancer (especially colorectal cancer with some evidence for lung and breast cancer, too) may reduce risk of cataracts
Vitamin B_3 (niacin) RDA: 16 mg (m) 14 mg (f) TUL: 35 mg (from supplements only)	fish liver red meat poultry mushrooms	reduces risk of cancer reduces risk of cardiovascular disease
Vitamin B_5 (pantothenic acid) AI: 5 mg	organ meat fish eggs meat (red meat and poultry) mushrooms	reduces risk of cardiovascular disease may improve non-alcoholic fatty liver disease accelerates wound healing improves rheumatoid arthritis symptoms inhibits premature graying and maintains hair color

	Best Food Sources	Links to Health
Vitamin B_6 (pyridoxine) RDA: 1.3 mg TUL: 100 mg	fish liver poultry red meat hearts of palm	reduces risk of cardiovascular disease reduces risk of late-life depression reduces risk of some forms of cancer (especially colorectal cancer, esophageal cancer, and stomach cancer) lowers inflammation regulates sex hormones reduces PMS symptoms reduces risk of kidney stones
Vitamin B_7 (biotin) AI: 30 mcg	liver and kidneys eggs mollusks nuts and seeds mushrooms	improves hair and nail health important during pregnancy may improve multiple sclerosis symptoms may reduce risk of Alzheimer's disease and type 2 diabetes, but more research is needed
Vitamin B_9 (folate) RDA: 400 mcg	legumes organ meat leafy vegetables seaweed beets	essential for fetal development reduces cardiovascular disease risk reduces colorectal cancer risk reduces age-related cognitive decline and Alzheimer's disease risk
Vitamin B_{12} (cobalamin) RDA: 2.4 mcg	organ meat shellfish fish red meat eggs	reduces risk of stroke may reduce breast cancer risk, but more research is needed essential for fetal development reduces risk of dementia including Alzheimer's disease reduces risk of depression important for neurological health

	Best Food Sources	Links to Health
Vitamin C RDA: 90 mg (m) 75mg (f) TUL: 2,000 mg	leafy greens tropical fruit citrus cruciferous veggies tomatoes	reduces risk of cardiovascular disease improves mental health reduces risk of type 2 diabetes reduces risk of neurodegenerative disease including Alzheimer's disease reduces risk of some forms of cancer (especially stomach and breast cancer) improves immune health improves eye health reduces risk of gout
Vitamin D RDA: 15 mcg (600 IU) TUL: 100 mcg (4,000 IU)	fish shellfish mushrooms liver eggs	reduces risk of cancer reduces risk of autoimmune disease reduces risk of cardiovascular disease improves bone health improves immune health important during pregnancy reduces risk of inflammatory bowel disease improves gut microbiome composition reduces risk of type 2 diabetes reduces risk of neurodegenerative disease including Alzheimer's disease and Parkinson's disease improves atopic dermatitis reduces risk of obesity
Vitamin E RDA: 15 mg TUL: 1,000 mg	nuts and seeds olives avocado vegetable oils berries	important for immune health improves eye health may reduce risk of prostate cancer, but more research is needed reduces risk of cardiovascular disease slows cognitive decline and Alzheimer's disease progression

	Best Food Sources	Links to Health
Vitamin K AI: 120 mg (m) 90 mg (f)	leafy vegetables green vegetables natto liver egg yolk	essential for blood clotting reduces risk of cardiovascular disease reduces risk of osteoporosis and bone fracture
Choline AI: 550 mg (m) 425 mg (f) TUL: 3,500 mg	eggs organ meat fish red meat shellfish	important during pregnancy supports digestive health reduces risk of cardiovascular disease

RE: retinol equivalent

RDA: recommended dietary allowance

AI: adequate intake

TUL: tolerable upper limit

m: male

f: female

*Only recommended dietary allowances for adults aged nineteen to fifty are shown. Except where otherwise noted: (m): recommendations for adult males; (f): recommendations for adult females. Visit Nutrivore.com for other age groups as well as recommendations for pregnant and lactating people.

CHAPTER 8

Phenomenal Phytonutrients

The final frontier of nutritional sciences is the exploration of the health effects of phytonutrients, which are biologically active, nutritive compounds in plants (derived from the Greek *phyton* meaning "plant," so literally *plant nutrients*), at least ten thousand of which have been identified.[1] Phytonutrients are responsible for giving many fruits and vegetables their rich colors, distinctive flavors, and unique scents, like the deep red of tomatoes, the bitterness of Brussels sprouts, or the pungent aroma of garlic.

The first class of phytonutrients to be identified was flavonoids (the largest subclass of polyphenols that we now know encompasses at least six thousand chemicals), which were originally given the name "vitamin P" in the 1930s when it was discovered that flavonoids isolated from lemon peel protected against one of the known symptoms of scurvy, fragile capillaries (our smallest blood vessels).[2]

Flavonoids then went through a reputational rough patch—first they lost their vitamin status in the 1950s once it was deemed that they were nonessential, then in the 1970s, they became suspected of being carcinogens (compounds that cause cancer).[3] Their redemption arc started in the late 1980s, when their cancer-preventive properties were identified, and continued into the 1990s once it was discovered that flavonoids strongly protected against heart disease as well. Their good name finally restored, flavonoids are now recognized as very important nutrients for reducing risk of cancer (especially lung and colorectal cancer), reducing risk of cardiovascular disease, and lowering inflammation.[4]

Most of what we know about phytonutrients was learned only in the last four decades, with new studies being published all the time that further expand our understanding of this underrated class of nutrients. There's a lot left to learn about phytonutrients—only a few hundred of them have been studied in detail so far. There's also a large body of irrefutable evidence showing that phytonutrients are a big reason unprocessed plant foods—including fruits, vegetables, whole grains, nuts, seeds, pulse legumes, herbs, spices, cacao, tea, and coffee—are found to be disease protective in study after study.

Phytonutrients are very commonly strong antioxidants (although, not ubiquitously). You've probably heard that term before (I know I've used it already several times in this book) but might not really know what an antioxidant is. Antioxidants are chemicals that neutralize hazardous metabolic by-products called *reactive oxygen species*, which also go by the aliases *oxygen radicals* and *free radicals*.[5] Reactive oxygen species are unstable molecules that contain oxygen and that react very easily with other molecules; for example, oxidizing and damaging DNA, RNA, and proteins. Reactive oxygen species are a normal result of our metabolism—they even have some important cellular signaling roles—and our bodies produce antioxidant enzymes in addition to relying on antioxidant compounds from our diets (like phytonutrients, vitamin C, and vitamin E) to counterbalance their production. The thing that's associated with cancer, cardiovascular disease, osteoporosis, neurodegenerative diseases, and other diseases associated with aging is something called *oxidative stress*, referring to an imbalance where the amount of reactive oxygen species produced exceeds the capability of the cell to mount an effective antioxidant response.

Science has only scratched the surface of all the amazing health benefits phytonutrients have to offer us—we'll talk about a few of the most broadly applicable in this chapter.

SORE? LEVERAGE THE PAINKILLING PROPERTIES OF ANTHOCYANINS

Approximately one fifth of Americans suffer from chronic pain, and for 8 percent of Americans, chronic pain limits their ability to work, socialize, engage in recreation, and/or perform self-care activities.[6] In addition, chronic pain increases risk of opioid dependence, anxiety, depression, and poor quality of life. Healthy dietary patterns—including eating more fruits, vegetables, and seafood—addressing nutrient shortfalls, and making sure vitamin D levels are normal have all been shown to help alleviate chronic pain.[7] And one class of phytonutrients—called *anthocyanidins and anthocyanins* (which I will refer to as *anthocyanins* for the remainder of this section)—in particular may be especially helpful.

Anthocyanins are a class of flavonoid polyphenols known to reduce inflammation, improve serum lipids and glucose metabolism, and support brain and eye health.[8] They are uniquely and specifically capable of both crossing the blood-brain barrier and localizing in areas of the brain involved in learning and memory, including the hippocampus. And, most relevant to our current discussion, they have pain-relieving properties due to an affinity for certain "pain-sensation" cell membrane receptors in the brain. Plus, they are about as potent as NSAIDs like ibuprofen for reducing inflammation (through the same mechanism, too, inhibiting activity of two enzymes, cyclooxygenase-1 and cyclooxygenase-2), which also helps to alleviate pain.[9]

Most of the clinical trials looking at the pain-relieving properties of anthocyanins have examined delayed-onset muscle soreness—that feeling of sore, tight muscles the day or two after a hard workout—for which the benefits are very impressive. In fact, a 2021 meta-analysis showed that anthocyanins improve all facets of recovery after a workout, including reducing delayed-onset muscle soreness, reducing inflammation, increasing antioxidant capacity, and increasing strength![10] The authors further point out that anthocyanins are more effective than many other therapeutic recovery interventions, including massage, cold water immersion, and compression garments. So adding anthocyanins to your pre- or postworkout shake or electrolyte beverage—or better yet, including anthocyanin-rich foods in your daily diet, with a specific focus on your meal closest to your workout—is a great idea!

There's also a growing collection of studies evaluating the benefits of anthocyanins in arthritic pain.[11] In a 2017 crossover design study, obese patients with osteoarthritis had significant decreases in knee pain scores and markers of inflammation after consuming a freeze-dried strawberry drink containing sixty-six milligrams of anthocyanins daily for three months, compared to a placebo.[12] A 2016 study showed that just six weeks of anthocyanin-rich pomegranate juice (two hundred milliliters per day) reduced stiffness and improved physical function of osteoarthritic knees compared to the control group.[13] And a 2016 study in patients with rheumatoid arthritis showed that 250 milligrams per day of anthocyanin-rich pomegranate extract decreased disease activity and joint pain compared to the control group.[14]

Anthocyanins are responsible for the beautiful deep red, blue, and purple hues of many fruits and vegetables, most notably berries, but also red cabbage, radicchio, pomegranate, and purple carrots and sweet potatoes.

CATECHINS CAN REDUCE RISK AND ALLEVIATE SYMPTOMS OF AUTOIMMUNE DISEASE

Let's look at how another class of flavonoid polyphenols, catechins, can help regulate the immune system in autoimmune disease, which is estimated to affect between 7.6 and 9.4 percent of the population.[15] Autoimmune disease is a broad category of at least 140 different conditions in which the immune system gets confused and learns to attack a protein or tissue in the human body. Some of the most common autoimmune diseases are alopecia areata, celiac disease, Hashimoto's thyroiditis, inflammatory bowel disease, multiple sclerosis, psoriasis, rheumatoid arthritis, Sjögren's syndrome, and type 1 diabetes.

Catechins have been shown to help regulate blood pressure, support weight loss, enhance the activity of antioxidant enzymes, exhibit neuroprotective activity, and are potent modulators of immune function.[16] The best-studied catechin is epigallocatechin gallate (EGCG), abundant in green tea, which is twenty-five to a hundred times more powerfully antioxidant than either vitamin C or vitamin E. EGCG is known to directly affect immune function in a way that is beneficial in autoimmunity, helping to bring various immune cells into a healthier relative balance.[17] In addition, EGCG and other catechins are strongly anti-inflammatory.[18]

While supplementation with green tea catechins has yielded lackluster results for generalized inflammation in clinical trials, results have been more promising in autoimmune disease clinical trials.[19] For example, a 2020 study showed that regular green and black tea consumption decreased disease activity in patients with rheumatoid arthritis.[20] Specifically, patients who regularly drank three or more cups of tea per day were 61 percent more likely to have low disease activity, with jasmine tea having the strongest association. A 2017 double-blind study of patients with systemic lupus erythematosus showed that green tea extract (five hundred milligrams taken twice daily for twelve weeks) significantly reduced disease activity while increasing physical health, general health, and vitality compared to a placebo control.[21] A 2023 study in patients with multiple sclerosis showed that a combination of EGCG and coconut oil supplementation for four months improved gait speed and balance.[22] And a 2022 study of people with multiple sclerosis showed that regular tea drinkers tended to have lower symptom severity, whereas coffee drinkers tended to have higher symptom severity.[23]

Regular tea drinkers also have reduced risk of developing autoimmune disease in the first place. A 2019 study showed that the more tea you drink, the lower your risk of developing rheumatoid arthritis—a 17 percent reduced risk with four or more cups of tea daily.[24] (This study showed no benefit to rheumatoid arthritis risk from coffee consumption.) A 2019 meta-analysis showed that tea consumption reduces risk of ulcerative colitis.[25] And a 2023 study showed that tea consumption reduces the risk of developing multiple sclerosis.[26]

There are many other health benefits to drinking two or three cups per day, including reducing cardiovascular disease risk, reducing risk of some forms of cancer, improving bone mineral density, reducing risk of type 2 diabetes, and reducing risk of depression![27] In fact, a 2022 study

Coffee Lovers, Rejoice!

Coffee is such a concentrated source of phytonutrients—most notably chlorogenic acid, cafestol, and kahweol—that it has an incredibly high Nutrivore Score of 6,832! And the good news for coffee lovers is that a number of research studies show that drinking coffee in moderation could legitimately provide a range of health benefits, including reducing the risk of certain cancers, type 2 diabetes, Parkinson's disease, Alzheimer's disease, cardiovascular disease, gout, gallstones, and depression, along with protecting against antibiotic-resistant bacterial infections and a variety of liver diseases. It can even reduce muscle soreness after a workout, and boost your mood and focus.

There are also studies that show that drinking coffee every day can have a life-extending effect. In fact, a 2017 meta-analysis found that drinking three or four cups per day was associated with a 17 percent reduction in all-cause mortality, a 19 percent reduction in cardiovascular disease mortality, a 15 percent reduction in cardiovascular disease incidence, and an 18 percent reduced risk of cancer.[28]

Unfortunately, it's not all rainbows and sunshine—coffee does increase the risk of some adverse health effects, such as poor pregnancy outcomes (pregnancy loss, preterm birth, and low birth weight) and bone fracture in females. And coffee can disrupt sleep if you drink too much of it or drink it too late in the day, which can cause a vicious cycle of not getting enough sleep, so you drink more coffee, which then disrupts your sleep more, so you drink even more coffee.[29] So make sure that you're not using coffee as a crutch to make up for poor sleep habits.

showed that drinking tea (three to six cups per day) reduces all-cause mortality by about 20 percent.[30]

In addition to tea—white, green, black, oolong, and pu-erh—catechins can also be found in apples, grapes, cocoa, lentils, and some herbs like rosemary, thyme, and mint. Most herbal teas are not high in catechins—options that do have a good amount include dandelion, rose hip, chamomile, hawthorn, lemon verbena, and rooibos—but are still packed with antioxidant phytonutrients and are a healthy choice.[31]

BETALAINS WILL HELP YOU REACH YOUR FITNESS GOALS

Whether you're just starting your fitness journey, or you're an athlete looking to improve performance in your chosen sport, or anything in between, let's talk about why adding betalains to your regime can help you reach your fitness goals.

Betalains, of which there are about eighty that are well characterized, are a class of red to yellow pigments found only in certain plants, including beets (in which they were first identified), chard, amaranth, cactus pear, pitahaya (dragon fruit), and some species of wild mushrooms. Interestingly, even though they appear to have very similar functions, anthocyanins and betalains have never been found together in the same plant.

Betalains demonstrate a variety of health-promoting biological activities, most notably as powerful antioxidants.[32] They have cancer-preventive properties, inhibiting growth and inducing apoptosis of a variety of malignant cell types in addition to preventing DNA damage. They lower serum glucose levels, decrease the postprandial glucose response and insulin secretion (even in people consuming three hundred grams of carbohydrates together with 250 milliliters of beet juice), and protect against complications of diabetes, such as kidney injury.[33] Betalains improve lipid profiles, including reducing total cholesterol, triglycerides, and LDL cholesterol, while increasing

HDL cholesterol. In a 2019 clinical trial of obese people, consuming twenty-eight grams of freeze-dried red beet leaves resulted in improved serum lipids as well as weight loss.[34] Furthermore, betalains have liver-protective effects and improve detoxification via increased phase 2 detoxifying enzymes. Animal models demonstrate neuroprotective properties of betalains as well, with potential benefit for neurodegenerative diseases including Alzheimer's and Parkinson's disease. And betalains have anti-inflammatory effects through similar pathways to anthocyanins.

Is there anything betalains can't do? They can even deliver more bang for our workout buck! Betalains improve endurance, performance, and exercise recovery.[35] A 2017 study in male and female triathletes showed that taking a betalain-rich concentrate of beets (versus a placebo) for a week helped them run a 10K faster, even though there was no change to average heart rate or perceived exertion.[36] And when the athletes came back the following day to test recovery by running a 5K, they still ran faster and had lower levels of markers of muscle damage and lower subjective fatigue. In a similar 2016 study, male competitive runners ran for half an hour at a controlled speed on a treadmill followed by a 5K run, again after a week of supplementation with a betalain-rich concentrate of beet or a control.[37] After the week of betalains, the runners had a 3 percent lower heart rate and 15 percent lower rate of perceived exertion on the treadmill, and ran their 5K faster, in addition to having reduced markers of muscle damage. Similar results have been found in recreational runners[38] and cyclists.[39] And while betalains don't seem to improve sprints, they do improve performance in some types of high-intensity interval training.[40]

Betalains can also help you kill it at the gym. In a 2022 study of physically active women, taking a single two-ounce shot of beet juice two and a half hours before a back squat test improved velocity and power—the women also jumped higher in a countermovement jump test.[41] In a 2020 study of healthy men, a shot of beet juice taken two hours before resistance training helped them get more reps per set of back squats.[42] And a similar 2020 study showed that beet juice increased velocity, power, and repetitions in bench press, too.[43]

And finally, you don't need to be already fit to benefit from betalains. A 2017 study in sedentary adults showed that fifty milligrams of beet concentrate taken two and a half hours before walking on a treadmill for thirty minutes increased their step count and burned more calories compared to the control group.[44]

You probably already noticed that beet juice or concentrate is the go-to for betalain studies, and that's because you just can't beat the betalain content of beets! Of course, if you don't like beets, there are other options—here's the betalain content per serving of the few foods that contain this awesome class of phytonutrients.

Betalain Content of Fruits and Vegetables

Food	Serving Size (measured raw)	Nutrivore Score	Betalains (mg per serving)
Beets	1 cup	2,013	245.7
Bulgur	1 ounce	542	120.3
Prickly pears	1 cup	881	90.6
Dragon fruit, red flesh	1 cup	800	32.2
Rainbow chard	2 cups	6,573	4.2
Swiss chard	2 cups	6,198	2.4
Amaranth grain	1 ounce	207	0.3

CAROTENOIDS IMPROVE AGE-RELATED EYE DISEASES AND VISION

During the 1940 Blitzkrieg of London, the Royal Air Force was able to repel the German fighters during the citywide blackouts thanks to the development of a new, secret radar technology. One RAF night fighter ace, John Cunningham, was nicknamed "Cat's Eyes" after he shot down twenty enemy planes, nineteen of which were at night. But to keep the technology under wraps, the Ministry of Information told newspapers that Cat's Eyes' impressive performance was due to an overabundance of carrots. And behold, the old wives' tale that eating carrots will improve your vision was born—but perhaps even more fascinatingly, there's actually science behind this one.

There are two common diseases of the eye associated with aging for which poor night vision is one of the earliest symptoms.[45] Cataracts, where the normally clear lens of the eye gets cloudy, affects a whopping 92.6 percent of people aged eighty and older;[46] and age-related macular degeneration, where the retina deteriorates, affects 42.6 percent of people aged eighty-five and older.[47] Carotenoids, which give fruits and vegetables vibrant red, orange, and yellow pigmentation, can both prevent and reverse these common eye diseases.

Across studies, eating foods high in carotenoids reduces the risk of head and neck cancers, supports vision health, reduces inflammation, and protects against metabolic syndrome and type 2 diabetes.[48] Meta-analyses show that the more carotenoids we eat, the lower our risk of cardiovascular disease, cancer, and all-cause mortality.[49] These benefits can be attributed to carotenoids having strong antioxidant properties and helping facilitate communication between cells by promoting the synthesis of connexin proteins, which create gap junctions in cell membranes that allow small molecules to be exchanged (which is part of how cells "talk" to each other). Most of us are familiar with beta-carotene, but there are actually more than six hundred different carotenoids out there. And when it comes to vision and eye health, the ones you want to pay attention to are lutein and zeaxanthin.

Lutein and zeaxanthin are known as macular pigments.[50] Due to their high concentration in the retina and their ability to filter harmful blue-light rays, lutein and zeaxanthin play a major role in maintaining eye health, protecting critical parts of the eye from light-induced oxidative damage. As a result, they've been implicated in prevention and treatment of age-related macular degeneration, protecting against cataracts, and reducing the risk of retinitis pigmentosa. A 2014 meta-analysis showed that high intake of lutein and zeaxanthin reduced risk of cataracts by 27 percent and 37 percent, respectively.[51] Consumption of lutein- and zeaxanthin-rich foods is more protective against progression of age-related macular degeneration rather than preventing it from occurring altogether—high intake of these carotenoids reduces early symptoms by just 4 percent, and late symptoms by an impressive 26 percent.[52]

Even better, increasing lutein and zeaxanthin can, at least partially, reverse these eye diseases even after they've started. A 2003 study showed that lutein supplementation in people with cataracts improved visual acuity and decreased the chances of needing surgery—cataract progression was not observed in 80 percent of the patients in the lutein group compared to just 20 percent of subjects in the placebo group over two years.[53] A 2019 meta-analysis showed that lutein supplementation could substantially improve visual acuity by 28 percent and contrast sensitivity by 26 percent in patients with age-related macular degeneration.[54] So it's never too early or too late to increase carotenoid intake for eye health!

When it comes to lutein and zeaxanthin, carrots are mediocre at best, with only 328 micrograms per one-cup serving. So if better vision at night is the goal, Cat's Eyes would have done better to chow down on spinach instead. If you're specifically looking to up your intake of carotenoids to support vision and eye health, leafy greens, peas, zucchini, and pumpkin will all give you more lutein and zeaxanthin bang for your buck.

The table below summarizes the lutein and zeaxanthin content of some of the best food sources. It doesn't matter if you eat these foods raw or cooked, but you'll better absorb the carotenoids from fruits and vegetables if you consume them with some fat, whether by adding salad dressing or enjoying them as part of a balanced meal.

Lutein and Zeaxanthin Content of Vegetables and Fruits

Food	Serving Size (measured raw)	Nutrivore Score	Lutein and Zeaxanthin per Serving
Spinach	2 cups	4,548	7,320 mcg
Peas	1 cup	431	3,600 mcg
Zucchini	1 cup, chopped	1,477	2,630 mcg
Kale	2 cups, chopped	4,233	2,620 mcg
Romaine lettuce	2 cups, shredded	2,128	2,180 mcg
Pumpkin	1 cup, cubed	1,036	1,740 mcg
Brussels sprouts	1 cup	2,817	1,400 mcg
Broccoli	1 cup, chopped	2,833	1,270 mcg
Pistachios	1 ounce, shelled	265	822 mcg
Eggs	100 grams (2 large)	355	503 mcg

REDUCE CANCER RISK WITH ORGANOSULFUR COMPOUNDS

With approximately 1.9 million new diagnoses and 610,000 deaths each year, cancer is the second leading cause of death in the United States, after cardiovascular disease.[55] Cancer develops when a complex hodgepodge of genetics and environmental factors combine to cause a cell to divide uncontrollably. There are many forms of cancer, broadly classified as hematologic cancers (affecting blood cells) and solid tumors (affecting any other tissue in the body). Treatment options vary by cancer type and how quickly it's growing and spreading, but generally include surgical removal, radiation treatment, and drug treatments, like chemotherapy and immunotherapy.

Despite the many claims to the contrary that you may have read in books or on the internet, no nutrient, food, diet, cleanse, detox, supplement, enema, positive mindset, or any combination thereof has ever been shown to cure cancer. In fact, eschewing cancer treatment in favor of unproven alternative medicine approaches can reduce five-year survival rates by up to 60 percent.[56] However, there are many nutrients and foods that can reduce your risk of developing cancer in the first place. Chief among them are two classes of plant organosulfur compounds:

1. glucosinolates—a group of more than a hundred bitter-tasting phytonutrients responsible for the distinctive pungency of cruciferous vegetables, also known as the cabbage family.
2. thiosulfinates—a group of at least nineteen aromatic phytonutrients responsible for the distinctive pungency of allium vegetables, also known as the onion family.

Glucosinolates (or more specifically, their biologically active metabolites, including isothiocyanates, thiocyanates, and indoles) reduce cancer risk through several pathways, including upregulating genes involved in protecting against DNA damage, inflammation, and oxidative stress, as well as increasing the activity of phase 2 detoxification enzymes (such as quinone reductase and glutamate cysteine ligase) that help remove toxic substances and carcinogens from the body.[57]

A variety of epidemiological studies have shown that eating five or more servings of cruciferous vegetables per week reduces risk of cancer.[58] A 2017 systematic review evaluating fruit and vegetable intake showed that eating a hundred grams of cruciferous vegetables per day (about one serving), on average, led to a 16 percent decrease in total cancer risk.[59] Numerous studies have found that overall cruciferous vegetable consumption is associated with lower risk of specific cancers, too, including:

- bladder cancer (up to a 20 percent lower risk)[60]
- breast cancer (up to a 15 percent lower risk)[61]
- colorectal cancer (up to an 18 percent lower risk)[62]
- endometrial cancer (up to a 21 percent lower risk)[63]
- gastric cancer (up to a 19 percent lower risk)[64]

- lung cancer (up to a 25 percent lower risk)[65]
- ovarian cancer (up to an 11 percent lower risk)[66]
- pancreatic cancer (up to a 21 percent lower risk)[67]
- prostate cancer (up to a 10 percent lower risk)[68]
- thyroid cancer (up to a 13 percent lower risk)[69]

Glucosinolates are found in all cruciferous vegetables such as cabbage, broccoli, kale, turnips, and bok choy.

Thiosulfinates similarly exert their cancer-protective effects by modulating important enzymes (like the cytochrome P450 superfamily and glutathione S-transferases) that help detoxify carcinogens and prevent DNA adducts from forming (a segment of DNA bound to a cancer-causing chemical).[70] Thiosulfinates additionally are able to stop cancer cells from proliferating (cell division), and even induce apoptosis (programmed cell death) in malignant cells.[71]

Eating alliums reduces risk of cancer, with the strongest evidence for stomach, colorectal, esophageal, and prostate, and emerging evidence for oral, larynx, renal, breast, ovarian, and endometrial cancer.[72] In a 2011 meta-analysis, the highest allium consumers saw a 46 percent reduced risk of gastric cancer—for every twenty grams per day (about the same as a single large garlic clove), risk of gastric cancer decreased by 9 percent.[73] In a 2006 study, eating onions seven times per week or more reduced risk of oral cancers by 84 percent, laryngeal cancer by 83 percent, esophageal cancer by 88 percent, colorectal cancer by 56 percent, breast cancer by 25 percent, prostate cancer by 71 percent, kidney cancer by 38 percent, and ovarian cancer by 73 percent, compared to never eating onions.[74] People who cooked frequently with garlic also saw reduced risk of each of these cancer types, although the effect was typically smaller (between 10 and 57 percent reduced risk).

Garlic is the most concentrated source of thiosulfinates. In fact, a tablespoon of garlic (about three cloves) has more thiosulfinates than an entire cup of any other allium, and about ten times more thiosulfinates than a cup of onion! But all alliums contain thiosulfinates and are healthy choices.

Thiosulfinates in Common Alliums

Food	Serving Size (measured raw)	Nutrivore Score	Thiosulfinates (mg per serving)
Garlic	1 tablespoon	5,622	81.4
Shallots	1 cup, sliced	740	75.3
Leeks (bulb and lower leaf-portion)	1 cup, chopped	1,128	47.7
Welsh onions	1 cup, sliced	1,704	32.5
Chives	¼ cup, chopped	3,531	8.4
Onions, spring, or scallions (includes tops and bulb)	1 cup, sliced	1,932	8.1
Onions	1 cup, sliced	380	7.5

And of course, glucosinolates and thiosulfinates deliver a variety of other health benefits.

Glucosinolates have been shown to improve glycemic control in patients with obesity and poorly controlled type 2 diabetes as well as reducing hepatic gluconeogenesis (production of glucose in the liver).[75] They have powerful anti-inflammatory effects, delay progression of osteoarthritis, and protect against cardiovascular disease. Some glucosinolate metabolites, like sulforaphane, have additionally shown efficacy for neurodegenerative diseases, including Alzheimer's disease, Parkinson's disease, and multiple sclerosis.

Thiosulfinates are also excellent for reducing cardiovascular disease risk, by lowering total cholesterol and LDL cholesterol, by inhibiting the enzymes involved in cholesterol and fatty acid synthesis, and by reducing platelet clumping and abnormal clot formation. And for example, the allicin in garlic is so good at preventing thrombosis that it has been pitted head to head against anticoagulant medications like Plavix, where garlic pills were shown to be equally effective.[76] Eating garlic is also associated with reduced risk of type 2 diabetes and Alzheimer's disease.[77] (Of course, garlic is not a substitute for medical intervention—if you're on an anticoagulant medication, talk to your doctor before increasing your garlic intake or making any changes to your medications or diet.)

WANT TO MAXIMIZE PHYTONUTRIENTS? SPICE IT UP!

Herbs and spices are any savory, aromatic, edible plant used to flavor or garnish food (or in some cases, for their medicinal properties). Their distinctive aromas and flavors come from their high concentration of various phytonutrients, so an excellent way to benefit from a wide array of phytonutrients is to season your food liberally.

Herbs have been important to virtually every human culture long before recorded history, and even show up on cave paintings in France dating as far back as 25,000 BCE. Ancient Egyptians began writing about herbs by the twenty-eighth century BCE, and by 700 BCE, Greek merchants were trading marjoram, sage, and thyme in markets in Athens. (Hippocrates, the "father of medicine," later catalogued four hundred different herbs being used at the time!)

Today the health benefits attributed to herbs and spices, thanks to their particularly high concentration of phytonutrients, are incredibly vast. For example, one of the many benefits of cinnamon is improving insulin sensitivity and reducing fasting blood sugar in females with PCOS.[78] Among ginger's many useful qualities is reducing nausea and vomiting associated with surgery, elective C-sections, chemotherapy, motion sickness, and pregnancy.[79] Rosemary also delivers many benefits, including improving memory and sleep quality while lowering anxiety and depression.[80] We have the best coverage when we embrace a diversity of herbs and spices and use them liberally in our cooking.

A serving of dried herbs and spices is defined as one tablespoon, whereas a serving of fresh herbs is defined as a quarter cup. Eating just a fraction of this amount daily benefits our health. For example, a 2022 study added a mere 6.6 grams per day per 2,100 calories of herbs and spices (that's about one teaspoon of seasonings throughout the whole day) to the diets of adults with risk factors for cardiovascular disease, with a crossover design comparing to a 3.3 grams of herbs and spices phase as well as a less than 0.5 grams herbs and spices phase.[81] After four weeks consuming the higher level of herbs and spices—a mix of cinnamon, coriander, ginger, cumin, parsley, black pepper, garlic, turmeric, onion powder, paprika, chili powder, rosemary, cilantro, oregano, basil, red pepper, thyme, bay leaf, cardamom, sesame seeds, sage, poppy seeds, dillweed, and allspice—the participants had significant improvements in gut microbiome composition including growth of bacteria associated with reduced cardiovascular disease risk. A 2021 study by the same research group showed reductions in blood pressure after a single day of higher intake of herbs and spices.[82] And a follow-up 2022 study showed reduced markers of inflammation after four weeks of the higher spice diet.[83]

All in all, this makes a compelling case for aiming for at least a teaspoon per day of dried herbs and spices, equivalent to a tablespoon of fresh, added to our meals. That's just two servings of herbs and spices cumulative per week.

EAT THE RAINBOW, REVISITED IN CHART FORM

There's a huge range of phytonutrients to benefit from. The pigments that give different fruits and vegetables their characteristic colors are phytonutrients. And each one of these classes of phytonutrients has distinctive benefits—even the ways in which different classes of phytonutrients reduce cardiovascular disease or cancer, for example, tend to be additive rather than interchangeable—which is why "eating the rainbow" is important for ensuring that we consume a wide variety of these beneficial compounds.

The most common pigment-associated phytonutrients and their benefits are summarized in the table below.

Phytonutrients: What and Why

Color	Phytonutrients	Benefits	Example Foods (and Nutrivore Scores)
Red	beta-cryptoxanthin lycopene anthocyanins	antioxidant anti-inflammatory reduces risk of some cancers reduces risk of osteoporosis reduces risk of cardiovascular disease reduces risk of Alzheimer's disease	red bell peppers: 1,358 tomatoes: 983 strawberries: 762 rhubarb: 598 pomegranate: 256 cherries: 171
	betalains	antioxidant anti-inflammatory reduces cancer risk reduces cardiovascular disease risk supports liver health improves insulin sensitivity may reduce risk of neurodegenerative disease	rainbow chard: 6,573 beet greens: 3,259 beet: 2,013 prickly pear: 881 red dragon fruit: 800 amaranth: 207
Orange and Yellow	alpha-carotene beta-carotene lutein zeaxanthin chalcones flavonols	antioxidant anti-inflammatory reduces risk of cardiovascular disease reduces risk of cancer improves insulin sensitivity supports immune function improves vision and eye health	pumpkin: 1,036 carrots: 899 sweet potatoes: 379 pineapple: 358 mango: 341 banana: 185
Green	chlorophyll glucosinolates lutein zeaxanthin	antioxidant anti-inflammatory strongly reduces cancer risk reduces cardiovascular disease risk improves vision and eye health	spinach: 4,548 broccoli: 2,833 Brussels sprouts: 2,817 asparagus: 1,385 green bean: 605 kiwi: 453

Color	Phytonutrients	Benefits	Example Foods (and Nutrivore Scores)
Blue and Purple	anthocyanins anthocyanidins tannins	antioxidant anti-inflammatory mediates pain improves memory and cognition reduces cancer risk reduces cardiovascular disease risk improves vision and eye health prevents dental caries	radicchio: 2,471 purple cabbage: 1,369 blackberries: 743 plum: 521 eggplant: 563 blueberries: 396
White and Brown	flavones glucosinolates thiosulfinates tannins	antioxidant anti-inflammatory reduces cancer risk reduces cardiovascular disease risk prevents dental caries	turnips: 1,954 mushrooms: 1,872 cauliflower: 1,585 onion: 380 parsnips: 372 white potatoes: 273

Part 3

NUTRIVORE IN PRACTICE

I feel much more motivated to choose a particular path, even if I anticipate that following that path will be harder, when I understand *why* that is the preferred path to take. The more complete my understanding, the higher my motivation, and often the less effort that harder path will seem to take. And while this applies to all areas of my life (hello, PhD in medical biophysics), nowhere has it been more apparent than in my own health journey over the last dozen or so years. Knowing the science behind why a particular food is good for me has always been the key to getting me to eat it, although it definitely helps if I also enjoy it. Fortunately for me, there are very few foods that I truly dislike, and I'm a good cook, so finding ways to prepare healthy foods that cater to my own tastes has been relatively easy. Stick a pin in that, because we'll come back to it.

One of the biggest revelations for me over the last decade-plus of being a science communicator on nutrition and health topics on the internet is that people engage with diet and nutrition information in three ways.

First, there are many others out there who, like me, need to know the science behind things, and in as much detail as possible. For us, the scientific legitimacy of Nutrivore is incontrovertible, and we can geek out indefinitely over all the cool things nutrients do in our bodies. If you read straight through part 2, and maybe at one point put the book down to excitedly share a fascinating snippet with a friend, family member, or roommate, then there's a pretty good chance that you're one of these need-to-understand people. You probably already have a good sense of what a Nutrivore diet looks like day to day, based on everything you've learned so far, although there's still plenty of nerdtastic tidbits for you coming in this final part.

Of course, there's yet another huge group of people who are satisfied to know that the science to support something exists but would rather focus on the practical application. Whether you read part 2 in its entirety or jumped around to read about just those nutrients related to your own health challenges, you're eager to get to the good stuff. You want to know what the best foods are to eat, how to combine foods in order to reach your Nutrivore goals, and how to find nutrient-dense foods on a budget. Well, you're in luck because in this part, I will give you a straightforward plan to follow so you can apply Nutrivore principles to your diet without sweating the details.

And the last group of people are those with high epistemic uncertainty with regard to diet and health, and whose trust I have had to earn with every page thus far. You probably belong to this group if you've tried many different diets, cleanses, and/or supplement regimes, and you aren't sure if those things didn't work or if you didn't do it right. You may even be worn out, skeptical that any diet can help you reach your goals or make you feel better. You may have read my promises that yes, you can eat a healthy diet and still have a treat, and felt conflicted or disbelieving. And some of the science behind certain nutrients or foods may have contradicted what someone else told you, leaving you feeling frustrated that no one gave you this information before. This last part is for you most of all, because I know how badly you need Nutrivore to be it, the lasting solution. Not only will I provide you with tangible guidance on what foods to eat in what quantities but I'll also bust the most common myths about food quality and "toxins" so you can move forward with Nutrivore with confidence.

And what about preparing healthy and nutrient-dense foods in delicious and satisfying ways? I've got you covered there, too. First of all, I want to assure you that you don't need to eat a food you hate. There is no one food that will make or break your diet—we've talked about this in the context of quality-of-life foods—that slice of chocolate cake—

but it's also true about nutrition powerhouse foods like liver, kale, and oysters. If you hate one or all three of those, you can still get all the nutrients your body needs from the foods you eat while omitting them from your diet. We'll also talk about taste adaptation in this part—just because you find a food to be gross now does not necessarily mean you'll dislike it forever. Some yucks can turn into yums, although even if that doesn't happen, I will repeat: That's totally okay. And finally, I will share fifteen nutrient-dense snack suggestions plus a dozen mix-and-match recipes, providing you with near endless options for tasty, balanced, and nutritious Nutrivore breakfasts, lunches, and dinners.

CHAPTER 9

Nutrivore Foundational Foods

The easiest path to Nutrivore is to have the foundation of the diet be a wide variety of nutrient-dense whole and minimally processed foods, including selections from all of the nutritionally distinct food families, which I call the *Nutrivore foundational foods.* We've covered all of these foods (and then some) in the previous four chapters, so here I will compile that information into one place while summarizing the scientific studies that provide us with some guidance on how many servings of each Nutrivore foundational food family we need to support overall health.

I use the term "food family" to denote a more granular approach to food groups. So instead of the usual five food groups (vegetables, fruit, dairy products, protein foods, and grains), I divide foods into a few dozen categories where each member is much more closely related nutritionally, such as cruciferous vegetables (the cabbage family), mushrooms, shellfish, citrus fruits, and pulse legumes each as their own food family. You can view every member of a food family as nutritionally interchangeable—swapping broccoli for Brussels sprouts, or lemons for limes, or oysters for mussels, for example. I deem a food family to be nutritionally distinct when it offers nutrients that are difficult or impossible to get from other food families.

I want to acknowledge up front that if you're used to thinking of foods as belonging to four or five food groups, the list of a dozen Nutrivore foundational foods is going to feel long at first. But by paying attention to those foods that form the foundation of our diet in this more granular way, we can ensure that we're getting all the nutrients our bodies need *without tracking*.

That's right, paying attention to the twelve Nutrivore foundational food families means you don't need to weigh, measure, log, track, or obsess over the foods you eat. You don't even need to pay attention to the Nutrivore Score of individual foods if you don't want to. Variety is key to getting all the nutrients we need in synergistic quantities for optimal health. The Nutrivore foundational foods are really just those groups of foods that offer something special nutritionally, because when it comes to food choices, the more different ones we make within food subgroups, the better.

THE TWELVE FOUNDATIONAL FOOD FAMILIES

Foods benefit our health by supplying us with nutrients our bodies can use as biological constituents or for biological processes. Foods that supply a wide range of important nutrients, or alternatively, a large amount of a nutrient that's harder to get, quantitatively improve health, for example, by reducing risk of chronic disease. When determining which foods form the foundation of Nutrivore, we first look at what nutrients those foods contain that are hard or impossible to get from other sources. Then we look at the vast variety of studies evaluating how varying intake levels of those foods affect health outcomes, the most relevant of which is all-cause mortality, but also cardiovascular disease and risk factors, cancer prevention, risk of developing and worsening type 2 diabetes, and risk of neurodegenerative disease.

The nutritionally distinct Nutrivore foundational foods are:

vegetables in general
cruciferous vegetables
root vegetables
leafy vegetables
mushrooms
alliums

fruit in general
citrus fruits
berries

pulse legumes
nuts and seeds
seafood

These food families each have something uniquely beneficial to offer us and we maximize both our nutrient density and health benefits when we focus on these foods as the foundation of our diet.

But this does not mean these are the only foods to eat on Nutrivore; it just means that getting all the nutrients your body needs from the foods you eat will be easiest when you prioritize these foods in your diet. You can then round out your diet with whatever other foods you choose. There are plenty of other food families with nutritional merit; they just aren't amazing enough to be elevated to foundational food status. This is also why we've been building nutrient awareness, so you know how to adapt Nutrivore principles to fit your preferred diet. Again, there's no one magic food that will guarantee great health, and there's no food that you have to eliminate completely in order to be healthy (unless of course, you're allergic or intolerant).

If you know that you're cutting out all food sources of essential nutrients—whether due to dietary preference, religious dietary practices, allergies or intolerances, or just because you can't stand them—it's best to work with your doctor, a registered dietitian, and/or a licensed nutritionist in order to identify any foods you can eat to fill those nutritional gaps or specific supplements you might need to take. For example, if you're vegan, you may need vitamin B_{12} supplements; if you're keto, you may need fiber and vitamin C supplements; and in both cases, you're likely to need vitamin D supplements (because most of us do). When in doubt, ask your health care provider.

With that preamble out of the way, let's go through each of the Nutrivore foundational foods one by one, and examine the studies that provide some guidance in terms of how many servings per day or per week to aim for to get all the health benefits these food families have to offer us.

Vegetables

There are huge benefits to be had from eating more vegetables. A 2014 meta-analysis showed that just three servings of vegetables per day reduced all-cause mortality risk by 25 percent.[1] A 2017 meta-analysis showed that consuming six hundred grams of vegetables daily (about five or six servings) reduced risk of all-cause mortality by 25 percent, of cardiovascular disease by 28 percent, and of cancer by 12 percent.[2] And a 2022 meta-analysis showed that consuming four or five servings of vegetables reduced risk of stroke, ischemic heart disease, and type 2 diabetes all by 23 percent or more.[3]

In general, aim for at least five servings of vegetables, and as much as you want above that amount. A serving is one cup (remember, that's about the size of your fist) for most raw vegetables and two cups (or two fists) for raw leafy veggies. Most vegetables will shrink to half a cup (or half a fist) when cooked. You don't need to weigh or measure your veggie servings—approximations are just fine. And yes, your

Do I Count Tomatoes as a Vegetable or a Fruit?

Ah, the age-old debate, are tomatoes a fruit or a vegetable? Botanically, tomatoes are a fruit, as are squash, cucumbers, peppers, green beans, eggplant, peas, okra, olives, and avocado. Culinarily, we treat all of these as vegetables, i.e., in savory applications. On Nutrivore, we use the culinary definitions of fruits and vegetables (and certain families, like berries) because they align with the nutrient content of these foods. For example, cucumber is nutritionally similar to celery, and winter squash is nutritionally similar to sweet potatoes. So it makes more sense to classify them as vegetables from a nutrition standpoint. In fact, scientific studies that look at the health benefits of vegetable consumption most often use the culinary definition of vegetables for classification purposes.

Fun historical fact: In 1893, the US Supreme Court unanimously ruled that an imported tomato should be taxed as a vegetable rather than as a fruit (which were taxed at a lower rate) in the case *Nix v. Hedden*. In the decision, the court acknowledged that a tomato is a botanical fruit, but prioritized what they called the "ordinary" definitions of fruit and vegetable. So, yes, in the grocery store, the kitchen, and the Supreme Court, tomatoes are a vegetable!

servings of cruciferous vegetables, root vegetables, leafy vegetables, mushrooms, and alliums also count toward your five-plus servings of total vegetables.

If eating five or more servings of veggies feels intimidating, you're not alone! In fact, the average vegetable consumption is a mere 1.64 cup equivalent of vegetables per day, which is about one third of optimal intake.[4] What's important to know is that every bit counts—you'll get way more health bang for your veggie serving buck going from zero to some than you will from going to quite a lot to even more—so it's okay to work up to that intake slowly over time.

Cruciferous Vegetables (The Cabbage Family)

A 2017 meta-analysis showed that eating a hundred grams of cruciferous vegetables (about one serving) per day on average leads to an 18 percent decrease in ischemic stroke, a 17 percent decrease in hemorrhagic stroke, and a 12 percent decrease in all-cause mortality and cardiovascular disease.[5] A 2019 meta-analysis turned up similar results, showing that for every hundred grams of cruciferous vegetables we consume daily, risk of cardiovascular disease decreased by 11 percent and risk of all-cause mortality decreased by 10 percent.[6] Plus, cruciferous vegetables were some of the most important fruits or vegetables to consume on a daily basis in this study (root vegetables and green leafy vegetables were also important, as were mixing up eating raw versus cooked vegetables).

All in all, a strong case can be made for aiming for one serving of cruciferous vegetables daily—two is even better. A serving is one cup (or one fist) measured raw, and two cups for leafy cruciferous veggies like kale. Most cruciferous veggies will shrink to about half a cup when cooked.

Leafy Vegetables

Greens offer a huge range of scientifically demonstrated health benefits. For example, a 2018 study showed that, among older and elderly adults, the highest intake of green leafy vegetables correlated with slower cognitive decline—an average of only 1.3 servings per day was associated with the equivalent of being eleven years younger in cognitive age.[7] A 2013 study showed that consuming 1.5 servings of leafy greens per day, versus 1.5 servings per week, was associated with a 17 percent lower risk of coronary heart disease.[8] A large prospective cohort study published in 2012 found that eating at least fifty-six grams (about two thirds of a serving) of leafy vegetables daily (compared to less than fifteen grams daily) was associated with a 30 percent lower risk of developing breast cancer over the course of eleven years.[9] A 1999 study showed that compared to infrequent consumption of salad vegetables, eating salad vegetables daily or near daily all year long was associated with an 84 percent lower risk of diabetes.[10] And a 2019 meta-analysis showed that for every hundred grams per day of leafy vegetables (about 1.3 servings), risk of all-cause mortality decreased by 22 percent.[11] Wow!

These studies make a strong case for a serving of leafy vegetables every day, and two servings daily would be even better! A serving is two cups (or two fists) measured raw, which shrinks to a third to half a cup when cooked.

Root Vegetables

A 2019 meta-analyses showed that for every hundred grams of root vegetables (about two thirds of a serving) we eat per day, we reduce risk of all-cause mortality by 24 percent.[12] That's huge, and in fact, the highest magnitude of benefit compared to all other vegetable and fruit families in this study. And a 2012 study that looked at the effect of fruit and vegetable intake on the incidence of type 2 diabetes showed that comparing highest with lowest average intake, among fruit and vegetable subtypes, only root vegetables protected strongly against diabetes, demonstrating a 13 percent reduced risk.[13]

All in all, a strong case can be made for eating at least one serving of root vegetables daily. A serving of root vegetables is one cup (or one fist), chopped and measured raw, which shrinks to about half a cup when cooked.

Alliums (The Onion Family)

A 2019 meta-analysis showed that, for every hundred grams of alliums we eat daily (about one serving), there is a 24 percent reduced risk of all-cause mortality.[14] But we don't need to eat that much alliums to benefit. A 2020 study showed that eating half a serving per day decreased cardiovascular disease by 21 percent compared to rarely eating alliums.[15] And a 2002 study found that men consuming a mere ten grams of alliums per day (only about one tablespoon!) were 49 percent less likely to develop prostate cancer than men consuming under two grams of alliums daily.[16]

A strong case can be made for aiming for three servings of alliums per week, and a serving per day would be even better. A serving of garlic is one tablespoon (or about the size of the top half of your thumb), or about three cloves. A serving of chives is a quarter cup, chopped (about a rounded palmful). A serving of all other alliums is one cup (about one fist), chopped, measured raw, which shrinks to about a half cup when cooked.

Mushrooms

A 2019 study showed that eating a hundred grams of mushrooms (about 1.3 servings) daily reduced risk of all-cause mortality by a whopping 26 percent.[17] And a 2021 study showed that eating any amount of mushrooms reduced all-cause mortality by 16 percent compared to no mushrooms.[18] So even a serving per week will be beneficial, but from an ergothioneine perspective, aiming for three servings per week is a better target to get the longevity benefits of the longevity vitamin. Of course, there's no maximum amount of mushrooms to eat, so if you want to eat a serving or even two daily, go for it! A serving is one cup (or about one fist) measured raw, and most mushrooms will shrink to about a half cup when cooked.

Fruit

A 2013 meta-analysis showed that consuming four grams of fiber from whole fruit, which is equivalent to one to two servings, reduced risk of coronary heart disease by 8 percent and risk of cardiovascular disease by 4 percent.[19] A 2017 meta-analysis showed that consuming 250 to 300 grams of fruit daily (about two servings) reduced all-cause mortality by 10 percent, with no additional benefit above that amount.[20] And a 2018 review concluded that two to three servings of fruit daily was optimal for reducing risk of cardiovascular disease, type 2 diabetes, obesity, chronic obstructive pulmonary disease, chronic constipation, and inflammatory bowel disease.[21]

In general, aim for two servings of fruit per day. It's okay to eat more fruit than that, but this is the sweet spot for the most health benefit. A serving is one cup (or a fist) for raw fruits. Most fruits will shrink to about half a cup (or half a fist) when cooked. And yes, your servings of citrus and berries also count toward total fruit.

Citrus

A 2006 study showed that people who consumed citrus fruit three to four times per week had an 8 percent lower risk of dementia, and people who consumed citrus almost every day had a 14 percent lower risk of dementia, compared to those who consumed citrus two or fewer times per week.[22] A 2017 meta-analysis found that high citrus consumption (compared to low) reduced risk of total stroke by 26 percent, ischemic stroke by 22 percent, hemorrhagic stroke by 26 percent, coronary heart disease by 9 percent, cardiovascular disease by 22 percent, and all-cause mortality by 10 percent.[23] This study showed that just two or three servings per week reduces all-cause mortality by 8 percent.

A strong case can be made for aiming for three servings per week of citrus fruits, and up to a serving per day. A serving is one cup, raw, or a fruit about the size of your fist.

Berries

A 2019 meta-analyses showed that for every 100 grams of berries (about two thirds of a serving) we eat per day, we reduce risk of all-cause mortality by 8 percent.[24] A 2018 meta-analysis showed that eating berries benefits cardiovascular disease risk factors, reducing total cholesterol, LDL "bad" cholesterol, triglycerides, and blood pressure, while increasing the level of HDL "good" cholesterol.[25] A 2002 study showed that the people who ate the most berries had a 26 percent lower risk of developing type 2 diabetes compared to the people who ate the fewest berries.[26] And a 2012 study showed that just two to four servings of berries per week reduced risk for Parkinson's disease by 23 percent compared to three or fewer servings per month.[27]

In general, eating two or more servings of berries per week is great for overall health, but again, there's no limit to the benefits of berries. A serving is one cup (or about one fist), measured raw.

Pulse Legumes

In a 2021 study, eating two and a half or more servings of legumes per week reduced all-cause mortality by 17 percent, and cardiovascular disease by 14 percent, compared to eating only two servings per month, also lowering cardiovascular disease mortality, cancer incidence, and cancer mortality.[28] A 2001 study showed that eating legumes four times per week reduced coronary heart disease risk by 22 percent and cardiovascular disease risk by 11 percent compared to eating them less than once per week.[29] And a 2014 meta-analysis likewise showed that four servings per week of legumes reduces coronary heart disease risk by 14 percent.[30]

Even a serving or two per week of pulse legumes—like lentils, chickpeas, soybeans, and black beans—is going to deliver health benefits, but the preponderance of evidence supports four servings per week as a great goal for optimal health. Of course, there's no maximum amount of legumes, so you can eat them up to every meal if you like. A serving of whole pulse legumes is half a cup cooked (about half of your fist), which is the equivalent of one ounce (or about one fifth of a cup) for raw, dried pulse legumes (like dried beans or lentils). A serving of tofu, tempeh, or natto is a quarter cup (about a rounded palmful).

Nuts and Seeds

A 2016 meta-analysis showed that a mere ten grams of tree nuts per day (or twenty-eight grams for total nuts, seeds, and peanuts) reduced risk of all-cause mortality by 18 percent, coronary heart disease by 27 percent, stroke by 11 percent, cardiovascular disease by 25 percent, cancer by 20 percent, respiratory disease mortality by 21 percent, neurodegenerative disease mortality by 19 percent, infectious disease mortality by 36 percent, and kidney disease morality by 34 percent.[31] And a 2015 meta-analysis calculated that twenty-eight grams of nuts and seeds per day was associated with a 27 percent reduced risk of all-cause mortality and a 39 percent reduced risk of cardiovascular disease mortality, and the highest nut and seed consumers saw a 14 percent reduced risk of cancer mortality.[32]

It really doesn't take much to see impressive health benefits with nuts and seeds; just three one-ounce servings per week are associated with huge effects. One ounce (twenty-eight grams) of nuts and seeds translates to about a quarter cup (about a level palmful) if they're whole or chopped, and to two tablespoons (about two top halves of your thumb) for nut and seed butters. Importantly, more is not better with nuts and seeds—studies show that benefits cap out at about an ounce per day.

Seafood

A 2021 meta-analysis showed that for every twenty grams (about three quarters of an ounce) per day of fish, risk of cardiovascular disease mortality decreased by 4 percent.[33] A 2019 meta-analysis showed that for every hundred grams of fish (just shy of one serving) we eat per day, we reduce risk of all-cause mortality by 8 percent.[34] And a 2017 meta-analysis showed that compared with little or no intake, modest fish consumption (forty grams, or about 1.5 ounces, per day) results in a 9 percent decrease in all-cause mortality.[35]

These studies make a compelling case for aiming for at least three servings of seafood per week, and up to every meal. A serving of seafood is four ounces (115 grams) raw, or about three ounces cooked, about the same size as your palm.

Where Are the Whole Grains?

Whole grains are certainly health-promoting foods and a good source of fiber, but they don't earn foundational food status on Nutrivore. That's because intervention studies, where people add whole grains to their diet for an amount of time to see how doing so affects their health, have shown conflicting or lackluster results.

In a 2016 study, overweight adults added 120 grams (about four servings) of whole grains to their diet daily for sixteen weeks. There was no benefit to cardiovascular disease risk factors—including blood pressure, LDL cholesterol, total cholesterol, and triglycerides—insulin sensitivity, weight, body fat percentage, or inflammatory markers.[36] A 2022 review of the effect of whole grains on cardiovascular disease, obesity, type 2 diabetes, and cancer concluded, "The role of the consumption of whole grains in disease prevention is promising but not conclusive, and more clinical trials and epidemiologic studies are needed."[37] On the other hand, a large body of scientific literature consistently shows that eating more pulse legumes provides these benefits—legumes deliver even more fiber per serving than whole grains, along with more vitamins, minerals, and phytonutrients.[38]

While not foundational, whole grains absolutely can fit into a Nutrivore diet, are certainly a better choice than refined grains, and can be an excellent and affordable choice to boost fiber intake.[39] Plus, there are some standout whole grains, most notably oats, which can reduce total and LDL cholesterol by up to 23 percent (while preserving or sometimes increasing HDL cholesterol) when consumed at levels of 35 to 120 grams per day (one to four servings).[40] And in more than a dozen studies, oat consumption has been shown to improve blood sugar regulation and insulin responses.[41]

FOOD GROUPS THROUGH THE NUTRIVORE LENS

A Nutrivore approach is inherently flexible, and the more nutrient-dense foods we choose, the more flexibility there is for incorporating quality-of-life foods in our diet. While all whole foods are great options, some do offer more nutrition than others. So let's look at the nutritional merits of common whole food families by examining both their nutrient and caloric contributions to our diets. You can find average Nutrivore Scores and energy density of all whole food families in appendix C.

The following graph shows the average nutrient density, as represented by the Nutrivore Score, of select food families on the x-axis, with energy density (calories per hundred grams) on the y-axis. The size of each circle is representative of the variability in nutrient density within that food family (the size is half of a standard deviation of the Nutrivore Scores).

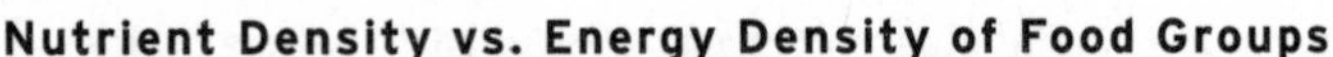

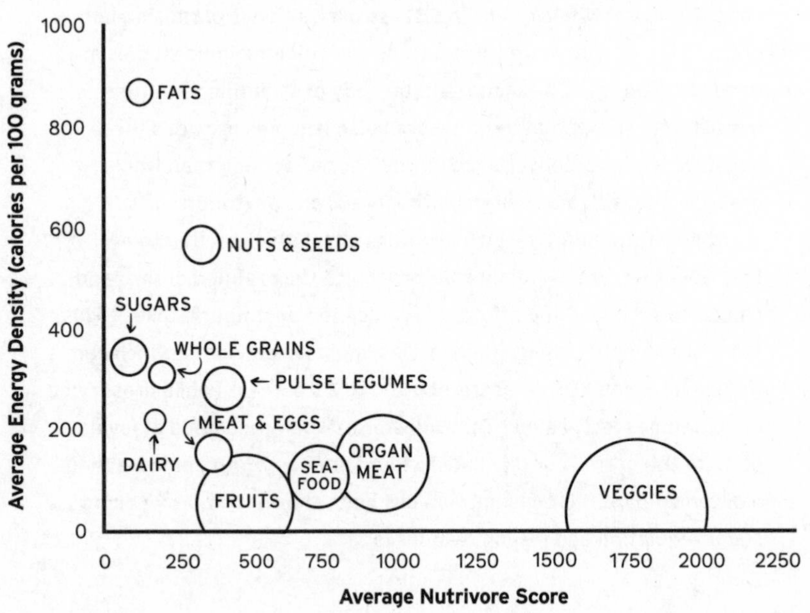

What does this graph tell us? Well, the farther to the right, the more nutrient-dense a food is, and the higher up, the more calories it has per gram. So vegetables, being far to the right and also very low down, are foods that offer a ton of nutrients and not very many calories, which helps to emphasize the importance of a vegetable-forward approach to the overall diet. On the opposite side of the spectrum, fats are high calorie and don't deliver a lot of nutrients per calorie. This doesn't mean that fats are bad, and as we've already covered, there are many that are extremely health promoting. Instead, it gives you a sense of the proportions of these foods to eat, relative to each other, vegetables in abundance and fats in more moderate amounts.

There are some other interesting insights to glean from this graph. For starters, organ meat and seafood are the clear winners in terms of protein foods—many of them rival the most nutritionally impressive vegetables in terms of nutrient density, despite the fact that they are more energy dense. In contrast, dairy has the lowest average nutrient density of the protein foods. This doesn't mean that we need to avoid dairy—it's our most concentrated food source of calcium after all—but rather emphasizes that it would be best not to rely solely on dairy products as our protein food, since that would contribute much fewer nutrients to the total diet than if we vary our protein sources more and include some organ meat and seafood.

Another interesting revelation from this graph is that whole grains have the lowest nutrient density among starchy foods and are second only to nuts and seeds in terms of caloric density of whole foods—we would get a lot more nutrition if we swapped at least some servings of grains for other starchy foods like legumes, root vegetables, and winter squash. Again, this doesn't mean we need to avoid grains but rather that it's important to make sure excess grain servings aren't displacing more nutrient-dense options.

It's also easy to see that adding sugars and fats to a recipe or meal tends to add a lot of calories but not much in the way of valuable nutrition, so they are best used with that in mind. But I will once again emphasize that there are no "yes foods" and "no foods" with a Nutrivore approach.

LEARNING TO LIKE HEALTHY FOODS

If you're still feeling intimidated by some of the new-to-you foods highlighted throughout this book, let me emphasize that it takes only a few weeks for our taste buds to start adapting to big shifts in our diets. Studies looking at taste adaptation to one of a low-sugar, low-salt, or low-fat diet have shown that over the course of a few weeks (four to twenty-four, depending on the study, with adaptation to lower salt intake seeming to take the longest), participants develop a preference for the healthier foods they've been eating.[42] This is attributable to our taste buds becoming more sensitive.

Food familiarity and flavor association with positive experiences (e.g., feeling good physically, the food tasting good, or eating in a positive social environment) is another key driver of food preference.[43] Studies show that with repeated exposure to foods that we innately dislike, we can not only lose our aversions to those foods but actually develop a preference for them.[44] In fact, we can learn to like new flavors after trying them as few as four or five times. What does this mean? If you aren't enjoying the new healthy foods you're adding to your diet, don't give up! The more of these healthy foods you eat, the more likely it is that you'll start to enjoy them.

Another way to increase adaptation to new foods is to pair them with foods you love. A 2015 study looked at ways to increase children's liking and willingness to consume Brussels sprouts through associative learning.[45] Basically, that means they investigated whether they could get kids to eat more Brussels sprouts by repeatedly pairing them with flavors that the children liked. Children (aged three to five) were given Brussels sprouts (bitter) and cauliflower (nonbitter), new-to-them veggies, either plain, with cream cheese, or with sweetened cream cheese. While mere exposure to veggies was not very successful (80 percent of the children given Brussels sprouts plain disliked them at the end of the study), an impressive 72 percent of the kids who ate their veggies with cream cheese (sweetened or unsweetened) liked them, and they ate more veggies overall than the kids who received theirs plain. What does this mean for you? If you aren't a fan of Brussels sprouts (or any other nutrient-dense food), try pairing them with one of your favorite foods or with a dip or dressing that you like. In no time at all, you may be looking forward to eating this nutrient-dense albeit bitter veggie.

It's okay to sneak nutrient-dense foods you don't like into recipes where you won't taste them. For example, you might add some vegetable puree to a muffin recipe, or add a tiny bit of ground liver to your ground beef before making burgers, or add pureed black beans to your brownie batter. These are strategies that parents sometimes use to sneak healthier foods into their kids' diets, but there's nothing wrong with making these types of recipes for yourself.

And if you just can't bring yourself to eat a certain food, no worries! As we've covered already, there's no one food that will make or break your diet.

NUTRIVORE FOUNDATIONAL FOODS CHEAT SHEET

Here's a handy-dandy summary of how many servings we'd ideally consume, plus a dozen example foods, of each of the twelve Nutrivore foundational food families. More extensive food lists for all the food families can be found at Nutrivore.com. And remember, it's okay to work up to these serving goals over time!

Nutrivore Foundational Foods: Serving Goals and Examples

Vegetables: Aim for Five-Plus Servings Daily	Fruit: Aim for Two to Three Servings Daily
• artichoke	• apple
• asparagus	• banana
• avocado	• dragon fruit
• broccoli	• grapes
• carrot	• kiwi
• celery	• mango
• chard	• orange
• cucumber	• papaya
• peas	• peach
• peppers	• plum
• tomato	• strawberries
• zucchini	• watermelon

Cruciferous Vegetables: Aim for Seven-Plus Servings Weekly

- arugula
- bok choy
- broccoli
- Brussels sprouts
- cabbage
- cauliflower
- collard greens
- kale
- kohlrabi
- radish
- rutabaga
- watercress

Citrus Fruits: Aim for Three-Plus Servings Weekly

- Buddha's hand
- citron
- clementine
- grapefruit
- kumquat
- lemon
- lime
- mandarin
- orange
- pomelo
- tangelo
- tangerine

Root Vegetables: Aim for Seven-Plus Servings Weekly

- beet
- carrot
- cassava
- jicama
- parsnip
- potato
- pumpkin
- rutabaga
- sweet potato
- taro
- turnip
- winter squash

Berries: Aim for Two-Plus Servings Weekly

- acai
- blackberry
- blueberry
- cranberry
- goji
- huckleberry
- lingonberry
- loganberry
- mulberry
- raspberry
- salmonberry
- strawberry

Leafy Vegetables: Aim for Seven-Plus Servings Weekly

- chard
- collard greens
- dandelion
- endive
- kale
- lettuce
- mizuna
- mustard greens
- radicchio
- sorrel
- spinach
- watercress

Pulse Legumes: Aim for Four-Plus Servings Weekly

- black bean
- black-eyed pea
- chickpea
- fava bean
- kidney bean
- lentil
- lima bean
- navy bean
- mung bean
- peas (split)
- pinto bean
- soybean

Mushrooms: Aim for Three-Plus Servings Weekly

- boletus
- button mushroom
- chanterelle
- cremini
- lion's mane
- maitake
- morel
- oyster mushroom
- portobello
- shiitake
- white mushroom
- wood ear mushroom

Alliums: Aim for Three-Plus Servings Weekly

- chives
- Egyptian walking onions
- elephant garlic
- garlic
- kurrat
- leek
- onion
- ramp
- scallion
- scapes
- spring onion
- shallot

Nuts and Seeds: Aim for Three to Seven Servings Weekly

- almonds
- Brazil nut
- cashew
- chia
- coconut
- flax
- peanut
- pecan
- pistachio
- pumpkin seeds
- sunflower seed
- walnut

Seafood: Aim for Three-Plus Servings Weekly

- clam
- cod
- crab
- halibut
- mussels
- oyster
- salmon
- sardine
- shrimp
- tilapia
- trout
- tuna

CHAPTER **10**

Busting Myths About What, When, and How to Eat

I've spent most of this book explaining the value of nutrients and the foods that contain them, and I've discussed the benefits of a balanced, nonrestrictive approach to diet. But I would be remiss if I didn't also address the most prevalent myths and misconceptions that may still be coloring your food decisions. I want to make sure that you can apply your newfound nutrition knowledge to a healthy relationship with food, and that you can adopt a Nutrivore diet without breaking the bank.

Myths about food quality, toxins, and antinutrients perpetuate healthism: the erroneous belief that a person's health is entirely their responsibility, and that good health has moral value. Healthism creates unrealistic standards and fuels the belief that only specific, often expensive, foods are deemed healthy, or that a costly supplement regime is a health necessity. The cacophony of food fearmongering out there may have you feeling confused about what foods are safe to eat, and pressured to conform to rigid notions of what constitutes "good" or "clean" eating. In this melee of conflicting information, it's easy to become discouraged and find yourself in that vicious cycle of guilt, stress, and ultimately, unhealthy eating habits.

The various rationales put forth by diet gurus for cutting out whole foods, and sometimes entire food groups, just don't hold water. These typically focus on how an isolated food compound may be harmful in one specific circumstance, such as avoiding eating tomatoes because their solanine is inflammatory in animal and cell culture models of colitis.[1] Just because one compound in a food is harmful to one biological system, that doesn't mean the whole food is bad for the whole us. In fact, tomato and tomato products overall reduce markers of inflammation.[2] A 2020 study found that the highest tomato intake (1.8 cups per day) was associated with a 14 percent reduced risk of total mortality, a 24 percent reduced risk of coronary heart disease mortality, and a 30 percent reduced risk of cerebrovascular mortality.[3] When you hear pitches for restricting foods that focus on how one specific component affects gut health, hormones, or inflammation, your best bet is to adopt a healthy dose of skepticism.

As you scan the grocery store shelves, the number of options you have for a single item (like olive oil, or canned tuna) is mind-boggling. And the price differential between the store brand and the one in the fancy packaging is even more so. So no wonder one of the most common questions I get is whether higher quality foods are worth the sticker shock. We're going to look at this from a nutrient-density perspective. The overarching theme here is that it matters much more what types of foods you're eating rather than whether each one of those foods is bargain basement or the pinnacle of food quality.

While it would take several encyclopedic volumes for me to cover every food-phobic myth out there, I'd like to address some of the most common ones in order to assuage your fears about food. If you have fallen for any of these food myths in the past, don't feel bad, because I did, too! It's taken me a great deal of research over the past few years, and a very open mind, to fully unpack and deprogram these misconceptions, which come from cherry-picked studies and logical-sounding explanations—they don't hold up under scrutiny and don't represent the scientific consensus. The great news is that by busting these myths, a Nutrivore diet becomes much more accessible and affordable.

FROZEN FOODS ARE GREAT OPTIONS

You may have heard that freezing foods for a long period destroys important vitamins and minerals, but actually the opposite is true!

Frozen veggies and fruit can be even more nutrient dense than fresh. Not only are they picked at peak ripeness, which maximizes nutrient density, but they're frozen quickly, which helps to preserve all their valuable vitamins, minerals, and antioxidants—yes, even over long-term storage. For example, raw fresh broccoli has a Nutrivore Score of 2,833, whereas frozen unprepared broccoli has a Nutrivore Score of 2,925. Fresh kale boiled with salt has a Nutrivore Score of 3,644, whereas frozen kale boiled with salt has a Nutrivore Score of 3,945. And raw cauliflower has a Nutrivore Score of 1,585, whereas frozen is nearly identical at 1,574.

Frozen vegetables, fruit, meat, and seafood all tend to be cheaper than fresh, and because they won't go bad as long as they stay frozen, buying them can help to reduce food waste. Frozen foods also usually come preprepared (washed, trimmed, chopped, preportioned, etc.), so they can also save time in the kitchen. And frozen foods almost always have detailed cooking instructions on the packaging, which is convenient and reduces risk of undercooking.

Of course, not all frozen foods are created equal—some options are heavy on breading and sauces that are high in added sugars and sodium, and some options qualify as being ultraprocessed. So read ingredients labels and apply the same criteria (and balanced mindset) as you would buying foods from any other aisle in the grocery store.

CANNED FOODS ARE HEALTHY AND SAFE

While flavor preferences are subjective, when we actually crunch the numbers, we see that canning has a minimal effect on nutrient density, compared to other cooking techniques, across food groups. For example, the Nutrivore Score of raw spinach is 4,548, and canned spinach has a Nutrivore Score of 4,117, still impressively high. Canned green beans have a Nutrivore Score of 588 (and an impressive 661 if you include the liquid), compared to 605 when fresh. And canned pink salmon has a Nutrivore Score of 752 compared to 625 when fresh. The exception here is fruits canned in syrup, since the added sugar contributes calories and not much nutrition. For example, peaches canned in light syrup have a Nutrivore Score of 81 compared to 295 for fresh peaches and 319 for peaches canned in water.

What about the elephant in the room: BPA in canned foods? Yes, bisphenol A has estrogenic activity, meaning that it can act like estrogen in our bodies. Toxicology studies show that high doses of BPA—on the order of a hundred thousand micrograms per kilogram of body weight per day—cause reduced gestational and postnatal body weight gain, negatively affect the ovaries (increased cystic follicles, depleted corpora lutea, and antral follicles), and negatively affect hormone levels (increased serum estradiol and prolactin and decreased progesterone).[4] Based on toxicology studies, the US Food and Drug Administration limit for BPA exposure is set to fifty micrograms per kilogram of body weight per day, and the European Food Safety Authority limit is set to four micrograms per kilogram of body weight per day. However, while controversial even among scientists and causality has yet to be established, there are newer studies indicating potential harm to our health at much lower exposure levels of BPA, in the range of 2.5 micrograms per kilogram of body weight per day, so the limits set by regulatory agencies are under review.[5]

The good news is that average human exposure is much less than these levels.

A large 2011 nationally based urine biomonitoring study with broad demographics concluded that median aggregate human BPA exposures in the United States from all routes of exposure were 0.034 micrograms per kilogram of body weight per day.[6] A 2015 study showed that on average, we're exposed to 0.013 micrograms per kilogram of body weight per day of BPA from our diets, almost all of which comes from canned vegetables.[7] That's great news!

But what if you eat a lot of canned foods, like *a lot*? Even in that case, you still don't need to worry. A 2011 study had participants consume canned foods at each of three meals during a day, while blood and urine samples were collected approximately hourly all through that day until the next morning (a twenty-four-hour period).[8] This study showed that BPA is efficiently eliminated from the body—the half-life of BPA in humans is three to six hours—and estimated the participants' BPA exposure averaged 0.27 micrograms per kilogram of body weight per day.

The preponderance of evidence currently is that we don't need to feel guilty about buying canned foods. They're safe and similarly nutritious as compared to fresh. Most of the time, opt for canned foods without added sugars (this does lower the nutrient density) or really high levels of sodium (to make it easier to keep sodium intake in check)—noting once again that there are no "bad foods" on Nutrivore and every food can have a place in a healthy diet.

BUT AREN'T ANIMAL FOODS BAD?

Nope! Despite the claims you might have heard to the contrary, large prospective studies show that eating animal foods, when you control for other dietary factors, overall has a neutral effect on long-term health. For example, a 2022 study in more than ninety-five thousand health-conscious Seventh-day Adventists followed for about ten years evaluated the relative risk of total mortality for people who consumed 25 percent or more of their calories from meat, fish, dairy products, and eggs, compared to those who consumed 0.4 percent or less of their calories from these animal foods. There was no difference in total mortality between people following vegetarian versus nonvegetarian diets.[9] A 2016 study of more than sixty thousand people in the United Kingdom followed for fifteen years also showed no difference in all-cause mortality risk between vegetarians and vegans, pescatarians (people who eat fish but not meat), and regular meat eaters.[10] This study very interestingly did a breakdown of cause-specific mortality, and showed the various diets each had health trade-offs—for example, pescatarians had a higher risk of circulatory diseases but a lower risk of malignant cancer.

Among animal foods, red meat, in particular, is demonized for its link to cardiovascular disease and cancer. But the link between red meat and health detriments isn't actually clear-cut in the scientific literature.

Many of the studies demonizing red meat put processed meats and red meat in the same food category, but when they are analyzed separately, the stronger association with negative health outcomes is with processed meats, not red meat. For example, a huge 2017 meta-analysis that incorporated data from 123 studies showed that red meat actually *decreases* risk of coronary heart disease up to intakes of about sixty-five grams per day (the equivalent of eating four 3.5-ounce servings per week), whereas the risk was higher with any intake of processed meats.[11] And a 2010 meta-analysis criticized the World Cancer Research Fund for lowering its recommended limit of red meat consumption to seventy-one grams (2.5 ounces) per day for exactly this reason, the fact that many studies combine red meat and processed meat, meaning there isn't a strong scientific underpinning for this recommendation.[12]

Many of the studies showing red meat is harmful are observational, even the meta-analysis showing benefit of moderate red meat consumption I just mentioned. It's thought that associations between red meat and cancer or cardiovascular disease are an example of what's called the *healthy user bias*. The idea is that people who eat less red meat also have a lot of other health-promoting behaviors, like eating more vegetables, not smoking, and being physically active. Because red meat has been demonized for so long, people who make a lot of day-to-day choices geared at improving their long-term health tend not to eat very much of it. While studies perform advanced statistical analyses to try to account for as many of these other factors as possible, there's typically a residual effect—it's impossible to account for every confounding variable.

Interventional studies, where study participants substitute red meat for something else in their diet and then health outcomes are measured, show that it might not matter how much red meat you consume if the rest of your diet is diverse, nutrient dense, and abundant in vegetables. In fact, a 2019 review of interventional studies concluded that the evidence is not strong enough to recommend reducing red meat *or* processed meat consumption at all![13]

Taken altogether, this research indicates that red meat absolutely can fit into a healthy diet, and it may even be beneficial to consume some red meat, three or four servings per week. And while eating more plant foods—especially vegetables, fruits, and legumes—is definitely a plus when it comes to supporting health, we don't need to avoid animal foods.

IT'S TOTALLY OKAY TO EAT NONORGANIC FOODS

It's a complete myth that organic foods are much better for you than conventional foods, from both a safety perspective and a nutrient density perspective.

While occupational exposure to pesticides definitely can cause health problems, the amount of pesticide residue in our foods—yes, even the Environmental Working Group's Dirty Dozen—is far below the level we need to worry about. A 2020 systematic review, the largest performed to date with its inclusion of thirty-five studies, evaluated the health effects of organic versus conventional foods and concluded that no definitive statement could be made on whether organic foods improve health.[14] This review looked at studies that showed that organic food consumption reduced risk of infertility, birth defects, allergic sensitization, ear infections, preeclampsia, metabolic syndrome, overweight and obesity, and non-Hodgkin lymphoma, but was extremely critical of these results since the effects were well within the range easily explained by healthy user bias.

People who regularly consume organic foods are much more likely to be health-conscious females who are physically active, eat a higher ratio of plant to animal foods, eat more whole foods, and eat few if any ultraprocessed foods.[15] They're also more likely to be in a higher income bracket and have achieved a higher level of education, very important social determinants of health. These people are not healthier because they eat more organic foods, they're healthier *and* they eat more organic foods.

Many of the individual studies examined by the systematic review did not account for different types of foods being eaten on an organic versus conventional arm of a study. Sure, when people are on an organic diet they have higher antioxidant capacity, but this can be easily explained by the fact that they were also eating more fruits and vegetables. The benefits can be explained by higher diet quality, not the fact that the diet was organic.

And lest we think the authors of this systematic review just have an ax to grind against organic food, other research groups have concluded the same in their systematic reviews: organic foods are neither safer, nor healthier, than their conventional counterparts.[16] Organic and conventional foods—whether we're talking about produce, meat, dairy, legumes, eggs, grains, etc.—are equal in their health effects.

It's also a myth that organic fruits and vegetables are much more nutritious than conventional. Of course, there are no complete nutrition datasets for organic produce, but using the nutritional comparison studies that have been done (typically evaluating differences in seven or eight nutrients), I crunched some numbers for you.[17] (Briefly, to do this comparison, I replaced the nutrient values in the Nutrivore Score calculation, amalgamating data from four studies, to differentiate any effect from organic growing practices.) The results are completely underwhelming! Some nutrients are enhanced in organic produce, increasing overall nutrient density, but sometimes the reverse is true, decreasing overall nutrient density. And for all but tomatoes, the difference is within 10 percent.

Nutrient Density of Organic vs. Conventional Fruits and Vegetables

Food	Nutrivore Score (Conventional)	Nutrivore Score (Organic)	Percentage Difference
Carrots	932	1,026	+10%
Tomatoes	1,056	839	-20%
Lettuce	1,896	1,968	+4%
Spinach	4,287	4,410	+3%
Potatoes	265	253	-5%
Cabbage	2,034	2,184	+7%
Strawberries	1,070	1,044	-2%

If you're surprised and wondering why organic fruits and veggies aren't more nutrient dense, science can answer this question very easily. It turns out that the quality of the soil, what fertilizer if any is used, and other growing conditions have larger effects on crop nutrient density than the chemicals they're treated with.[18] And these factors vary farm to farm, region to region, and season to season. So you're likely still getting more nutrient-dense versions of fruits and veggies when you shop for in-season produce from local farmers' markets or farm stands, since family farms tend to use regenerative farming practices that improve soil quality. But if farm-fresh produce isn't accessible to you, it's not something to worry about.

All in all, whether you buy organic foods should be a personal choice motivated by preference and not by any expectations of increased nutrient density or better health. I find that organic produce tends to be fresher and higher quality in my local grocery stores, so unless it's cost prohibitive, I usually buy organic. When conventional looks better than organic when I'm shopping, that's what I go for.

No, Our Produce Isn't Depleted of Nutrients

A myth that is often used to try to push you to buy expensive vitamin and mineral supplements is that fruits and vegetables are empty shells compared to what they were in our grandparents' time, all due to industrial farming practices that deplete soil. The basis for this sales tactic is an oft-cited 2004 paper that compared USDA food composition data in forty-three crops in 1950 versus 1999 showing modest declines in some nutrients (increases in others, and no change in yet others)—but these results have since been misrepresented and exaggerated online.[19] A 2017 critical review argued that soil is not depleted and showed that these small changes in nutrient content are all well within the natural variation of nutrient levels in vegetables, fruits, and grains.[20] The authors further calculate that common nutrient shortfalls could be easily remedied by eating the recommended daily servings of vegetables and fruits, even assuming the lowest levels measured for these nutrients—yep, Nutrivore to the rescue again!

MEAT, DAIRY, AND EGG QUALITY: IS IT WORTH THE PRICE?

Is it worth the premium price for meat, dairy, and eggs that boast of being organic, hormone-free, non-GMO, grass-fed, pasture raised, etc.? There aren't health effect studies beyond the ones we already talked about comparing organic to conventional foods, but we can answer this question through the lens of nutrient density, even though we only have limited nutrition data to look at.

In general, yes, there are some nutrients that are enhanced in organic meat, dairy, and eggs, as well as in grass-fed beef and dairy, pasture-raised pork and chicken, and eggs from pastured hens—but the difference is not as big as the internet would lead you to believe. For example, a 2009 analysis showed that grass-fed beef has more calcium, magnesium, potassium, vitamin B_1, vitamin B_2, omega-3 fatty acids, and conjugated linoleic acid than conventional beef.[21] A 2019 study showed that grass-fed dairy products contain more vitamin A, vitamin E, carotenoids (beta-carotene and lutein), and conjugated linoleic acid, but lower levels of calcium, magnesium, and phosphorus.[22] Free ranging and pasture access doesn't affect nutritional value in poultry or pork very much—there is a small increase in vitamin E and omega-3 fatty acids—although it does improve the flavor and texture of the meat.[23] A 2016 meta-analysis comparing the nutrition of organic versus nonorganic meat highlighted the healthier fat composition of organic meat as the main difference, with more omega-3 fatty acids and lower saturated fats.[24] And when laying hens have access to forage so they can scratch for bugs and eat a diversity of plants, their eggs contain more carotenoids and flavonoids, which is responsible for the characteristic deeper yellow to orange color of their yolks—other nutrients in eggs are remarkably consistent across different farming practices.[25]

How much does this affect the overall nutrient density? We only have complete enough datasets to look at two cuts of beef and ground bison.

Nutrient Density of Grass-Fed vs. Conventional Red Meat

Food	Nutrivore Score (grass-fed)	Nutrivore Score (conventional)	Percentage Difference
Ground beef (85/15)	208	197	+6%
Striploin steak	371	209	+78%
Ground bison	322	208	+55%

It's likely that grass-fed meat being much leaner, and therefore lower calorie, compared to its conventional counterpart is the main reason for the differences in nutrient density—lower energy density means more nutrient per calorie. When the amount of fat is held steady, as in 85/15 ground beef, the difference in overall nutrient density is underwhelming. And while there isn't sufficient data to calculate their Nutrivore Scores, we can expect the differences to be even smaller for dairy products, poultry, pork, and eggs, based on the smaller number of nutrients that are affected by different feed and living conditions—although they're likely also a little more nutrient dense than conventional. Is this a big enough difference in nutrition to be worth the premium price? That's for you to decide.

And what about raw milk? There is no meaningful difference in the nutrient content between raw and pasteurized milk, and the purported benefits you may have heard about are quite simply not supported by scientific evidence.[26] Drinking raw milk increases risk of serious and life-threatening infections like campylobacter, cryptosporidium, *E. coli*, listeria, brucella, and salmonella.[27]

SEAFOOD SAFETY, SUSTAINABILITY, AND SELECTION

In terms of seafood safety, there are so many myths it's hard to know where to start! Seafood has a bad rap for being bursting with mercury, microplastics, and other toxins—none of these are actually a concern.

For the vast majority of fish, mercury is not an issue thanks to the selenium also found in seafood.[28] Methylmercury (the organic form that is a potent neurotoxin) harms us by binding with and deactivating our selenoenzymes. Most typically consumed varieties of fish contain much more selenium than methylmercury.[29] This is good for the fish (they don't die from mercury exposure) and even better for us because selenium-bound methylmercury is not efficiently absorbed by our bodies. Any methylmercury that is absorbed is already bound to selenium, so it can't interfere with our selenoenzymes. The only exceptions are those top-predator fish from contaminated waters in which the methylmercury bioaccumulation is higher than their selenium content, which is a fairly short list: king mackerel, marlin, pilot whale, shark, tarpin, tilefish, and swordfish, although data is mixed on swordfish and several studies show that swordfish is okay.

Microplastics—small particles of plastic less than five millimeters in size and all the way down to microscopic (less than one micron) in size—are ubiquitously polluting our environment and may eventually pose a health risk to humans.[30] While much hullabaloo has been made about microplastics found in fish, currently fish represent a small minority of our exposures.[31] The most pessimistic estimates of microplastic exposure from seafood consumption are about 54,000 particles per year, compared to 458,000 microplastic particles per year if you drink mainly tap water, and 3,569,000 microplastic particles per year if you drink mainly bottled water, not to mention many other sources of exposure.[32] Microplastics are a pollution problem that needs to be solved globally, but currently it's unclear whether they harm our health (at least at current exposure levels) and they certainly aren't a reason to avoid eating seafood.

As for other pollutants like dioxins, radioactive isotopes, and PCBs, which are of concern due to their carcinogenic properties, fish is actually much lower than other foods (including beef, chicken, pork, dairy products, and vegetables). And yes, this is even true for "bottom feeder" shellfish—most are filter feeders rather than the dirty scavengers they are portrayed as—which have some of the lowest levels of pollutants of all seafood.

If you are worried about antibiotic use in farmed fish, you'll be relieved to know that this is tightly regulated in the United States, Canada, and the European Union.[33] If antibiotics are used, there is a mandatory withdrawal period (a different amount of time for different antibiotics) before the fish can be harvested to make sure there are no antibiotic residues in the fish you eat. There have thankfully only been a few reported cases of antimicrobial residues in farmed fish from North America and Europe due to noncompliance. And if you've been told to avoid farmed seafood when the label says "color added," this is another myth. This label simply means that a beneficial carotenoid (for the fish and for us) called astaxanthin was added to the fish feed—it's the exact same thing that gives wild fish (like salmon, rainbow trout, Arctic char, and red bream) and shellfish (like krill, shrimp, and lobster) their distinctive orange-pink-red color, but in the wild, it's biomagnified from red algae.

There have been a few European studies showing a U-shaped response curve to fish consumption, where moderate fish consumption reduces all-cause mortality and cardiovascular disease risk but higher fish consumption increases risk. The authors of these studies have postulated that this may be due to increased exposure to the above toxins. However, this isn't seen in studies of North American or Asian cohorts, where fish is equally as likely to contain these toxins but where there's a linear relationship between health and fish intake—the more fish the better. The authors of a rigorous 2017 meta-analysis proposed an alternate explanation for a U-shaped dose-response curve in Europe but a linear or curvilinear dose response elsewhere in the world: method of preparation.[34] Traditional preparations of fish in many parts of Europe include deep-frying, pickling, or salting, and it may be this high-salt and/or trans fat intake to blame for the higher all-cause mortality seen with higher fish consumption. These studies do highlight that when upping your fish intake, it's best if you eat fish prepared in a variety of ways—baked, steamed, poached, grilled, stir-fried, pan-seared, and as sushi or sashimi—and not always reach for the battered fish and chips.

So yes, seafood is safe to consume, whether farmed or wild-caught. Of course, in either case, it's beneficial to seek out sustainable seafood. Fish, shellfish, and marine algae are considered renewable resources because they naturally reproduce to replenish their populations—but if we harvest beyond certain limits, we can damage or deplete their populations, which is not sustainable.

It's a myth that there's no such thing as sustainable seafood. In fact, the United Nations' Food and Agriculture Organization (FAO) has estimated that 66 percent of fisheries are sustainable, and that they contribute 78.7 percent of the product to the market of dietary seafood. And, if managed carefully, our oceans are amazing ecosystems that can recover and replenish, if given the chance. Several species of fish have rebounded in population after regulatory oversight and control tactics, including the widely eaten tuna fish.

When seeking out sustainable seafood for your meals, the main certification to look for is the MSC label, which stands for Marine Stewardship Council and ensures that your catch was performed using methods that will not harm or deplete the natural supply of fish. Other labels and notes that indicate sustainably sourced seafood include the Monterey Bay Aquarium, the Blue Ocean Institute, and the Tuna Tracking and Verification Program (TTVP).

Phew, that one was a doozy of a myth collection to bust! Now that we've established that seafood is safe and healthful to eat, let's address the question of selection: Is wild-caught better?

In general, wild-caught seafood is more nutrient dense than farmed, although how much so depends greatly on the specific fish or shellfish in question. The following table summarizes those seafood options for which I have complete-enough nutrient datasets to compare wild versus farmed—you can see that the increase in nutrient density ranges from negligible to a whopping 83 percent difference.

Nutrient Density of Wild-Caught vs. Farmed Seafood

Food	Nutrivore Score (wild-caught)	Nutrivore Score (farmed)	Percentage Difference
Eastern oysters	3,049	2,974	+3%
Atlantic salmon	868	673	+29%
Coho salmon	724	636	+14%
Rainbow trout	645	644	+0%
Crayfish	616	578	+7%
Catfish	559	305	+83%

So yes, you are most often going to get more nutrients per bite from wild-caught seafood, but it's important to emphasize here that even farmed seafood includes some of the most nutrient-dense proteins we can possibly choose. If farmed is accessible and affordable to you, you're making a nutrient-dense choice to feel good about.

EXTRA-VIRGIN OLIVE OIL VS. VEGETABLE OILS

It's a common misconception that most olive oils you can buy at the grocery store are fake or poor quality. The origin story of this myth is a 2010 non-peer-reviewed report by researchers at the University of California, Davis, which found that 69 percent of imported oils and 10 percent of Californian oils marked as extra-virgin olive oil (EVOO) failed to meet the usual criteria for this label. The findings showed that many of these oils were cut with less expensive olive oil, and some were even cut with vegetable oils (mainly canola and soybean). It's worth noting that an attempt to repeat this report did not show the same results.[35] Nevertheless, stricter regulations have been put in place in the EU and California, so you don't have to worry about your EVOO being mislabeled. And even more important, the oils that were being used to cut the extra-virgin olive oil are also healthy options.

That's right: There's nothing wrong with vegetable oils. The reason you might have heard that they're inflammatory is because they're rich in linoleic acid, the essential omega-6 polyunsaturated fatty acid. Omega-6 fats contribute to proinflammatory pathways, so in theory, we regulate inflammation when we balance our intake with anti-inflammatory omega-3s. But, while this is plausible from a mechanistic angle, a wealth of recent research in humans has not borne this out.

Most studies have shown a neutral or even protective effect of linoleic acid (and the vegetable oils rich in it) on inflammation, cardiovascular health, and all-cause mortality. For example, a 2014 meta-analysis found that over time, participants with the highest intake of linoleic acid (up to a whopping 10 percent of total calories) had a 15 percent lower risk of experiencing a heart disease event, and a 21 percent lower risk of dying from heart disease compared to the lowest intake (more like 1 percent of total calories).[36] A 2020 meta-analysis looking at tissue levels of linoleic acid (a potentially more reliable indicator of intake than dietary recalls) found a strong linear relationship between higher linoleic acid concentrations and *reduced* cardiovascular disease, cancer, and all-cause mortality.[37] The people with the highest levels had a 13 percent lower risk of all-cause mortality, 13 percent lower risk of cardiovascular disease mortality, and 11 percent lower risk of cancer mortality than the people with the lowest levels. And, a 2012 meta-analysis found no association between linoleic acid intake and any inflammatory markers, contradicting the theory that linoleic acid contributes to cardiovascular disease by increasing inflammation.[38]

Olive oil does have the edge over vegetable oils when it comes to supporting health. A huge 2021 prospective study showed that substituting butter or margarine with corn oil, canola oil, and olive oil all lowered all-cause mortality and cause-specific mortality, including from cardiovascular disease, type 2 diabetes, cancer, respiratory disease, and Alzheimer's disease.[39] Olive oil had the highest magnitude of benefit (4 percent reduction in cardiometabolic mortality for every tablespoon daily), followed by canola oil (2 percent reduction), and corn oil (1 percent reduction). So from a health perspective, olive oil still wins, which is why I talked about its heart-health benefits in depth in chapter 5. But if you can't afford, don't have access to, or just don't like it, you're still going to enjoy overall benefit from other vegetable oils.

While we're on the subject of olive oil, it's a myth that cooking with olive oil destroys all of its heart health benefits. In fact, thanks to its vitamin E content, olive oil is very stable under heating conditions.[40] But as with all fats, it's best to stay below the smoking point while cooking—for olive oil, that's typically about 410 degrees Fahrenheit, which is higher than most cooking applications.

Fun fact: The intense peppery taste at the back of your throat when you consume high-quality extra-virgin olive oil is thanks to the high concentrations of a polyphenol called oleocanthal. Of course, you're getting all the benefits of oleic acid no matter what kind of olive oil you choose, so don't feel bad if the cheaper refined stuff suits your budget better.

THE MYTH OF PLANT TOXINS

Let's take a moment to address the various myths about plant foods, typically ascribed to plant "toxins," "defense chemicals," or "antinutrients" like phytates, oxalates, lectins, goitrogens, and phytoestrogens. These myths about "toxic superfoods" are ones you likely have encountered if you followed Paleo, keto, plant paradox, low-oxalate, carnivore, or similar diets in the past. (If you haven't encountered these myths before, think of this section as an inoculation against plant food phobias for the future.)

Let's first correct the record on antinutrients, specifically the prevalent idea that they leach valuable nutrients from your body. Compounds like phytates and oxalates are considered antinutrients because they are naturally found in food as salts—i.e., complexes with minerals like calcium, copper, iron, and zinc—which hinders the minerals they're bound to from being absorbed in our gastrointestinal tract. For example, vegetarians and vegans may need to consume more dietary zinc because the zinc in their diets comes predominantly from higher-phytate foods, which reduces its absorption.[41] But blocking nutrient absorption is a far cry from depleting our bodies' stores, which just isn't the case.[42] In addition, our gut bacteria do metabolize phytates and oxalates for us, making a large proportion of the minerals bound to them bioavailable.[43]

Although phytates are viewed in a negative light due to their antinutrient properties, they appear to have some impressive health benefits, potentially thanks to their molecular similarity to a vitamin-like compound called myoinositol, which is known to improve insulin sensitivity and reduce anxiety. For example, a 2013 study showed that high phytate levels lowered the risk of osteoporosis in menopausal females.[44] A 2018 study showed that higher consumption of phytates reduced hemoglobin A1c in type 2 diabetics.[45] And a 2019 study in people with hyperuricemia (high uric acid levels in the blood, which can cause gout and kidney disease) showed that supplementing with phytates reduced fasting serum uric acid levels.[46]

Oxalates are often blamed for kidney stones (and other health problems for which there is no established connection in the scientific literature), with rumors online that eating too much spinach can cause calcium oxalate kidney stones in as little as two weeks. However, studies show inconsistent effects of dietary oxalates on urinary oxalates—most of the oxalates in our urine are ones our bodies produce. A 2008 study concluded that "The impact of dietary oxalate on urinary oxalate appears to be small. For many stone formers, restricting dietary oxalate may be a relatively ineffective intervention to reduce urinary oxalate excretion."[47] And in a 2002 study, healthy females consumed 150 grams—about five cups—of spinach daily for three weeks.[48] Not only did the study participants *not* develop kidney stones but they also had lower levels of oxidative stress. If you are prone to kidney stones, talk to your doctor for personalized recommendations, and remember that the best thing you can do is hydrate.

Lectins are a vast collection of carbohydrate-binding proteins and glycoproteins that are ubiquitous in nature and found in a wide variety of commonly consumed foods.[49] Because a few lectins can have a negative health impact in some circumstances—for example, gluten triggering gastrointestinal symptoms in people with celiac disease and nonceliac gluten sensitivity;[50] or phytohemagglutinin being responsible for food poisoning from eating undercooked kidney beans[51]—this entire class of molecules has been dismissed by some diet gurus. A growing collection of studies are identifying *beneficial* effects of some lectins—such as inhibiting cancer metastasis and tumor growth, improving serum lipids and blood sugar regulation in diabetes, and antimicrobial effects that could be leveraged in the development of new antiviral medications—so we just can't paint this entire class of molecules with the same brush.[52] Plus, proper food preparation inactivates many lectins—for example, soaking, sprouting, fermenting, and/or boiling pulse legumes can reduce the lectin content to near zero.[53] Lectin-rich foods like pulse legumes, whole grains, fruits, vegetables, nuts, and seeds offer consistent and impressive health benefits, as we've already discussed ad nauseam, which would just not be the case if their lectins were as harmful as the claims imply.

You may have read that you shouldn't eat cruciferous vegetables because their glucosinolates (or, more specifically, glucosinolate metabolites called isothiocyanates) are goitrogens, i.e., compounds that interfere with thyroid hormone synthesis. However, a variety of studies have shown that this concern is unfounded, even in the context of iodine deficiency. For example, in a 2019 study, participants were given a broccoli sprout extract rich in isothiocyanates, or a placebo, daily for twelve weeks—there was absolutely no change to thyroid hormones (free T4, thyroid stimulating hormone, and thyroglobulin) nor the percentage of participants who met the diagnostic criteria for autoimmune thyroid disease.[54] Yes, cruciferous vegetables, even raw, are safe for people with thyroid problems.

Phytoestrogens are phytonutrients with a structure similar enough to estrogen that they can bind to estrogen receptors in our body, modulating estrogen activity. There are four main classes: isoflavones, which are abundant in soy and many pulse legumes; coumestrol, which is found in soy; lignans, which are high in flaxseed, sesame seed, other seeds, and grains; and stilbenes, which are abundant in grapes, berries, and nuts. There's just no truth to claims that phytoestrogens, especially the isoflavones in soy, will cause gynecomastia (aka "man boobs"), lower sperm counts, or cause any other "feminizing" effects in males.[55] Nor does soy affect onset of puberty[56] or female fertility.[57] In fact, consuming phytoestrogens is associated with many health benefits, including cognitive improvements and reducing risks of osteoporosis, cardiovascular disease, type 2 diabetes, breast cancer, ovarian cancer, prostate cancer, and bowel cancer.[58]

Of course, all of these plant compounds are subject to even more fanciful myths that have no basis in fact, but I hope this breakdown of the most common myths gives you peace of mind about consuming plant foods and a cynical view of any other anti–plant food propaganda you encounter.

THE DOSE MAKES THE POISON

The adage "the dose makes the poison" can be traced back to Paracelsus, considered the father of toxicology, who defended his use of chemicals in medicine (like using mercury to treat syphilis and arsenic to treat skin rashes) when he wrote in 1538 his famous dictum: "What is there that is not poison? All things are poison and nothing is without poison. Solely the dose determines that a thing is not a poison."[59] While none of Paracelsus's remedies are in use today, thankfully, the importance of dose continues to underly the field of toxicology, i.e., the study of how chemicals adversely affect health—everything is a poison in a large enough quantity. As an extreme example, you need water to live, and dehydration can cause a variety of health problems such as bladder infections and kidney stones, yet it is possible to die from drinking too much water in a short period of time—in one report, drinking six liters of water over three hours was deadly.[60]

Many ingredients found in modern foods are disparaged because they are toxic in large quantities; for example, the tumult regarding artificial food dyes, preservatives, artificial and natural flavors, and flavor enhancers like monosodium glutamate. But while some people can have legit allergies or intolerances to these compounds, these additives aren't bad for us in the quantities we normally consume. I could write yet another whole book examining the extensive scientific evidence that dispels prevalent myths about food additives, but for the sake of brevity, let me just briefly touch on two hot-button issues.

Despite five decades of research, a causal link between artificial food dyes and hyperactivity in children still has not been established.[61] Food dyes, like most additives, have acceptable daily intake (ADI) levels established, which is an estimate of the amount of a substance in food or drinking water that can be consumed daily over a lifetime without presenting an appreciable risk to health. When it comes to food dyes, some people do exceed the ADI, with the top contributors to high food dye intake being juice drinks, soft drinks, icings, and ice cream cones.[62] Although it's still unclear if this has any negative effect, it is prudent not to exceed the ADI for food dyes (or anything else). An easy way to accomplish this is to follow Nutrivore principles, like making sure at least 80 percent of your calories come from whole and minimally processed foods.

If you've heard of monosodium glutamate (MSG) as something to avoid and the culprit behind "Chinese restaurant syndrome," it may surprise you to learn that this myth has xenophobic origins.[63] Again, despite more than fifty years of research, no causal link between MSG consumption and symptoms such as headache, asthma attack, runny nose, rashes, and flushing has been established.[64] Additionally, MSG is naturally found in many foods—including tomatoes, mushrooms, soy sauce, seaweed, anchovies, miso, yeast spreads (like vegemite and marmite), and cheeses—which were never scorned like the crystalline powder used as a food additive. In fact, a compelling case has been made for embracing MSG because its umami flavor helps to reduce sodium intake.[65] The ADI of MSG is not specified and doses of up to five grams in a single meal have revealed no adverse effects in humans.[66]

My point is that even the most villainized of food additives aren't something to worry about in the context of a diet that focuses mostly on whole foods. Yes, you can even let go of your value judgments of foods laden with additives as "bad foods" because the dose really does make the poison. Once again, we come to the refrain that no one food will make or break your health.

DOES IT MATTER WHEN YOU EAT?

It's ideal to eat three meals per day spaced about five hours apart. This might not jibe with some of the advice you may have read on the internet, so let's review some of the scientific evidence for different eating patterns in terms of timing, specifically the benefits of breakfast and where snacks may fit in.

Breakfast Really Is the Most Important Meal of the Day

If you're a fan of skipping breakfast in favor of intermittent fasting, then I have some bad news. Most studies in humans have shown that intermittent fasting (whether via alternate-day fasting or a time-restricted feeding period) doesn't provide any additional benefit compared to other diets, with metabolic and cardiovascular benefits attributable solely to the weight lost during the study. The advantage of intermittent fasting is that it's a structure that helps many people cut calories that doesn't feel too restrictive. But like so many diets, it comes at a significant health cost.

Studies routinely show that eating breakfast is super beneficial for our health. A 2019 meta-analysis showed that people who skip breakfast have a 22 percent increased risk of developing type 2 diabetes than people who eat breakfast every day, even after accounting for BMI.[67] And the more days of the week you skip breakfast, the higher your risk. Skipping breakfast four or five times per week increases your risk of type 2 diabetes by a whopping 55 percent! Another 2019 meta-analysis showed that people who regularly skip breakfast are 21 percent more likely to develop cardiovascular disease, or die from it, than people who eat breakfast every day.[68] The authors also calculated that people who regularly skip breakfast have a 32 percent higher risk of all-cause mortality compared to people who eat breakfast every day. That's a huge effect. And a 2020 study showed that people who never eat breakfast have a 2.7 times higher risk of depressive symptoms than people who always eat breakfast.[69]

Why is eating breakfast so good for us? It turns out that it's an important regulator of our circadian rhythm (how our body knows whether it's day or night) and of our hypothalamic-pituitary-adrenal axis (which controls reactions to stress, like fight or flight). So we have a healthier stress response and better-regulated cortisol levels when we routinely eat breakfast. This in turn regulates appetite and cravings later in the day. A 2002 study showed that people who regularly skip breakfast have higher morning cortisol levels that fall off more slowly than people who always eat breakfast.[70] Breakfast skippers also had higher spikes of cortisol after lunch. A 2015 study showed that women who regularly skipped breakfast had disrupted cortisol rhythm, hypothalamic-pituitary-adrenal axis overactivation, and elevated blood pressure, even though they had the same levels of perceived stress as the women who always eat breakfast.[71]

What about Skipping Other Meals?

A 2023 study showed that eating just one meal per day increased risk of all-cause mortality by 30 percent and risk of cardiovascular disease mortality by 83 percent compared to eating three meals per day.[72] Eating two meals per day also increased risk—while it didn't have as big an effect as skipping breakfast, skipping lunch increased all-cause mortality by 12 percent and skipping dinner increased all-cause mortality by 16 percent. This study also showed that it was optimal to go about five hours (give or take half an hour) between meals.

If you love, love, love intermittent fasting, it's better to skip dinner rather than breakfast.

When Is It Okay to Have a Snack?

Pop culture wisdom may tell you that eating six to eight small meals daily will help you lose weight, but studies don't bear this out.[73] So if there's no advantage to skipping meals and no advantage to grazing, what is optimal? From a health perspective, sticking with three balanced meals per day is best. But if you're going to go longer than five and a half or six hours between meals, or if you have certain health conditions like reactive hypoglycemia, or if you're a child or adolescent, then you may need a snack. What to eat for a snack is discussed on page 69, and fifteen snack recipes can be found in chapter 12.

While a morning or afternoon snack may be appropriate for you, a 2021 study highlighted that evening snacks aren't good for us—this is likely because they rev up our metabolism before bed, which lowers our sleep quality.[74] It's best not to eat for at least two hours before bedtime, and having your last meal of the day four to five hours before going to bed is even better.

RAW VS. COOKED FOODS

Does it matter if we eat foods raw or cooked? And does it matter how we cook them? Yes and no. Let's delve into some details.

Cooking depletes some nutrients and causes others to form. Cooking improves the digestibility and bioavailability (how well our bodies actually digest, absorb, and use them) of many nutrients, but inactivates some beneficial enzymes, kills probiotic organisms, and changes the quality of the fiber in foods. It's not as simple as either raw or cooked being better but rather a trade-off that demonstrates the benefits of both.

Boiling broccoli about halves its vitamin C content, and boiling chard depletes nearly all of its vitamin C.[75] But lycopene increases when tomatoes are cooked or sun-dried. A 2021 study showed that fresh tomatoes had 2,573 milligrams lycopene per one hundred grams fruit, while tomato paste had 28,764 milligrams, boiled tomato sauce 13,895 milligrams, ketchup 12,062 milligrams, and spaghetti sauce 12,700 milligrams.[76] That's a big difference! And, studies comparing the effect of raw versus cooked fiber on the gut microbiome show that they feed different probiotic strains.[77] A 2019 meta-analysis showed that both raw and cooked veggies are independently beneficial—for every hundred grams of raw or cooked vegetables, all-cause mortality risk decreased by about 10 percent—meaning we benefit most when we include both in our diets.[78]

When we compare the Nutrivore Score of raw versus cooked foods, we see that there isn't typically a huge difference in the total amount of nutrients per calorie—some foods increase a little, some decrease a little, it's really all a wash in the end. For example, fresh green beans have a Nutrivore Score of 605—boiling reduces their nutrient density a little (they end up with a Nutrivore Score of 516), while microwaving increases their nutrient density a little (they end up with a Nutrivore Score of 622). Broccoli increases in nutrient density when boiled—raw, broccoli has a Nutrivore Score of 2,833, and boiled, it has a Nutrivore Score of 2,914. Same for white mushrooms, which go from a Nutrivore

Score of 1,872 raw to 1,876 when boiled, although they lose a little nutrient density when stir-fried (Nutrivore Score of 1,783) or microwaved (Nutrivore Score of 1,691). Sockeye salmon also loses a smidge of nutrient density, going from 750 raw to 719 when cooked with dry heat methods. And the aforementioned tomatoes increase in nutrient density, going from 983 for fresh red tomatoes, to 1,019 when cooked, to 1,309 when canned.

Altogether, it's best to mix up raw versus cooked, but the biggest take-home message here is that however you enjoy that healthy food, that's the best way to prepare it!

Microwaves, Grills, and Deep Fryers, Oh My!

Did you twitch a little when I mentioned microwaving green beans and mushrooms above? Let's bust some more myths!

Not only is microwaving completely safe—the hazards typically ascribed to microwaves are either based on heresy or on weak, nonreplicated, and debunked science—plenty of studies show we have better nutrient retention with microwaving than other cooking methods. For example, a 2009 study of the health-promoting compounds in broccoli showed that out of five different cooking methods (steaming, boiling, stir-frying followed by boiling, stir-frying alone, and microwaving), microwaving resulted in the second-lowest chlorophyll loss, retained more vitamin C than stir-frying or boiling (or a combination of the two), and retained more carotenoids than boiling and the combination of stir-frying and boiling.[79] And a 2007 study showed that cauliflower, broccoli, potatoes, frozen corn, and frozen peas retained more vitamin C, vitamin B_6, calcium, and magnesium when cooked in the microwave compared to traditional cooking methods.[80]

So yes, you can enjoy the convenience of microwaving foods, whether to cook or reheat, and let go of any worries that this is somehow bad for you; it just isn't. Still, it's important to never heat or store food in plastic containers that are not intended for food. Single-use containers, like yogurt tubs, tend to warp or melt in the microwave, which may allow for plastic chemicals to leach into your food. Make sure to check the instructions on frozen dinners or bagged veggies for microwave suitability of the packaging.

Think you have to give up your favorite barbecue dish to be healthy? I'm happy to report this isn't the case either, but it's a little bit more complicated than simply busting a myth. That's because grilling, frying, and other high-temperature cooking methods cause the production of heterocyclic amines (HAs) and polycyclic aromatic hydrocarbons (PAHs), both known to be mutagenic, causing changes in DNA that may increase your risk of cancer. Although human studies show a very modest increased cancer risk (think 2 to 6 percent for highest consumers) and some show no effect, it's safe to say we should try to mitigate the potential detriments of HAs and PAHs.[81] One way to do that, of course, is to stick with gentle cooking methods (hello, slow cooker!) instead of charring our meat to smithereens. Fun fact: A 2023 study showed that air frying resulted in the lowest production of HAs compared to pan frying or cooking in an infrared cooker or electric oven.[82]

But if you love a well-done burger, guess what can counteract these meat mutagens? Phytonutrients! Various studies show that marinating or adding spices—like turmeric, garlic, ginger, rosemary, cinnamon, and chilis—to meat before cooking reduces the formation of HAs.[83] And including cruciferous vegetables like Brussels sprouts and broccoli in your regular diet can negate much of the cancer-causing effects of HAs in the body.[84]

What about deep-frying? Whether or not deep-fried foods are harmful is still a matter for debate. Some big studies show increased risk for coronary heart disease, while others show no effect.[85] This likely has more to do with the type of fat being used for deep-frying and the overall quality of the diet than it has to do with deep-frying itself. For example, a huge 2012 study in Spain, where olive or sunflower oil are more commonly used for deep-frying, showed no harm.[86] In contrast, a 2014 study showed that Americans who consume deep-fried foods daily had a 21 percent increased risk for coronary heart disease compared to people who eat fried foods less than once per week.[87] Notably, the people who ate the most fried foods in this study also had the overall lowest quality diets, the lowest vegetable and fruit consumption, the highest sugar-sweetened beverage consumption, and they had the lowest physical activity and were the most likely to smoke. While sophisticated statistical analyses try to take all of these into account, it's possible that healthy user bias explains these results, meaning that the people who ate less fried food had a constellation of other healthy behaviors that we can't fully account for in the mathematical modeling.

Certainly a case can be made that it matters more what the overall quality of your diet looks like than whether or not any of the healthy foods you eat are fried. A case can also be made to only eat deep-fried foods occasionally, or make them at home with healthier oil options.

You're Allowed to Enjoy Food

The most important message here, though, is that you're allowed to prepare foods in a way that you enjoy. Somewhere along the line, diet culture taught us that we need to eat vegetables plain, fighting our gag reflex the whole way, in order for it to count. But that's just not true! You can add fruit to a salad and honey to its dressing to balance the flavor of bitter greens; you can toss roasted Brussels sprouts in some balsamic vinegar, maple syrup, pecans, and bacon to build a balanced and delicious dish; you can dunk carrot and celery sticks into your favorite dip; and you can make vegetable tempura or fried okra. Adding a flavor you like to veggies you're unenthusiastic about so you enjoy eating them is a great trade every time. And studies back this up. A 2019 study looked at how emphasizing the tastiness of vegetable dishes versus the health benefits in college cafeterias showed that, sure enough, expecting a positive taste experience increased how much vegetables students served themselves, but it also increased how much they ate.[88] A secondary finding of this study was that we eat more vegetables when they are prepared in ways that we enjoy the flavor.

All in all, what foods you're eating is more important than how you're preparing them. So go ahead and make that broccoli however it tastes best to you.

CHAPTER 11

Applying Nutrivore Principles

As we wrap up an epic amount of information on the value of nutrients and the foods that contain them, we're ready to shift our focus to tools and strategies to make eating a Nutrivore diet easy, stress-free, and satisfying. Now we get to put all your new knowledge to work for you.

In this chapter, we're going to examine Nutrivore in practice, what it looks like to eat a Nutrivore diet every day. We have covered several super-useful Nutrivore tools already: the Nutrivore Score (chapter 3 and appendix D); the Nutrivore Meal Map (chapter 4); and the Nutrivore foundational foods (chapter 9). I have one more essential and efficient tool to help you successfully apply Nutrivore principles to your diet: the Nutrivore Weekly Serving Matrix. It's a simple-to-use and flexible weekly checklist that pairs with the Nutrivore Meal Map, and that is designed to help you maximize nutrient density without having to use a food tracking app or analyzing micronutrients, all while eating the right amounts of all the Nutrivore foundational foods.

We'll also discuss other aspects of implementation, like shopping for Nutrivore foods on a budget and the benefits of building Nutrivore into a lifelong healthy habit. So if you have any lingering questions, I hope to address them all in this penultimate chapter. Let's start with distilling all the information we've covered so far into eight simple action steps.

EIGHT EASY STEPS TO NUTRIVORE CHEAT SHEET

Use the simple steps below as a guide to easily make following a Nutrivore approach a healthy part of your everyday eating.

1. **Eat mostly whole foods.** Aim to get at least 80 percent of your calories from whole and minimally processed foods. This is easier if you prepare most of your meals at home.
2. **Choose as much variety as possible.** Aim to eat twelve or more different foods daily and thirty-five or more different foods throughout the week.
3. **Cover half your plate with a variety of fruits and vegetables.** Aim for five or more servings of vegetables and two servings of fruit daily, choosing from all five of the color families (red, orange and yellow, green, blue and purple, and white and brown) and mixing up whether they are raw or cooked.
4. **Cover one quarter of your plate in a starchy food and another quarter of your plate in a protein food.** This is an easy way to balance macronutrient intake while upping your intake of important micronutrients. Merge these two quarters when you choose a whole food plant protein like lentils.
5. **Choose healthy fats.** Opt for seafood, nuts, seeds, avocados, and olives as meal components, and olive oil, avocado oil, and vegetable oils to cook and dress your foods.
6. **Meet Serving Targets for Nutrivore Foundational Foods.** Throughout the week, aim to eat seven servings of cruciferous vegetables, seven servings of root vegetables, seven servings of leafy vegetables, three servings of mushrooms, three servings of alliums, three servings of citrus, two servings of berries, four servings of pulse legumes, four servings of nuts and seeds, and three servings of seafood. Examples of each of these food families can be found on pages 189–91.
7. **Don't Sweat Food Quality.** It matters much more what foods you eat than the quality of those foods, so it's totally okay to go

for the more affordable option. Frozen and canned vegetables; canned beans and seafood; frozen and unsweetened, canned fruit; nonorganic foods; farmed seafood; conventional meat; and eggs are all healthy choices.

8. **Progress Is Better Than Perfection.** There are no "bad foods" on Nutrivore. You don't need to feel guilty about eating a food that isn't particularly nutritious, and instead can celebrate the choices you make that are focused on nutrients. And it's okay to work up slowly to your serving goals.

THE NUMBER ONE WAY TO BE A NUTRIVORE: COOK AT HOME

Over the last few decades, we've gotten used to eating more and more meals outside the home. About half of Americans eat two or more meals prepared outside the home each week, with 16 percent of us eating five or more weekly meals away from home.[1]

Meals you make at home are typically much more nutrient dense than those you eat out of the home. For example, a 2021 analysis in adolescents showed that eating out of the home two or more times per week, compared to eating out less than twice weekly, lowered their intake of choline, vitamin D, potassium, magnesium, fiber, phosphorus, folate, and iron as well as total vegetables, beans, and greens.[2] A similar 2022 study in adults showed that eating out of the home more than twice per week resulted in reduced consumption of foods high in fiber, such as greens and beans, total fruits, whole fruits, and whole grains.[3]

And of course, those less nutritious meals eaten outside of the home add up, and are reflected in health outcomes. A 2021 study calculated that people who ate two or more meals away from home per day (which would typically mean one meal or fewer prepared at home each day) had a 49 percent increased risk of total mortality, an 18 percent higher risk for cardiovascular mortality, and a 67 percent higher risk for cancer mortality compared to people who ate most of their meals at home (less than one meal per week out).[4]

The good news is that meals you make yourself from whole food ingredients are almost always cheaper than prepared or restaurant options while delivering a lot more nutrition—yes, this has even been shown in studies![5] And while you may be operating within a tight budget, saving money on prepared foods, fast food, takeout, and dine-in can more than offset the typically higher costs of vegetables, fruit, and seafood.

Preparing your own food is one of the most important aspects of improving the nutritional quality of your diet. When you shop for and cook your food yourself, you have complete control over which ingredi-

Tips for Eating Nutrivore in Restaurants

Of course, it's absolutely fine to eat in a restaurant or even get fast food once in a while. If it's truly an occasional treat, go ahead and enjoy it, no holds barred. If you eat out more frequently, here are some tips to up the nutrient density of any meals eaten outside of the home:

1. Look for grilled, baked, steamed, or boiled options on the menu.
2. Seafood is almost always more nutrient dense than meat or poultry.
3. Look for menu options that include lots of vegetables.
4. Look for options with legumes, whole grains, fruit, and other more nutrient-dense foods.
5. Swap fries for a side salad or veggies. Or add a side salad or veggies in addition to fries.
6. Choose water to drink. Or have one glass of your favorite beverage and water afterward instead of refills.
7. Take home leftovers. Restaurants are notorious for serving multiple portions, so instead of feeling pressured to clean your plate, bring home what you don't finish for a wonderful leftover meal the next day.

ents are used. You can think of your food choices in terms of the nutrition your body needs and plan your meals to ensure that you're getting the full complement of nutrients throughout the week. Plus, you have the opportunity to cater to your own tastes, so you can make sure that every meal is full of flavors you love.

But what if you don't know how to cook from scratch? This is definitely part of the learning curve for many people. My recommendation is to find accessible recipes in a cookbook or online (like the dozen mix-and-match options in the next chapter, and all the recipes on Nutrivore.com), and just jump in. The best teacher is experience when it comes to cooking. If time and skills are a challenge, save your recipe adventures for the weekend when you have more time and try to cook double or triple batches to enjoy leftovers all week. It will get easier, I promise. You've got this.

NUTRIVORE ON A BUDGET

Here's a crazy statistic: According to a 2023 analysis, 73 percent of the US food supply is ultraprocessed, and on average, those ultraprocessed foods are 52 percent cheaper than their minimally processed counterparts.[6] In the 2019 study I discussed way back in chapter 1, where study participants spent two weeks eating a diet that was 83 percent of calories either from ultraprocessed foods or from unprocessed foods, the ultraprocessed food diet was $45 per week cheaper ($151 per week for whole foods per person versus $106 per week for ultraprocessed foods per person).[7] Yes, only about one quarter of the foods you can buy at the grocery store are whole foods, and they cost more. Dang!

Plus, the popularity of diets that demonize specific foods while lionizing others propels classism in diet and health—food elitism increases the cost of healthy foods, so you need greater income to access them.[8] In fact, simply identifying a food as healthy, whether based in scientific evidence or clever marketing, drives up its cost.

In 2006, restaurants began incorporating quinoa into their menus as an "ancient grain." Quinoa subsequently took consumer markets by storm, dubbed "the miracle food of the Andes" and included in Oprah Winfrey's twenty-one-day "cleanse" diet in 2008. By 2013, the price of quinoa had increased 600 percent, making it unaffordable to many Peruvian and Bolivian people for whom quinoa had long been a traditional food. In 2013, large-scale farms in Peru began replacing other commercial crops with quinoa, and when production subsequently overshot demand, the price of quinoa declined sharply—the results were devastating for small Andean farmers. Was quinoa worth the hype? In a 2018 clinical trial, healthy overweight men consumed quinoa daily for four weeks, but there was no change in cardiovascular disease risk factors, and the small decrease in blood glucose and LDL cholesterol was no different from the control group, which consumed 100 percent refined wheat bread.[9]

Even accounting for foods with inflated price tags but middling nutrient density, when you spend more money on food, the nutritive quality of your diet tends to be higher. A 2021 study showed that the people with the highest diet quality (as measured by the Healthy Eating Index; see page 13) spent 22 percent more on food per person per day, compared to the people with the lowest Healthy Eating Index.[10]

It would be negligent of me to teach you how to be a Nutrivore and omit this very important skill: how to shop for Nutrivore foods on a budget.

Of course, all the usual tips and tricks for budgeting apply, like shopping around for the best price, taking advantage of sales and coupons, and buying in bulk. I'm writing this section after a whole chapter of busting myths about food quality because an important way to get more nutrient bang for your buck is to stop paying that premium price for organic, grass-fed, pasture-raised, wild-caught, cold-pressed, non-GMO, all-natural . . . and many other buzzwords on labels. Now you know that frozen and canned are great options, and almost always cheaper than fresh. And you also know that if olive oil is too expensive, there's nothing wrong with buying canola or corn or whatever vegetable oil fits your budget. You also don't need to fork out for trendy "superfoods" like acai, goji berries, maca root, camu camu, spirulina, wheatgrass, or any other miracle cure du jour—there's nothing wrong with any of these foods, but you're not missing out if they don't fit your budget or preferences.

A really important strategy for eating Nutrivore on a budget is to reduce (and ideally eliminate) food waste.

First, you want to make sure you're eating or freezing any leftovers within four or five days, after which it's safer to toss. And you want to make sure you're using up the foods you buy before they go bad. Note that expiration dates and best-by dates don't mean the food is unsafe to eat after that date. Canned foods will last years and years in your pantry—as long as the can isn't dented or bulging, and hadn't been heated much above room temperature at any point (like sitting in the hot camper for a week before being returned to the pantry), it should still be safe to eat. Foods can last indefinitely in your freezer—even though they may get dry and that freezer-burned flavor, they're still safe to eat. In this case, preparing that finally thawed food with lots of seasoning can camouflage the taste of freezer burn. A great resource if you aren't sure is the USDA FoodKeeper app, which is free, and will also tell you how long foods will keep in various conditions (like fridge versus freezer).

Meal planning is a great way to eliminate food waste—even just making a rough plan of what you're going to eat each day before you go to the store will help you to avoid buying any extra food that might go bad before you get to it. If you know you're only going to need one onion for the week ahead, it will save you money to buy a single onion compared to buying a bag of them and risking the rest of the bag rotting or sprouting before you have a chance to use them. Meal planning is also a great way to reduce unscheduled trips through the drive-through or fast casual restaurants—if you know it's Taco Tuesday and you already have everything at home to make some killer tacos, it'll be easier to drive right on by Chipotle.

Have a good idea of how long different produce lasts so you can make sure it fits into your meal plan before it's likely to go bad. For example, heartier greens like kale usually last longer in the fridge than more delicate greens like lettuce, so planning to eat your lettuce within a few days of purchasing and saving your kale for later in the week is another great strategy to eliminate food waste. And if you think you won't get to it before it goes bad, you can also freeze it for later. Yes, you can even freeze lettuce—it won't be good for salad, but it'll taste delightful in a soup or smoothie.

And finally, don't throw out food scraps that can be used for something! For example, save the bones from your bone-in meat to make homemade bone broth with it. (I keep a freezer bag in my freezer and add bones to it as we go, then make a big batch of broth once the bag is full; see page 251.) You can also keep veggie scraps, the ends of carrots, celery, and the outer peel and ends of onion in the freezer to make veggie broth or use as aromatics in your bone broth. (I also keep a freezer bag to throw my veggie scraps into to save up for broth.) It's super easy to make homemade apple cider vinegar with apple cores and peels. And there are lots of recipes that use stale bread, sour milk, Parmesan rind, citrus peels, used coffee grounds, even banana peels (which you can make into banana bread!). A quick Google search for "recipes that use food scraps" will deliver a wealth of options. These might not all work for you, and that's totally okay—I just compost my used coffee grounds instead of making anything with them—but the more ways you find uses for food scraps, the less goes to waste.

Most (and Least) Cost-Effective Nutrivore Foods

Yet another approach to Nutrivore on a budget is looking at which foods deliver the most nutrients per dollar. To figure this out, I tracked down average US retail prices per pound for one hundred common food items and then calculated, using the Nutrivore Score and energy density of these foods, a measure of nutrients per dollar. I then divided the results into five cost categories, symbolized by one to five dollar signs ($). One $ means those foods give you the most nutrients for your dollar spent, and five $$$$$ means those foods give you the least nutrients for your dollar spent. Remember, there are no bad foods (even expensive foods that also don't deliver a lot of nutrients). This list is designed to help you prioritize which foods to buy when following Nutrivore on a budget.

Prices do vary by region, season, and of course, there's inflation. So please consider that large price differences between what you see in the grocery store today and the national average retail price I used to perform this analysis could change which category a food ends up in. To illustrate, as I write this, eggs have recently about tripled in price. (I hope, future reader, that the price has come back down for you, because at the time of this writing, I still have sticker shock every time I go grocery shopping.) Eggs would have ended up in the one $ category if I had done this analysis just a few months ago, but today, they're in the three $$$ category.

But just thinking about food by this metric gives a fascinating new perspective. If you're on a really tight budget, you might want to look at just those foods that are both inexpensive and in the one $ or two $$ categories, rounding out with your go-to budget-stretching foods.

Nutrition vs. Cost of One Hundred Common Foods*

Food	Nutrivore Score	Price per Pound	Value
Coffee	7,036	$7.48	$
Radish	5,863	$1.01	
Garlic	5,622	$3.17	
Spinach	4,548	$2.90	
Kale	4,233	$2.04	
Tea	3,286	$2.12	
Broccoli	2,833	$2.01	
Brussels sprouts	2,817	$2.97	
Green cabbage	2,034	$0.87	
Cauliflower	1,585	$1.66	
Mussels	1,564	$4.68	
Chili peppers	1,234	$1.59	
Pumpkin	1,036	$0.65	
Cocoa powder	1,024	$6.90	
Carrots	899	$1.21	
Papaya	636	$0.99	
Watermelon	405	$0.37	
Dry beans	389	$1.24	
Pineapples	358	$0.73	
Turkey, whole	299	$1.85	
Chicken legs	297	$0.78	
Nuts and seeds	276	$6.02	
Potatoes	272	$0.80	
Milk	224	$0.43	
Bananas	185	$0.56	
Coconut	179	$1.07	
All-purpose flour (fortified)	70	$0.55	

Food	Nutrivore Score	Price Per Pound	Value
Herbs and spices	1,080	$14.47	$$
Clams	1,046	$4.68	
Squash	670	$1.63	
Cantaloupe	457	$0.78	
Avocado	251	$2.38	
Bread, whole wheat	215	$2.53	
Chicken, whole	205	$2.32	
Sweet corn	202	$0.80	
Bread, white	128	$1.94	
Rice, white	66	$1.32	
Oysters	2,255	$11.97	$$$
Lettuce, romaine	2,128	$2.81	
Leeks	1,128	$4.20	
Artichokes	771	$3.06	
Plums	521	$2.09	
Kiwis	453	$2.11	
Oranges	418	$1.24	
Onions	380	$1.15	
Grapefruit	361	$1.24	
Eggs	355	$3.45	
Mangos	342	$1.29	
Chicken, thigh	288	$2.33	
Ham	214	$2.76	
Butter	57	$2.81	

Food	Nutrivore Score	Price Per Pound	Value
Mushrooms	1,872	$4.34	$$$$
Asparagus	1,385	$2.99	
Crab	1,211	$12.58	
Peppers, sweet	1,094	$2.58	
Tomatoes	983	$2.08	
Salmon	868	$15.05	
Strawberries	762	$2.71	
Green beans	605	$2.59	
Eggplant	563	$1.63	
Lemons	477	$1.95	
Peas	431	$5.35	
Limes	344	$1.36	
Pork	315	$4.96	
Ground turkey	295	$4.04	
Peaches	295	$1.71	
Clementines	291	$1.46	
Chicken, breast (boneless)	288	$4.98	
Ground chicken	282	$3.79	
Grapes, Thompson Seedless	271	$2.09	
Pomegranate	256	$2.71	
Tangerines	238	$1.46	
Honeydew	228	$0.96	
Lamb	215	$7.24	
Apples	213	$1.66	
Chicken, wings	174	$3.44	
Ground beef	165	$4.52	
Olives, black	164	$2.89	
Olives, green	160	$2.89	
Cheese, cheddar	126	$5.92	
Bacon	122	$5.24	
Sour cream	82	$1.97	

Food	Nutrivore Score	Price Per Pound	Value
Lobster	839	$17.01	$$$$$
Celery	767	$2.01	
Blackberries	743	$6.28	
Dill pickles	593	$2.89	
Shrimp	535	$8.90	
Raspberries	491	$7.62	
Cucumbers	472	$1.29	
Blueberries	396	$4.61	
Orange juice	301	$2.89	
Cranberries	288	$2.72	
Steak	283	$10.99	
Apricots	260	$3.20	
Nectarines	222	$2.03	
Yogurt	184	$2.21	
Cherries	171	$3.14	
Figs	158	$6.72	
Pears	145	$1.54	
Ice cream	86	$5.92	
Sugar, white	1	$0.88	

*Calculations were made using average national prices compiled by the US Bureau of Labor Statistics in March 2023.

Are Food-Based Supplements a Nutrivore Cheat Code?

While expensive, veggie powders, fruit powders, greens powders, mushroom extracts, liver pills, oyster pills, fish oil, bone broth protein, and various other "superfood" supplements are absolutely a valid strategy for increasing your intake of nutrient-dense foods that you otherwise might not be able to get enough of, due to either flavor preference or other factors. Note that the quality of these types of food-based supplements varies greatly from manufacturer to manufacturer, and some are deceptively labeled (promising effects that aren't supported by the scientific literature or including a lot of added ingredients that you may or may not need). But there are great options for all of the above, too—you can find my up-to-date recommendations for products and brands on Nutrivore.com.

As a general rule, your biggest question will be, "What is the fresh, whole food equivalent of a serving?" This isn't always easy to figure out, depending on the information on the label of the product you're considering. The most reliable conversion will be by calories, if you know how many there are in a serving (for example, a scoop or a capsule) of a single-ingredient product. Let's say one scoop of kale powder has ten calories. You can then Google "how much is ten calories of kale" and get the answer: twenty grams. From there, you can Google "how many grams in a cup of kale" and get the answer: sixty-seven. You now know your scoop of kale powder is about the same as one third of a cup of raw kale (or one sixth of a serving). When you don't have calories, you can look at any other nutrient you have on the label, maybe fiber content or vitamin A, and follow the same logic to do a conversion. For freeze-dried powders, you're usually looking at about a ten-to-one ratio, so if you're consuming two grams of freeze-dried liver in four capsules, for example, that's usually going to be the equivalent of twenty grams fresh, or about three quarters of an ounce.

These are realistic examples, and I use them to emphasize that the fresh equivalent is often a lot less than you think it is, making these products much more costly than eating the actual food. Of course, that trade may absolutely be worth it to you, and that's awesome if that's the case!

THE NUTRIVORE WEEKLY SERVING MATRIX

The Nutrivore Weekly Serving Matrix makes it super easy to put the Nutrivore philosophy into practice, regardless of which dietary template you follow. It's quite simply a checklist to keep track of your daily and weekly servings of Nutrivore foundational foods (using the targets established in chapter 9), other foods known to improve health, and dietary diversity.

The idea behind the Nutrivore Weekly Serving Matrix is to track the healthiest foods you eat, not every single thing you eat. Whenever you eat, check off every checkbox that applies for each component of your meal or snack. If a food doesn't fit a checkbox, you're still allowed to eat it, you just don't need to track it. You can use visual approximations to estimate serving sizes, so you don't need to weigh or measure anything. It takes me all of thirty seconds to fill mine out each meal, so this is a much easier way to keep track of your nutrient intake than any app or food journal.

The Nutrivore Weekly Serving Matrix has three main sections. Let's go through each of them.

The first section is built around the Nutrivore Meal Map as a gentle reminder of how to craft a balanced meal. Here you'll find checkboxes for protein foods, starchy foods, total vegetables, and total fruit. If you choose a root vegetable for your starchy food, go ahead and check both your starchy food checkbox and a vegetable serving checkbox (and a root vegetable checkbox in the third section). If you choose a whole food plant protein like lentils for your protein food, merge your protein and starch quarters of your plate and check both your protein food box and your starchy food box (and a pulse legume box in the third section).

The second section is where you keep track of dietary diversity and eating the rainbow. In the Eat the Rainbow section, check a checkbox every time you eat a serving of vegetables or fruits from each color family. As a goal, aim for at least two or three different fruits and veggies of each color during the week—every day is even better, which is why there are seven checkboxes for each color family.

For Total Dietary Diversity, count all whole or minimally processed foods that you consume at least half a serving of cumulative throughout the week and write it down on the lines provided. Your goal is thirty-five different whole foods per week, and you have forty lines to use to keep track. Unfortunately, refined foods or ingredients don't count here, only the whole or minimally processed version of that food. For example, you wouldn't count cornstarch as corn, but you can count canned creamed corn or cornmeal as corn. Go ahead and count different varieties of fruits and veggies (since we know that red leaf lettuce and green leaf lettuce have different phytonutrient profiles) toward dietary diversity. However, different cuts of meat from the same animal don't vary enough nutritionally to count them separately, unless you're eating organ meat. So for example, if you eat chicken thigh one night and chicken breast the next for dinner, that's only one Total Dietary Diversity line item, i.e., chicken. But if you also make chicken liver mousse during the week, you get to write in "liver" on an additional line.

What about foods you eat in small quantities, like spices or ingredients in baked goods? As long as you get at least half of a serving cumulative throughout the week (so one and a half garlic cloves total during the week, or one and a half teaspoons of cinnamon, for example), it counts.

The third section is Nutrivore Foundational Foods Weekly Servings and Bonus Servings—simply check the appropriate box when you eat a serving of a food that qualifies. If you eat a food that belongs to two foundational food families, check both boxes that apply. For example, kale is both a leafy vegetable and a cruciferous vegetable, and turnips are both a root vegetable and a cruciferous vegetable.

Bonus Servings are for tracking additional nutrient-dense, health-promoting foods (like organ meat, tea, fermented foods, and sea vegetables) that didn't make the cut as foundational foods. These are the types of foods that pack a huge nutrient punch, so eating them earns you more wiggle room for quality-of-life foods. Because the scientific evidence just isn't there to support categorizing them as foundational, they're totally optional. This section is also where all you nutrient go-getters can keep track of any servings of foundational foods you eat beyond the weekly goal. For example, if you eat six servings of legumes during the week, you can check off the four boxes in the Foundational Foods Weekly Servings section, plus two boxes in the Bonus Servings section.

When you eat a food, you'll often check off a box in all three sections of the Nutrivore Weekly Serving Matrix. For example, let's say you eat an orange for a snack. In the first section, you'll check off a Total Fruits checkbox. In the second section, you'll both check off an orange plus yellow checkbox under Eat the Rainbow and write in "orange" under Total Dietary Diversity (provided it's the first orange you eat this week). And in the third section, you'll check off a citrus fruit serving checkbox under Foundational Foods Weekly Servings.

When in doubt, don't overthink it. If you aren't sure if a food counts toward a checkbox, or if how much you ate equals a serving or not, use your best judgment—and it's okay to guess! And if a checkbox section doesn't align with your dietary preferences or is for a food family that you're allergic to or intolerant of, feel free to ignore it.

MAKE NUTRIVORE A HABIT

You now have all the knowledge and practical tools you need to fully embrace Nutrivore principles. So let's wrap up with some cheerleading.

As with tackling any positive change, it helps to frame it in terms of habit formation. About 40 percent of the day-to-day actions we take aren't goal-directed behaviors (i.e., conscious decisions) but rather are behaviors driven by stimulus-response associations that are performed automatically requiring no conscious thought, i.e., habits.[11] The power of thinking of Nutrivore in terms of healthy habit formation is that the effort you put into diet changes now will pay off with ease and auto-

NUTRIVORE WEEKLY SERVING MATRIX

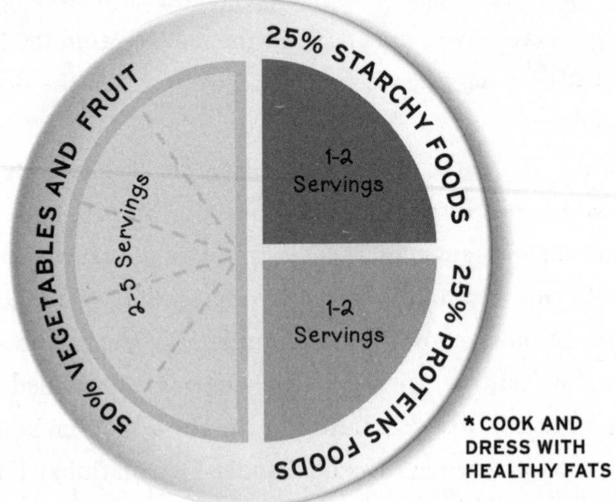

INSTRUCTIONS: EVERY TIME YOU EAT, CHECK EVERY BOX THAT APPLIES FOR EACH FOOD ON YOUR PLATE.

TOTAL VEGETABLES

AIM FOR AT LEAST 5 SERVINGS OF VEGETABLES DAILY

Can be any culinary vegetable

☐ ☐ ☐ ☐ ☐ ☐ ☐
☐ ☐ ☐ ☐ ☐ ☐ ☐
☐ ☐ ☐ ☐ ☐ ☐ ☐
☐ ☐ ☐ ☐ ☐ ☐ ☐
☐ ☐ ☐ ☐ ☐ ☐ ☐

Mix up whether your veggies are raw or cooked

TOTAL FRUIT

AIM FOR 2 SERVINGS OF FRUIT DAILY

☐ ☐ ☐ ☐ ☐ ☐ ☐
☐ ☐ ☐ ☐ ☐ ☐ ☐

TOTAL STARCHY FOODS

E.G., PULSE LEGUMES, WHOLE GRAINS, AND STARCHY VEGETABLES

Count starchy veggies like sweet potato both as a starch and a vegetable

☐ ☐ ☐ ☐ ☐ ☐ ☐
☐ ☐ ☐ ☐ ☐ ☐ ☐
☐ ☐ ☐ ☐ ☐ ☐ ☐

* If choosing whole-food plant proteins like lentils or edamame, merge the starch and protein quarters of your plate.

TOTAL PROTEIN FOODS

E.G., MEAT, SEAFOOD, BROTH, EGGS, DAIRY, AND PLANT PROTEINS

Adjust servings if you need more or less protein

☐ ☐ ☐ ☐ ☐ ☐ ☐
☐ ☐ ☐ ☐ ☐ ☐ ☐
☐ ☐ ☐ ☐ ☐ ☐ ☐

* 7+ daily servings of veggies and fruit is a great goal, but it's okay if you have to work up to it.

? ATE SOMETHING THAT DOESN'T FIT INTO A CHECKBOX?	That's okay! This Serving Matrix is for keeping track of the healthiest foods that are the foundation of a Nutrivore diet, rather than every single thing you eat.

EAT THE RAINBOW

AIM FOR AT LEAST 1 SERVING OF EVERY COLOR DAILY

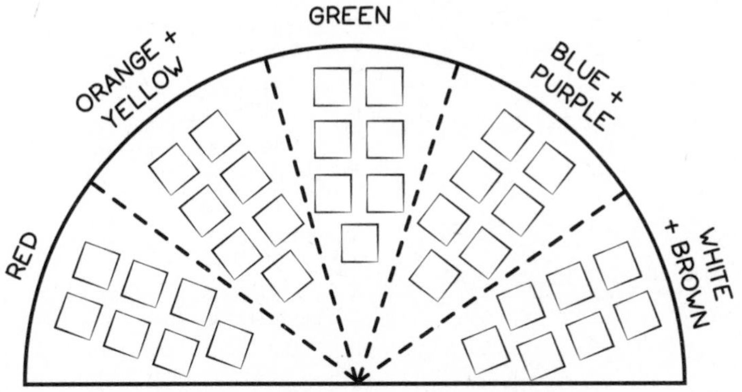

TOTAL DIETARY DIVERSITY

Count any whole or minimally processed food (even ones that aren't counted elsewhere on this Serving Matrix) that you eat at least half a serving of throughout the week.

1. __________
2. __________
3. __________
4. __________
5. __________
6. __________
7. __________
8. __________
9. __________
10. __________
11. __________
12. __________
13. __________
14. __________
15. __________
16. __________
17. __________
18. __________
19. __________
20. __________
21. __________
22. __________
23. __________
24. __________
25. __________

27. __________

26. __________

28. __________
29. __________
30. __________
31. __________
32. __________

33 __________

34. __________
35. __________
36. __________
37. __________
38. __________
39. __________
40. __________

To download a printable full-color version of the Nutrivore Weekly Serving Matrix, simply scan this QR code or visit: https://www.nutrivore.com/servingmatrixdownload

FOUNDATIONAL FOODS WEEKLY SERVINGS

7+ SERVINGS OF CRUCIFEROUS VEGGIES (e.g., cabbage, broccoli, kale) ☐☐☐☐☐☐☐

7+ SERVINGS OF LEAFY VEGGIES (e.g., lettuce, spinach, chard) ☐☐☐☐☐☐☐

7+ SERVINGS OF ROOT VEGGIES (e.g., sweet potatoes, carrots, beets) ☐☐☐☐☐☐☐

3+ SERVINGS OF ALLIUMS (e.g., onions, leeks, garlic) ☐☐☐

3+ SERVINGS OF MUSHROOMS ☐☐☐

3+ SERVINGS OF CITRUS ☐☐☐

2+ SERVINGS OF BERRIES ☐☐

4+ SERVINGS OF PULSE LEGUMES (e.g., black beans, lentils, chickpeas) ☐☐☐☐

4+ SERVINGS OF NUTS AND SEEDS ☐☐☐☐

3+ SERVINGS OF SEAFOOD ☐☐☐

DON'T FORGET TO DRINK ENOUGH WATER! ☐☐☐☐☐☐☐☐☐☐☐☐☐☐☐☐☐☐☐☐☐☐☐☐☐☐☐☐☐☐☐☐☐☐☐☐

Check for each 12–24 oz you drink

BONUS SERVINGS

PROGRESS > PERFECTION: REMEMBER THAT THESE ARE BONUS AND NOT MUST!

Additional VEGGIES ☐☐☐☐☐☐☐☐☐☐☐☐☐☐☐☐☐☐☐☐☐☐☐☐☐☐☐☐

Additional FRUIT ☐☐☐☐☐☐☐☐☐☐☐☐☐☐

Limit to 4 or 5 servings daily

Additional PULSE LEGUMES ☐☐☐☐☐☐☐☐☐☐☐☐☐☐

Additional NUTS & SEEDS ☐☐☐

Additional SEAFOOD ☐☐☐☐☐☐☐☐☐☐☐☐☐☐

SEA VEGGIES ☐☐

FERMENTED FOODS ☐☐☐☐☐☐☐

HERBS & SPICES ☐☐☐☐☐☐☐

EVOO, OLIVES & AVOCADO ☐☐☐☐☐☐☐

ORGAN MEAT ☐☐☐☐☐

TEA ☐☐☐☐☐☐☐☐☐☐☐☐☐☐

BROTH ☐☐☐☐☐☐

Serving Size Cheat Sheet

Here's a handy-dandy summary of serving sizes with visual approximation guides to make figuring out servings convenient.

1 tbsp	for	FATS, OILS, SPICES, AND DRIED HERBS	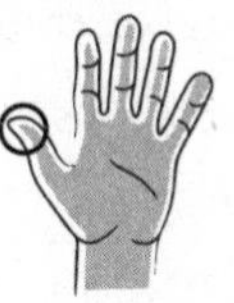	The top half of the thumb is approximately 1 Tablespoon
¼ cup	for	AVOCADO, OLIVES, COCONUT, TOFU, AND FRESH HERBS	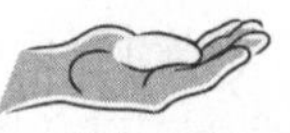	A rounded, cupped palm is approximately 1/4 Cup
½ cup	for	WHOLE GRAINS (measured cooked), LEGUMES (measured cooked), AND DRIED FRUIT	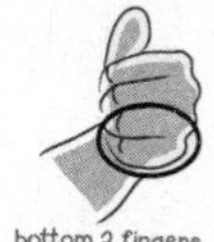	The bottom 2 fingers of a closed fist is approximately 1/2 Cup
1 cup	for	CHOPPED FRUITS, MOST VEGGIES (measured raw), BONE BROTH, MILK, AND YOGURT	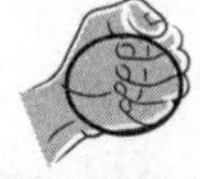	The 4 fingers of a closed fist is approximately 1 Cup
2 cups	for	LEAFY VEGGIES (measured raw)	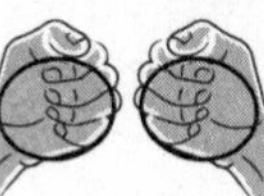	The 4 fingers of 2 closed fists is approximately 2 Cups
1 oz	for	NUTS AND SEEDS, WHOLE GRAINS (measured dry), PULSE LEGUMES (measured dry)	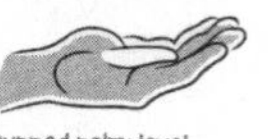	A level cupped palm is approximately 1 OZ
1.5 oz	for	CHEESE	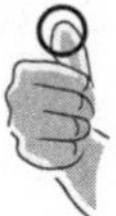 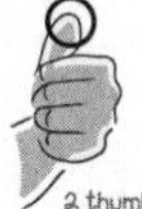	2 thumbs are approximately 1.5 OZ
3 oz	for	MEAT AND SEAFOOD (measured cooked)	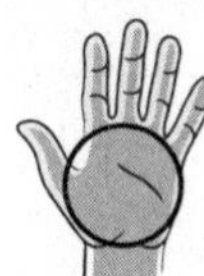	The palm is approximately 3-4 OZ (depending on size)
3.5 oz	for	ORGAN MEAT, RED MEAT, AND POULTRY (measured raw)		
4 oz	for	FISH AND SHELLFISH (measured raw)		

maticity in the future. While eating this way may feel like it's taking a lot of mental energy now, as you continue, the effort required will gradually diminish until, poof, one day, eating Nutrivore is as natural to you as brushing your teeth or tying your shoes.

I want you to remember that it's worth it to keep going, keep trying new foods and new recipes, keep working toward your serving goals, and keep finding ways to fit Nutrivore into your life. Depending on how big of a dietary shift this is for you, you might need to figure out solutions to a few common challenges. For example, maybe you need to find a few go-to recipes for quick weeknight meals when you're tired after a long day (the next chapter should help with that). Or maybe you need to keep some nutrient-dense breakfast foods in your freezer to quickly reheat on mornings you accidentally sleep in. Whatever your individual challenges are to implementing all aspects of Nutrivore, the energy investment you put in now to solving these challenges will pay dividends in terms of your health over the long term.

Keep going, it will get easier! You're worth it! You can do it! Rah-rah-rah!

CHAPTER **12**

Nutrient-Dense Master Recipes

Ready to get cooking Nutrivore meals? I've got you covered with this collection of twelve mix-and-match recipes featuring all the Nutrivore foundational foods that will yield hundreds of variations of nutrient-dense Nutrivore breakfasts, lunches, and dinners, followed by fifteen nutrient-dense snack suggestions. These recipes are more like flexible formulas to show you how to compose a balanced Nutrivore plate and allow you to pick your favorite options to cater to your tastes, budget, seasonality, and food availability. It's like a choose-your-own-adventure story, but with nutrition!

I've intentionally kept the cooking techniques simple with these recipes, and limited the requirements for any special equipment (one recipe uses a slow cooker and one uses a blender). So even the novice cook can make an awesome Nutrivore meal with a few simple ingredients and a bare-bones kitchen. *Bon appétit!*

Egg-cellent Frittata (or Egg Muffins)

YIELD: 6 TO 8 SERVINGS
TOTAL TIME: 45 TO 60 MINUTES

Frittata (or its mini version, egg muffins) is a great way to pack in the veggies at breakfast! While this is a time-consuming recipe, depending on how much chopping you need to do, it's also one that reheats beautifully—so you can make this on the weekend and then have leftovers for breakfast all week. If you have a thirteen- to fourteen-inch sauté pan, or two muffin pans, you can also double this recipe very easily and freeze leftovers.

12 large eggs

½ teaspoon salt, plus more to taste

¼ teaspoon black pepper, plus more to taste

2 to 3 tablespoons oil

CHOOSE ZERO TO TWO:

4 ounces bacon, sliced

4 ounces bulk sausage

4 ounces chopped ham

3 ounces grated cheese

¾ cup cottage cheese

CHOOSE TWO OR THREE:

1 onion, diced

8 ounces mushrooms, sliced

1 bell pepper, diced

4 cups spinach, roughly chopped

2 cups kale, tough stems removed and shredded

1 cup broccoli, diced

1 cup cherry tomatoes, halved

CHOOSE ONE (SEE TIP):

1 cup sweet potato, cubed and precooked

1 cup potato, cubed and precooked

1 cup winter squash, cubed and precooked

1 cup green plantain, cubed and precooked

OPTIONAL:

¼ to ½ cup chopped fresh herbs (parsley, cilantro, basil, oregano, chives, tarragon, thyme, marjoram)

Preheat oven to 425°F for frittata or 350°F for egg muffins. Whisk eggs with salt and pepper, set aside. If using cheese or cottage cheese, add to egg mixture after whisking.

Heat oil in a 10- to 12-inch skillet or sauté pan over medium-high heat (you'll need less oil if you're using fatty cuts of meat like bacon and sausage). Add meat and vegetables that will take longer to cook first (e.g., bacon, sausage, onions), and sauté, stirring frequently, until cooked, about 7 to 10 minutes.

Add faster-cooking meat and veggies (e.g., ham, mushrooms, bell pepper, broccoli, tomatoes), and cook, continuing to stir frequently, until al dente, about 3 to 5 minutes.

Add leafy greens, herbs (if using), and precooked root veggies last, cook until greens are wilted and root veggies are heated through, about 1 to 2 minutes. Taste and add salt and pepper, to taste.

If making a frittata, pour egg mixture over cooked meat and veggies in the pan. Move pan to the oven and cook until lightly browned on top and fully set, about 15 to 20 minutes. To test for doneness, insert a knife into the center of the frittata. If it comes out clean with no runny egg on it, your frittata is ready.

If making egg muffins, distribute meat and veggie mixture evenly across 12 wells of a muffin tin. Pour egg mixture over the top, mix a little with a fork. Bake until browned on top and fully set, about 20 to 25 minutes.

TIP: To precook your root vegetable, peel and cube, place in a pot with 1 inch of water, bring to a boil, and then reduce to a simmer. Simmer until you can pierce easily with a knife but not completely soft. Alternatively, you can steam in the microwave.

One of my favorite frittata combinations is to make this with 8 ounces bulk sausage, 1 onion, 1 bell pepper, 8 ounces sliced mushrooms, 1 cup diced broccoli, 1 cup potato, and fresh parsley. The Nutrivore Score of this variation is 383.

Never-Boring Breakfast Hash

YIELD: 4 SERVINGS
TOTAL TIME: 45 MINUTES

Breakfast hash is a great way to use leftover meat to make a hearty, nutrient-dense breakfast packed with veggies. Of course, you can also make hash with just about any ground meat or even kipper or hot-smoked salmon to get in a serving of fish. This is another one that you can make on weekends and reheat all week (frying a fresh egg each day if you choose).

1 to 2 tablespoons oil

CHOOSE ONE:

1 pound bulk sausage

1 pound ground beef, pork, chicken, or turkey

1 pound leftover shredded or pulled pork, beef, or chicken

6 to 8 ounces boned smoked kipper or hot-smoked salmon

CHOOSE ONE ALLIUM:

1 onion, diced

3 to 4 shallots, sliced

1 leek, sliced

CHOOSE ONE:

1 pound potatoes, cut into ½-inch or smaller pieces

1 pound sweet potato, cut into ½-inch or smaller pieces

CHOOSE 1 POUND TOTAL OF ONE OR MORE:

Green or red cabbage, shredded

Brussels sprouts, shredded

Carrots, diced

Mushrooms, sliced

Bell pepper, diced

Fennel, thinly sliced

Granny Smith apples, diced

½ cup water

½ teaspoon salt, plus more to taste

¼ teaspoon black pepper

OPTIONAL:

4 sunny-side-up fried eggs for serving

½ teaspoon dried oregano

½ teaspoon dried sage

¼ teaspoon cinnamon

2 to 3 garlic cloves, minced

¼ cup chopped fresh herbs (tarragon, basil, parsley, chives)

Add oil to a large skillet over medium heat, add ground meat and allium of choice and brown, stirring frequently to break it up, if needed. If using leftover pulled meat, add with potatoes, and if using kipper or smoked salmon, add with vegetables—and just brown the alliums in this step.

Add potatoes, and continue to cook, stirring frequently, for 5 to 7 minutes, until starting to brown but still firm.

Add vegetables, water, salt and pepper (omit if using preseasoned meat), and seasonings, if using, and cook 15 more minutes, stirring frequently, until vegetables and potatoes are cooked through. If hash starts to stick while cooking, add 1 or 2 tablespoons of additional water to deglaze the pan, and repeat as necessary.

Serve topped with a fried egg and garnished with fresh herbs, if desired.

One of my favorite breakfast hash combinations is to make this with 1 pound leftover shredded pork, 1 onion, 1 pound sweet potato, ½ pound shredded Brussels sprouts, ¼ pound mushrooms, and ¼ pound apple. The Nutrivore Score of this variation is 501.

Beyond Basic Breakfast Smoothie

YIELD: 1 SERVING
TOTAL TIME: 5 MINUTES

You just can't beat the ease of a breakfast smoothie, plus it's a great way to pack in nutrient-dense fruits and veggies first thing in the morning. I prefer to use frozen fruit when I make smoothies because they tend to be even more flavorful than fresh while keeping everything nice and cold.

1 scoop protein powder of choice

CHOOSE ONE (OR CHOOSE TWO BUT USE HALF THE AMOUNT EACH):

1 cup fresh or frozen berries (mixed or your favorite berry)

1 small fresh or frozen banana

1 cup diced fresh or frozen mango

1 cup fresh or frozen pineapple

CHOOSE ONE (OR CHOOSE TWO BUT USE HALF THE AMOUNT EACH):

2 cups kale, tough stems removed

2 cups collard greens, tough stems removed

2 cups chard

3 cups lettuce

3 cups spinach

CHOOSE ONE:

1 cup water

1 cup orange juice

1 cup carrot juice

1 cup milk of choice

1 cup unseasoned bone broth

OPTIONAL:

¼ avocado

¼ cup Greek yogurt

1 to 2 tablespoons fermented food (sauerkraut, kombucha, kefir)

1 to 2 tablespoons chia seeds

1 to 2 teaspoons honey or maple syrup

Place all the ingredients in a blender and blend on high for 1 to 2 minutes, until smooth. Add a little extra water or liquid of choice if it's too thick.

TIP: Nut butter also makes a great addition to smoothies if you use banana as your fruit and milk or water for your liquid. It doesn't pair as well with the other fruit and liquid options.

One of my favorite smoothies is frozen strawberries, kale, ½ cup each orange juice and bone broth, and ¼ avocado with whey protein powder. The Nutrivore Score of this variation is 557.

Hearty Any-Season Soup

YIELD: 6 SERVINGS
TOTAL TIME: 30 TO 50 MINUTES

This hearty soup is packed with your favorite nutrient-dense vegetables and cooks quickly thanks to using leftover or precooked meat. While it's the perfect comforting dish on a cold or cloudy day, there's no reason to enjoy soup only in winter. In fact, leftover soup makes a super healthy breakfast any time of the year!

6 cups broth (see tip), or more if you want a thinner soup

1 medium onion, diced

1 large carrot, diced

2 stalks celery, diced

CHOOSE ONE (OPTIONAL):

¾ cup rice (white or brown)

2 cups potato, cubed

2 cups sweet potato, cubed

CHOOSE ONE:

2 cups dried lentils

1 pound leftover or precooked meat (chicken, pork, beef, lamb, sausage), cut into bite-size pieces

1 pound ground meat, browned and drained of excess fat

CHOOSE TWO OR THREE:

4 cups collard, turnip, or mustard greens, shredded

6 cups spinach

1 cup peas (fresh or frozen)

8 ounces mushrooms, sliced

2 cups cauliflower, cut into small florets

2 cups artichoke hearts

OPTIONAL:

2 to 3 bay leaves

3 to 4 garlic cloves, sliced

¼ cup fresh herbs (rosemary, thyme, oregano, basil, parsley, chives, cilantro, dill)

2 or 3 chicken livers, chopped

Juice of 1 lemon or 1 to 2 tablespoons of apple cider vinegar

1 to 2 tablespoons tomato paste

Salt and black pepper, to taste

In a large pot, bring broth, onion, carrot, celery, and bay leaves and garlic, if using, to a simmer over medium heat. If using rice or lentils, add now. Cook until vegetables are soft and rice or lentils are cooked al dente, 10 to 35 minutes.

Add the vegetables (other than leafy greens or peas) and potatoes or sweet potatoes, if using. If adding a tough fresh herb like rosemary or thyme, add now, otherwise, add tender herbs (ones you would be happy to eat raw in a salad) with leafy greens and meat. If you're adding chicken liver, also add now.

Once the veggies are cooked to your liking (usually 10 to 20 minutes), add the meat, any leafy greens, peas, or tender herbs. If using lemon juice or tomato paste for flavor, add now. Cook 2 to 3 more minutes.

Taste and add salt and pepper, if needed.

TIP: Use leftover bones and kitchen scraps to make bone broth, at home. As you eat bone-in cuts of meat, save the bones in a container or bag in the freezer. Also save the peelings from celery, carrots, onion, garlic, and other vegetables in the freezer. Once you have enough, make broth. To make bone broth, put bones in a large pot and cover with water (water level should be an inch or two above the level of the bones). Bring to a boil, cover with the lid, and reduce to a low simmer. Simmer for 4 to 24 hours (12 hours to 4 days in a slow cooker, or 1 to 8 hours in a pressure cooker), checking water level a few times to make sure it's not dropping below the level of the bones (top off, if needed). Strain the bones. Add your veggie scraps (and optionally, herbs like rosemary, thyme, and bay leaf) and simmer for 1 hour. Strain veggie scraps. Season with salt to taste. Store in the fridge for up to 5 days or in the freezer for up to 6 months. You can also make veggie broth with just kitchen scraps and water, simmered for 1 to 2 hours.

One of my favorite ways to prepare this soup is with lentils, mushrooms, spinach, garlic, lemon juice, chicken livers, and fresh parsley to garnish. The Nutrivore Score of this variation is 871.

The Perfect Sandwich

YIELD: 1 SERVING
TOTAL TIME: 10 MINUTES

Yes, yes, I know, sandwiches are basic. But this recipe helps you take up not only the nutrient density of your sandwiches a notch (or three) but also their sophistication and flavor! With fresh meat instead of deli meat options, and a variety of toppings, you've got hot, cold, sweet, sour, crunchy, and soft all represented. The perfect sandwich for breakfast, lunch, or dinner.

2 slices bread or bun of choice, warmed or toasted

CHOOSE ONE OR TWO CONDIMENTS, TO TASTE:

Butter

¼ avocado, mashed

Mayonnaise (regular or Kewpie)

Mustard (hot, Dijon, grainy, or yellow)

Hummus

Cream cheese

Pesto sauce

Relish

Hot sauce

CHOOSE ONE PROTEIN:

4 ounces thinly sliced roast beef or pork, warmed if desired

4 ounces sliced grilled chicken, warmed if desired

4 ounces pulled pork or chicken, warmed if desired

3 ounces hot-smoked salmon, flaked, warmed if desired

4 ounces pan-seared or blackened whitefish (catfish, cod, haddock, tilapia)

1 can sardines, drained, panfried for 4 to 5 minutes

CHOOSE ONE OR TWO PICKLED VEGETABLES:

2 tablespoons pickled onion

2 tablespoons pickled carrot

2 tablespoons sliced dill pickles

1 or 2 tablespoons pickled jalapeños

2 tablespoons sauerkraut

OPTIONAL EXTRAS:

Sliced tomato

Sliced cucumber

Sliced radishes

Sliced red onion (rinse in cold water)

Sliced jalapeño

Bacon, cooked

Cheese, sliced

CHOOSE ONE GREEN (OR HALVE THE AMOUNT AND CHOOSE TWO):

1 cup arugula

1 cup iceberg, romaine, or butter lettuce

1 cup microgreens

1 cup alfalfa sprouts

Salt and black pepper, to taste

Spread condiment(s) over both slices of bread or bun. Place protein of choice on one half, and then top evenly with pickles, optional extras, and then greens. Season with salt and pepper. When placing second slice of bread or bun half on top, press firmly.

TIP: Yes, I've only included fresh meat options for the protein here, since deli meats are not covered in glory in the sciences. But remember, no one food will make or break your diet, so if you just have to use Black Forest ham or smoked turkey, that's totally okay!

One of my favorite sandwiches includes Dijon mustard, pan-fried sardines, sauerkraut, pickled onions, and microgreens on toasted whole wheat bread. The Nutrivore Score of this variation is 478.

Dynamite Dinner Salad

YIELD: 1 SERVING
TOTAL TIME: 10 MINUTES

Think salad is boring? Not so with this recipe! There are so many choices within each category that you can eat a different fancy salad every day of the month. Go ahead and get as sophisticated or as simple as you wish. Omit the protein to make this a side salad. This recipe includes making a homemade Italian vinaigrette—homemade dressings are easy to make and super flavorful, but you can sub your favorite store-bought dressing, too.

6 tablespoons extra-virgin olive oil

¼ cup apple cider or red wine vinegar

¼ teaspoon dried oregano

¼ teaspoon dried rosemary

¼ teaspoon dried marjoram

¼ teaspoon dried thyme

¼ teaspoon dried savory

1 garlic clove, crushed

Pinch of salt

Pinch black pepper

CHOOSE 2 CUPS OF LEAFY GREENS (OR YOUR FAVORITE PACKAGED MIX):

Arugula

Endive

Lettuce

Microgreens

Radicchio

Spinach

Watercress

CHOOSE ½ TO 1 CUP VEGGIE EXTRAS:

Cucumber, sliced

Fennel, thinly sliced

Red or green onion, sliced

Mushrooms, thinly sliced

Radishes, sliced or quartered

Sweet or hot peppers, sliced

Tomato, cubed

CHOOSE ½ TO 1 CUP FRUIT AND/OR STARCH:

Fresh fruit (apple, apricot, Asian pear, berries, citrus segments, fresh figs, halved grapes, mango, melon, pear, pomegranate seeds, peaches) or half the amount of dried fruit options (raisins, dried cranberries, dried apricots), diced

Canned cannellini beans, pinto beans, butter beans, chickpeas, or fava beans (drained and rinsed)

Roasted butternut squash, sweet potato, or fingerling or baby potatoes

Brown or wild rice, bulgur wheat, couscous, farro, buckwheat, or quinoa

CHOOSE ONE OR TWO PROTEINS:

3 ounces grilled or leftover chicken, sliced

3 ounces grilled or pan-seared steak, sliced

3 to 4 ounces salad shrimp

3 to 4 ounces grilled or poached salmon or trout

3 to 4 ounces canned salmon, tuna, or mackerel (drained)

1½ ounces cheese, cubed

½ to 1 cup edamame (boiled or steamed)

OPTIONAL FOR FLAVOR:

Avocado, cubed

Fresh herbs (basil, chervil, chives, cilantro, dill, fennel, mint, oregano, parsley, tarragon)

Hearts of palm, sliced

Canned artichoke hearts

Olives

Pickled vegetables

OPTIONAL FOR CRUNCH:

Crunchy chickpeas, mung beans, farro, bulgur, brown rice or quinoa (see Tips)

Croutons

Crumbled bacon

1 ounce nuts and seeds (sliced almonds, walnuts, pecans, sunflower seeds, pepitas, pistachios, pine nuts, chopped Brazil nuts)

Combine all the salad dressing ingredients in a bowl or jar and whisk or shake to fully combine.

Place all your chosen salad ingredients in a large bowl. (If you wish, you can leave out crunchy toppers to add at the end.)

Pour 2 to 3 tablespoons of salad dressing, or however you like it, onto your salad. Refrigerate the remainder of your salad dressing to save for another day, and use within three weeks.

Toss to fully coat. Add your crunchy toppers, if desired.

TIPS: To make crunchy chickpeas, quinoa, or grains: Combine 1 cup cooked grain or legume of choice with 2 tablespoons oil and ½ teaspoon salt. You can also add your favorite spice blend to kick it up a notch. Spread into a thin layer on a baking sheet and bake at 375°F, stirring every 10 minutes, until crispy. (This will take about 30 minutes for quinoa and up to an hour for chickpeas.) There are also store-bought versions if that's more convenient.

A salad combination I eat regularly includes 2 cups arugula, ¼ cup sliced cucumber, ¼ cup sliced red onion, ½ cup halved cherry tomatoes, ½ cup sliced Granny Smith apple, ¼ cup cannellini beans, 3 ounces grilled chicken, ½ cup canned artichoke hearts, ½ cup canned hearts of palm, and 2 tablespoons sliced black olives. The Nutrivore Score for this combination is 294.

Sheet Pan Fish Gremolata and Veggies

YIELD: 4 TO 6 SERVINGS
TOTAL TIME: 30 MINUTES

This is a simple dish fancy enough to serve for company, cooked on two sheet pans, one for the veggies and one for the fish. It's best with whitefish, but you can make this with fatty fish like salmon, too. If you're looking to save time, you can make the crumb topping ahead of time and keep it in the fridge or freezer until you need it.

1½ pounds whitefish filets (e.g., hake, sablefish, cod, sea bass, mahimahi, halibut, swordfish), cut into 4 to 6 pieces
4 tablespoons oil
¼ cup bread, panko, cracker, or plantain chip crumbs (see Tip)
¼ cup chopped fresh parsley
1 garlic clove, crushed
Finely grated zest and juice from 1 lemon
1 tablespoon butter, melted
¾ teaspoon salt, divided
⅜ teaspoon black pepper, divided

CHOOSE ONE OR TWO:

2 bunches asparagus, tough ends snapped off
1½ to 2 pounds green beans, trimmed
3 medium zucchini, angle cut into thick slices
2 sweet peppers, sliced into thick wedges
8 ounces snow peas, trimmed
2 large leeks, sliced

OPTIONAL:

1 pint cherry tomatoes, halved
1 cup walnut halves

Preheat oven to 425°F. Line one rimmed baking sheet large enough for the filets to be spaced at least an inch apart with tinfoil and spread

2 tablespoons oil over the top (alternately, use a silicone liner and skip the oil).

Mix crumbs with parsley, garlic, lemon zest, and melted butter.

Place fish fillets on prepared baking sheet. Drizzle with lemon juice and sprinkle with ¼ teaspoon salt and ⅛ teaspoon pepper. Evenly coat the top of the fish fillets with the crumb mixture.

Toss vegetables with remaining 2 tablespoons of oil, ½ teaspoon salt, and ¼ teaspoon pepper. Place on a second rimmed baking sheet large enough to allow the vegetables to form a single layer. Place cherry tomatoes and/or walnut halves around veggies, if using.

Place both baking sheets in the oven and bake for 15 to 20 minutes, until fish is fully cooked and veggies are starting to brown.

TIP: You can make your own crumbs by putting crackers, croutons, stale bread, or plantain chips in a plastic resealable bag and then pounding the outside of the bag with a kitchen mallet or rolling pin. You can also pulse in a food processor.

One of my favorite ways to make this dish is to use halibut and serve it with two bunches of asparagus, a pint of cherry tomatoes, and a cup of walnuts. The Nutrivore Score for this combination is 481.

Any-Day Roast and Veggies

YIELD: 8 TO 16 SERVINGS
TOTAL TIME: UP TO 3½ HOURS

Roasting a large cut of meat surrounded by vegetables is one of the simplest meals you can make, with very low hands-on time, and always delicious. There's no reason to make this only on Sundays, unless you're hoping to have leftovers all week. If you can't fit all your veggies into your roasting pan around your meat, place them on a sheet pan on a separate rack in the oven.

CHOOSE ONE:

1 or 2 whole chickens

1 pork loin roast

1 leg of lamb

1 tablespoon finely grated lemon zest

3 tablespoons finely chopped fresh oregano leaves, or 1 tablespoon dried oregano

3 garlic cloves, crushed

1 tablespoon finely chopped fresh mint leaves

1½ teaspoons salt, divided

¾ teaspoon black pepper, divided

CHOOSE ONE:

1½ pound potatoes

1½ pounds sweet potatoes

1½ pounds parsnips

1½ pounds turnips

1½ pounds beets

CHOOSE ONE OR TWO:

1½ to 2 pounds Brussels sprouts

1 bunch broccoli

1 head cauliflower

1½ to 2 pounds green beans

2 medium acorn squash, peeled and cut into quarters

6 large carrots

2 to 3 tablespoons oil

Roast Type	Oven Temperature	Roasting Time
Whole chicken (up to 6 pounds each)	350°F	20 minutes per pound (if cooking two, calculate with your larger chicken)
Pork loin (up to 5 pounds)	350°F	20 minutes per pound
Leg of lamb (up to 7 pounds)	325°F	25 to 30 minutes per pound for boneless 20 to 25 minutes per pound for bone-in (less time for medium rare, more time for medium)

Preheat oven as noted in table above.

Place meat in a large roasting pan and pat dry with paper towels. In a small bowl, combine lemon zest, oregano, garlic, mint, 1 teaspoon salt, and ½ teaspoon pepper, and season meat liberally. Place in the oven and roast for the amount of time indicated in the table above, until fully cooked to your liking.

Cut vegetables into large pieces, about 3 inches, leaving any veggies smaller than that whole. Toss with oil, remaining ½ teaspoon salt and ¼ teaspoon pepper.

With 50 minutes left in your meat cooking time, remove from oven and place vegetables all around the roast. (Place any veggies that don't fit on a sheet pan and cook on a separate rack in the oven.) Return to oven for remaining cooking time.

Let meat rest for 5 to 10 minutes before carving. During this time, if you want more browning on your veggies, you can return them to the oven and broil for 2 to 3 minutes.

TIP: Feel free to keep the seasoning as simple as you like. If you only want to use salt and pepper, that's totally fine! Or you can use your favorite seasoning blend.

My favorite is to roast a whole chicken and serve it with beets, Brussels sprouts, and carrots. The Nutrivore Score for this combination is 482.

DIY Stir-Fry

YIELD: 4 SERVINGS
TOTAL TIME: 30 TO 40 MINUTES

The biggest trick with stir-fries is to prep absolutely everything before you start cooking, including chopping vegetables, slicing meat, and measuring out all your sauce ingredients. In fact, most of the time investment in stir-fries is preparation. This is a high-heat cooking method, which can feel very frantic, but that's okay. Just make sure you are stirring almost constantly to avoid burning.

2 tablespoons soy sauce

1 tablespoon brown sugar

½ teaspoon sesame oil

¼ cup broth or orange juice

1 tablespoon cornstarch, arrowroot, or kudzu

3 to 4 tablespoons oil

½-inch piece fresh ginger, minced or grated

2 garlic cloves, minced

CHOOSE ONE:

12 ounces boneless, skinless chicken thigh, pork chop, or beef flank steak, sliced into very thin 2- to 3-inch strips

1 pound raw shrimp, shelled and deveined

1 pound squid, cut into rounds

14 ounces extra-firm tofu, excess liquid squeezed out and cubed

CHOOSE THREE OR FOUR:

1 onion, sliced

3 cups broccolini, cut into 3-inch pieces

8 ounces sliced mushrooms, or rehydrated dried mushrooms, any variety

4 cups bok choy or tatsoi, chopped

2 cups snow peas, trimmed

One 8-ounce can bamboo shoots

One 8-ounce can water chestnuts

OPTIONAL:

1 cup raw cashews or blanched almonds

Chili flakes, gochujang, or sriracha, for extra heat

3 green onions, sliced

2 teaspoons sesame seeds

Salt, to taste

Rice or noodles (egg noodles, soba, chow mein, lo mein, udon, rice noodles, etc.) for serving

In a small bowl or measuring cup, combine soy sauce, brown sugar, sesame oil, broth, and cornstarch and set aside.

Heat a wok or large frying pan on the stovetop over medium-high heat (just a notch lower than high heat). Add 3 tablespoons of oil to the hot wok, then add ginger and garlic, and cook, stirring constantly, for 1 minute.

Add protein of choice to the wok. Cook, stirring constantly, until fully cooked, about 3 to 5 minutes. Remove from the wok and set aside.

Add vegetables to the wok (if there isn't much oil left, add another tablespoon before adding your veggies). Add veggies that take longer to cook first (onion, broccolini, mushrooms) and then add veggies that are quick to cook or cut into very small pieces after larger veggies are most of the way cooked (bok choy, snow peas, canned veggies). If using nuts, add with faster-cooking veggies. Cook, stirring frequently, until vegetables are done to your liking, about 3 to 8 minutes. If the veggies are releasing a lot of liquid into the wok, turn the heat up to high.

Add your cooked protein back to the wok and add your sauce. Stir constantly until sauce has thickened, about 1 minute, then remove from heat.

Taste and season with salt, if needed.

Garnish with sliced green onion, sesame seeds, chili flakes, gochujang, and/or sriracha, if desired.

TIP: When stir-frying shrimp, you'll get a much better texture if you brine them first. To do this, stir 1 tablespoon salt into 4 cups cold water until dissolved. Pour over shrimp and let marinate for 5 minutes. Rinse shrimp and drain dry on paper towels.

One of my favorite ways to prepare this stir-fry is with shrimp, one can each bamboo shoots and water chestnuts, bok choy, and shiitake mushrooms (or any variety I have on hand), and served over brown rice. This variation has a Nutrivore Score of 673.

Slow Cooker Customizable Carnitas

YIELD: 8 SERVINGS
TOTAL TIME: 8 HOURS

Choose your meat, toppings, and whether you wrap it in a tortilla, place it in a taco shell, or serve it as a carnitas salad bowl! My favorite part of this meal, besides its deliciousness, is that it can simmer in the slow cooker all day. When serving, be generous with the veggies and condiments for the highest overall nutrient density.

CHOOSE ONE:

3 pounds chuck roast or brisket, cut into 4-inch pieces

3 pounds pork shoulder, cut into 4-inch pieces

2 pounds boneless, skinless chicken thighs

1 tablespoon ground coriander seed

1 tablespoon ground cumin

1 tablespoon dried oregano

2 teaspoons smoked sea salt

2 teaspoons chili powder

2 teaspoons paprika

½ teaspoon cayenne pepper

2 teaspoons granulated onion

2 teaspoons granulated garlic

1 teaspoon freshly ground black pepper

1 cup broth

Juice of 2 limes

CHOOSE ONE OR TWO:

Corn tortillas

Flour tortillas

Taco shells

Tortilla chips

Rice

Black beans

Refried beans

TO SERVE (PICK YOUR FAVORITES):

Small red onion, sliced and rinsed

Radishes, thinly sliced

Fresh cilantro, chopped

Iceberg or romaine lettuce, shredded

Cucumber, diced

Tomatoes, diced

Grated cheese

Guacamole

Sour cream

Salsa

Pico de gallo

Sliced or pickled jalapeño

In a slow cooker, combine meat of choice, spices, broth, and lime juice. Cook on high for 6 to 8 hours, until meat is so well cooked it falls apart, checking occasionally to make sure liquid level doesn't get too low (top off with a little water if it does). (You can also halve the amount of broth and cook in an Instant Pot or similar pressure cooker for 45 minutes on high pressure, allowing steam to naturally release for 15 minutes.)

Using a slotted spoon, transfer the meat to a large baking dish or rimmed sheet pan.

Using two forks, shred the meat.

Optional: Turn the broiler on high. Broil the shredded meat until the edges are crispy, 5 to 8 minutes.

Serve as burritos, quesadillas, tacos, or as a carnitas bowl with your favorite veggies and condiments.

I love to make these carnitas using pork shoulder and serve them as tacos in corn tortillas with a can of black beans, heated, and ¼ red onion, about ⅓ cup sliced radishes, ½ cup chopped tomatoes, ¼ cup fresh cilantro, and 2 cups shredded romaine lettuce. This combination has a Nutrivore Score of 319.

Sneaky Veggie Pasta

Pasta dishes tend to be very carb heavy, but not so with this recipe. This delicious pasta gets its rich and creamy sauce from blending overcooked vegetables in broth, and then adds more veggies to the dish itself.

4 tablespoons oil, divided

1 medium onion, diced

2 garlic cloves, sliced

1 celery root, peeled and diced (see Tip)

2 cups cauliflower florets and stems

2 cups broth

½ teaspoon salt, to taste

¼ cup shredded Parmesan or Romano cheese, plus more to serve (optional)

CHOOSE ONE (SEE TIP):

12 ounces penne

12 ounces rotini

12 ounces farfalle

CHOOSE TWO OR THREE:

8 ounces mushrooms, any variety, sliced

1 bunch asparagus, tough ends snapped off and diced

2 cups zucchini, sliced

2 cups broccoli florets

1 pint cherry tomatoes, halved

2 cups peas, fresh or frozen

6 cups spinach

CHOOSE ONE PROTEIN:

1 pound shrimp

1 pound mixed seafood

1 pound smoked salmon

1 pound grilled chicken

OPTIONAL:

Fresh basil, cut into chiffonade (see Tip), to serve

Grated cheese, to serve

In a large pot, heat 2 tablespoons oil over medium-high heat and sauté onion until starting to brown. Add garlic and cook for 1 minute. Add celery root, cauliflower, broth, and salt. Simmer uncovered until vegetables are overcooked and broth has reduced by half, about 15 to 20 minutes. Remove from heat and place in a blender. (For safety, do not fill your blender above halfway, and hold a tea towel over the lid while blending.) Blend until smooth, working in batches if needed. Stir in Parmesan, if using. Taste and add more salt, if needed.

Meanwhile, cook pasta according to package directions. Drain.

In a large skillet, heat remaining 2 tablespoons of oil over medium-high heat. Add vegetables (except peas and spinach, if using) and cook, stirring frequently, until al dente, about 5 to 8 minutes. Add protein and cook until fully cooked or heated through if precooked. (If a lot of water is released from vegetables or seafood, turn up the heat.) Add peas and spinach if using, stir to wilt the spinach or heat through the peas. Remove from heat.

In your pot, if it's big enough, or a large bowl, combine vegetable and protein mixture, sauce, and pasta. Gently stir to fully coat and combine. Taste and adjust seasoning if needed. Serve with basil and additional grated cheese, if desired.

TIP: If you can't find celery root, aka celeriac, you can substitute with one pound of parsnips, jicama, fennel bulb, kohlrabi, or turnips.

TIP: Lentil, edamame, or chickpea pasta are the most nutrient-dense options. They pack in even more protein and fiber and make this an incredibly satiating dish.

TIP: *Chiffonade*, which means "made of rags," is a technique used for cutting herbs or leafy vegetables. To chiffonade, stack the leaves evenly, roll them tightly to form a compact cylinder, slice the roll crosswise into thin slices, and then gently pull the slices apart into strips.

One of my favorite ways to make this pasta is with mixed seafood as the protein and mushrooms, asparagus, and peas as the veggies. This combination has a Nutrivore Score of 472.

T-*oat*-ally Great Muffins

YIELD: 12 MUFFINS
TOTAL TIME: 35 MINUTES

Make these muffins your own with your favorite additions to the basic oat muffin recipe. Try these muffin variations: nut, apple-spice, blueberry, raspberry, raisin-date, cranberry-almond, banana-coconut-macadamia, or chocolate chip. You don't even need to feel limited by the options here!

1 cup flour (see Tip)

1 cup rolled oats

½ cup brown, turbinado, date, or maple sugar

½ teaspoon sea salt

1 teaspoon baking powder

¾ cup water or milk

⅓ cup oil

3 large eggs

1 teaspoon pure vanilla extract

CHOOSE ONE:

1 cup chopped walnuts or pecans, ¼ teaspoon ground cinnamon, and ¼ teaspoon ground nutmeg

1½ cups fresh or frozen blueberries and ¼ teaspoon ground cinnamon

1½ cups fresh or frozen raspberries and 2 tablespoons finely grated orange zest

1 large Granny Smith apple, peeled, cored, and diced, plus ½ teaspoon ground cinnamon, ¼ teaspoon ground nutmeg, ¼ teaspoon ground cardamom, and a pinch of ground cloves

⅓ cup raisins, ⅓ cup dates (pitted and chopped), and 1 teaspoon ground cinnamon

1 cup fresh or frozen cranberries (chopped), 2 tablespoons finely grated orange zest, ½ cup sliced almonds, 2 additional tablespoons sugar, and replace water with orange juice

2 ripe bananas (sliced), ½ cup chopped macadamia nuts, and ½ cup coconut flakes

1 cup dark chocolate chips

OPTIONAL:

Additional 1 teaspoon ground cinnamon mixed with 3 tablespoons maple or brown sugar for topping

Preheat oven to 350°F. Grease the wells of a muffin pan, or use muffin pan liners.

In a large bowl, combine flour, oats, sugar, salt, and baking powder.

In a medium bowl, whisk together water, oil, eggs, and vanilla. Pour into dry ingredients and stir to incorporate. Fold in extras of choice.

Spoon batter into prepared muffin pan. Sprinkle cinnamon sugar topping over the top of each muffin, if desired.

Bake for 20 minutes, or until a toothpick inserted in the middle of a muffin comes out clean. Remove from oven and remove muffins from the pan immediately. (The easiest way to do this is to invert the pan over a cutting board.) Serve warm or let cool to room temperature.

TIP: You can use any flour or gluten-free flour alternative with these muffins, although follow package directions for conversions, if necessary.

The combination I make most often is with walnuts, cinnamon, and nutmeg. The Nutrivore Score for this combination is 221.

FIFTEEN NUTRIENT-DENSE SNACKS

Here are fifteen inspirational snacks that pack in nutrients for three hundred calories (give or take). Combine two and make it a meal!

1. Ants on a Log: Nutrivore Score 232

Cut 4 to 6 stalks of celery in half. Spread 2 tablespoons of peanut butter or your favorite nut butter into the concave part of the celery pieces. Make lines of raisins in the peanut butter to represent the ants, using 2 tablespoons of raisins and pushing them into the peanut butter.

2. Cantaloupe and Cottage Cheese: Nutrivore Score 254

Combine 1½ cups diced cantaloupe (about ¼ medium melon) and 1 cup cottage cheese in a bowl. Alternatively, you can fill the space in the cantaloupe melon where the seeds and pulp were with cottage cheese.

3. Lox and Watermelon: Nutrivore Score 626

Skewer cubes of watermelon with a small piece of cold-smoked salmon (lox) on toothpicks, using 3 ounces of lox and 2 cups of watermelon total. Add 2 tablespoons of chopped fresh mint leaves to garnish. (Alternately, you can slice watermelon to use like bread, or just place everything in a bowl and eat with a fork.)

4. Crackers and Pâté: Nutrivore Score 1,793

Spread ¼ cup liver pâté over 4 large or 8 small whole-wheat crackers and place ¼ cup peppery microgreens or arugula on the top.

5. Greek Yogurt with Berries and Walnuts: Nutrivore Score 307

Stir 1 teaspoon of honey into ¾ cup of Greek yogurt. Top with ½ cup berries of your choice and 1 ounce chopped walnuts (12 to 14 walnut halves).

6. Turkey Roll-Ups: Nutrivore Score 253

Lay 4 ounces (about 4 slices) of deli turkey on a cutting board and divide 2 teaspoons of mustard, 2 ounces of cheese (about 2 slices), 2 to 3 lettuce leaves, ½ cup sliced cucumber, and ¼ cup sauerkraut (or pickles, pickled onion, pickled carrot, etc.) evenly over the top of each turkey slice. Roll the turkey slice around the filling.

7. Veggies and Hummus Dip: Nutrivore Score 365

Cut 2 medium carrots (or use about 12 baby carrots) and 2 stalks of celery into sticks and dip into 6 tablespoons of hummus.

8. Hard-Boiled Eggs and Apple: Nutrivore Score 298

This one is as easy as can be. Simply eat 2 hard-boiled eggs and 1 medium apple (or any other piece of fruit you find convenient).

9. Avocado Rye Toast: Nutrivore Score 190

Toast 2 slices of rye bread. Mash ½ avocado over the top (¼ avocado on each slice) and season with salt and pepper to taste, or use your favorite seasoning blend. Top with ¼ cup of microgreens or alfalfa sprouts.

10. Deconstructed Caprese Salad: Nutrivore Score 319

Combine 2 cups of cherry tomatoes with 3 ounces of diced mozzarella cheese and 2 tablespoons of chopped fresh basil. You can skewer on toothpicks for a fun snack, eat with a fork, or use your hands!

11. Tuna Salad Collard Wrap: Nutrivore Score 561

Combine one 5-ounce can of tuna (drained) with 2 stalks of celery, chopped, 2 tablespoons of mayonnaise, and salt and pepper to taste. Remove the tough stems from 2 collard greens leaves. Divide tuna salad mix between the two collard leaves and then roll up like a burrito.

12. Pita and Baba Ghanoush: Nutrivore Score 260

Spread ½ cup baba ghanoush over 1 whole wheat pita. Alternatively, you can cut the pita into slices and dip into the baba ghanoush. Roasted red pepper dip and hummus are great spreads for this, too.

13. Sardines and Cucumber: Nutrivore Score 644

Drain a can of sardines. Add ½ cup sliced cucumber, 2 tablespoons of fresh, chopped dill, and the juice of half a lemon on the top. Mix and enjoy straight out of the can.

14. Homemade Trail Mix: Nutrivore Score 250

Combine ⅛ cup (2 tablespoons) each of walnuts and sunflower seeds (about ½ ounce each), ⅛ cup banana chips, 1 tablespoon dark chocolate chips, and 1 tablespoon coconut flakes.

15. Apple and Nut Butter: Nutrivore Score 212

Stir a dash (or three) of cinnamon into 2 tablespoons of your favorite nut butter. Slice 1 medium apple and use to dip in the spiced nut butter.

APPENDIX A

Seventeen Tips for Healthy and Sustainable Weight Loss on Nutrivore

If weight loss is a goal for you, that's okay! While the Nutrivore philosophy is weight inclusive and focused on health rather than on weight loss per se, you can still use a Nutrivore approach to lose weight. Indeed, many people do experience weight loss when they choose more whole and nutrient-dense foods, in part thanks to these foods being more satiating (you feel more full after fewer calories), and in part thanks to addressing important nutrient shortfalls. In fact, obesity is associated with key nutrient deficiencies, and studies show that increasing intake of vitamin A, vitamin B_1, vitamin B_3, vitamin B_5, vitamin B_6, vitamin D, biotin, coenzyme Q10, iron, carnitine, and creatine all facilitate healthy and maintainable weight loss.

Here are tips to lose weight in a healthy and sustainable way by focusing on healthy habits and taking a holistic approach to weight management.

1. Set realistic and healthy weight-loss goals. Many people chase that last ten or twenty pounds when they're actually already at a really healthy weight, and losing more weight would be less healthy. Instead of a number goal, think of a goal that is more reflective of health and how you feel, like the goal of having consistent energy throughout the whole day without vices like an afternoon coffee or sugar fix.
2. Think of weight loss in terms of forming lifelong healthy hab-

its, not dieting to lose weight within a certain time frame. This includes establishing new, healthier eating patterns as well as prioritizing important lifestyle factors. It can help to work on one healthy habit at a time, rather than focusing on weight loss.

3. Address any underlying health challenges (like hypothyroidism) and get help for disordered eating patterns (like food restriction or bingeing). You can also combine Nutrivore principles and all the healthy habits outlined here with medical weight loss.
4. Pay attention to your vitamin D. There's a strong association between low vitamin D levels and unintentional weight gain. Test regularly and supplement accordingly.
5. Get enough sleep every night, ideally eight or more hours, on a consistent schedule. This helps to regulate appetite and cravings, in addition to improving metabolic and overall health.
6. Live an active lifestyle (walking every day is a great way to go). This isn't about burning calories but rather about supporting metabolic health and regulating appetite and cravings.
7. Manage stress. High levels of stress increase appetite and drive cravings, along with contributing to insulin resistance.
8. Drink enough water. Some people mistake thirst cues for hunger cues, and eat a snack rather than supply what their body really needs, hydration.
9. Increase your protein intake. Studies show this helps preserve muscle mass through weight loss, which also helps to preserve your basal metabolic rate.
10. Include plenty of nonstarchy vegetables with your meals. These are packed with nutrients and fiber, while being low in calories, so can help you achieve a caloric deficit without weighing or measuring your food.
11. Eat some fermented foods and/or take a probiotic. Gut microbiome composition is closely tied to weight and metabolic health, even food cravings. Some studies have shown that people lose weight simply by taking a probiotic supplement.
12. Reduce foods that mess with your hunger signals (i.e., ultrapro-

cessed foods). Those foods that are way too easy to overeat, or that fill you up but then you're hungry an hour later, are not your friend. Note I said reduce, not eliminate. Remember that having an occasional treat is a valid strategy for helping you stay on track because food restriction can lead to disinhibition.

13. Aim for only a small caloric deficit. Slow, steady weight loss is the name of the game. Losing weight too fast causes increased hunger and decreased basal metabolic rate, making it harder and harder to stay in a caloric deficit.
14. Eat breakfast every morning, within an hour or two of waking. This helps to regulate your stress response and improve metabolic health, and studies show that regular breakfast eaters make healthier food choices later in the day. Ideally, your breakfast should include some protein and fiber.
15. Eat dinner on the early side, ideally about four hours before you go to bed. This improves sleep quality, and you're more likely not to be overly hungry by dinnertime. This also includes not snacking after dinner to keep yourself awake (go to bed instead).
16. Don't eat distracted. No TV, video games, or TikTok at the table, at least most of the time. Studies show most people eat more when they eat distracted, so this is an easy way to pay attention to your hunger signals and eat more intuitively. Family dinners are great and don't count as distracted eating.
17. Make sure you're meeting your nutritional needs from foods (aka Nutrivore!). As already covered, a number of nutrient deficiencies are associated with obesity, so addressing those can make a huge difference when your intention is healthy weight loss.

APPENDIX B

The Link Between Nutrients, Diseases, and Symptoms

The table to follow is a guide that's meant to help you understand the best-studied links between nutrients and your specific health challenges, including pointing you to where I discuss relevant links in more detail in part 2 of this book.

This table very specifically summarizes those nutrients for which shortfall increases risk of the disease developing or progressing, or increased symptom severity. Of course, not every possible link between a nutrient and a disease or symptom has been investigated in the scientific literature, so it's possible that new associations will be discovered. I have omitted nutrient deficiencies associated with disease in the case of the biology of the disease itself causing the nutrient deficiency. For example, deficiencies in iron, vitamin D, calcium, vitamin B_{12}, folate, and zinc are frequently observed in patients with celiac disease, but it is unclear whether dietary shortfall of any of these nutrients contributes to the etiology of celiac disease.

I know the urge will be to quickly scan this table for the nutrients that are relevant to your current symptoms, but the main takeaway here is that supporting health requires getting *all* the nutrients our bodies need from the foods we eat. If you just focus on the handful of nutrients relevant to today's health complaints, you could end up inadvertently causing new insufficiencies, increasing the risk of a new health problem down the line. You'll also see that for some conditions, the list of associated nutrient shortfalls is intimidatingly long—again emphasizing the limits of supplementation strategies and the value of a whole diet approach.

The Link between Nutrients, Diseases, and Symptoms

Disease/Symptom	Nutrients That Decrease Risk	
Allergies	alpha-linolenic acid fiber short-chain fatty acids taurine	vitamin A vitamin D vitamin E (see page 141) zinc
Asthma	alpha-linolenic acid arginine carnitine carotenoids choline conjugated linoleic acid coenzyme Q10 fiber glutamine	magnesium polyphenols short-chain fatty acids selenium vitamin B5 vitamin B9 (folate) vitamin D vitamin E (see page 141) zinc
Autoimmune disease		
Antiphospholipid syndrome	coenzyme Q10 vitamin D	
Autoimmune hepatitis	zinc	
Celiac disease	EPA and DHA vitamin C	
Crohn's disease	alpha-linolenic acid carnitine conjugated linoleic acid EPA and DHA	histidine selenium short-chain fatty acids vitamin D
Graves' disease	iodine selenium (see page 121)	vitamin D zinc
Hashimoto's thyroiditis	iodine iron selenium (see page 121)	vitamin D zinc
Inflammatory bowel disease	alpha-linolenic acid arginine conjugated linoleic acid cysteine EPA and DHA fiber (see page 90) glutamate glycine	selenium short-chain fatty acids taurine theanine tryptophan vitamin B9 (folate) vitamin D
Lichen planus	coenzyme Q10 selenium zinc	
Systematic lupus erythematosus	EPA and DHA vitamin D zinc	

Disease/Symptom	Nutrients That Decrease Risk	
Multiple sclerosis	alpha-linolenic acid conjugated linoleic acid coenzyme Q10 biotin	glucosinolates vitamin D zinc
Pemphigus vulgaris	selenium zinc	
Primary biliary cirrhosis	zinc	
Psoriasis	alpha-linolenic acid carotenoids conjugated linoleic acid	coenzyme Q10 selenium vitamin D vitamin E
Rheumatoid arthritis	alpha-linolenic acid conjugated linoleic acid coenzyme Q10 EPA and DHA gamma linolenic acid	glycine (see page 84) polyphenols (see page 152) vitamin B_5 vitamin D zinc
Type 1 diabetes	conjugated linoleic acid magnesium serine	vitamin B_3 vitamin D zinc
Ulcerative colitis	alpha-linolenic acid coenzyme Q10 EPA and DHA ergothioneine glycine	selenium short-chain fatty acids taurine vitamin D
Vitiligo	phenylalanine vitamin B_9 (folate)	vitamin B_{12} vitamin E
Bone and joint problems		
Osteoarthritis	betalains carnitine EPA and DHA glycine (see page 84) manganese magnesium	pyrroloquinoline quinone selenium vitamin E vitamin K zinc
Osteoporosis/ fracture risk	alanine calcium carotenoids copper fiber fluoride glucosinolates lysine magnesium	manganese polyphenols PPQ potassium selenium tryptophan vitamin D vitamin K (see page 142) zinc

Disease/Symptom	Nutrients That Decrease Risk
Cancer	
Bladder cancer	alpha-linolenic acid betalains glucosinolates (see page 160) selenium short-chain fatty acids vitamin A vitamin B_6 vitamin B_9 (folate) vitamin C vitamin D vitamin E
Brain cancer	carotenoids conjugated linoleic acid medium-chain triglycerides selenium vitamin B_9 (folate) vitamin C vitamin D vitamin E
Breast cancer	alpha-linolenic acid arginine betalains conjugated linoleic acid coenzyme Q10 copper EPA and DHA fiber gamma linolenic acid glucosinolates (see page 160) iodine linoleic acid magnesium polyphenols selenium stearic acid vitamin B_2 vitamin B_3 vitamin B_6 vitamin B_9 (folate) vitamin B_{12} vitamin C vitamin D vitamin E zinc
Cervical cancer	glucosinolates (see page 160) polyphenols vitamin A vitamin B_9 (Folate) vitamin C vitamin D vitamin E zinc
Colorectal cancer	alpha-linolenic acid arginine betalains calcium copper EPA and DHA gamma linolenic acid glutamine glycine histidine methionine oleic acid selenium short-chain fatty acids thiosulfinates (see page 160) vitamin B_2 vitamin B_6 vitamin B_9 (folate) vitamin C vitamin D
Endometrial Cancer	EPA and DHA fiber glucosinolates (see page 160) polyphenols vitamin A vitamin B_9 (folate) vitamin C vitamin E xarotenoids

Disease/Symptom	Nutrients That Decrease Risk	
Esophageal cancer	alpha-linolenic acid betalains EPA and DHA molybdenum	thiosulfinates (see page 160) vitamin B_6 vitamin B_9 (folate) vitamin C
Fibrosarcoma	stearic acid	
Kidney cancer	betalains calcium carotenoids selenium vitamin A	vitamin B_1 vitamin B_9 (folate) vitamin C vitamin D vitamin E
Laryngeal cancer	carotenoids EPA and DHA fiber selenium	vitamin C vitamin D vitamin E
Leukemia	betalains glucosinolates (see page 160) selenium	vitamin B_3 vitamin C vitamin E
Liver cancer	betalains carnitine conjugated linoleic acid copper glucosinolates (see page 160)	glycine linoleic acid methionine selenium vitamin E
Lung cancer	betalains carotenoids glucosinolates (see page 160) selenium	vitamin B_2 vitamin B_3 vitamin C vitamin D
Lymphoma	selenium vitamin B_3 vitamin C	vitamin D vitamin E
Mesothelioma	copper	
Oral cancer	carotenoids EPA and DHA fiber selenium	vitamin C vitamin D vitamin E
Ovarian cancer	polyphenols vitamin B_6	vitamin B_9 (folate) vitamin D
Pancreatic cancer	betalains glycine serine	vitamin B_9 (folate) vitamin C
Pharyngeal cancer	carotenoids EPA and DHA fiber	vitamin C vitamin D

Disease/Symptom	Nutrients That Decrease Risk	
Prostate cancer	alpha-linolenic acid betalains carotenoids conjugated linoleic acid glucosinolates (see page 160) linoleic acid	polyphenols selenium thiosulfinates (see page 160) vitamin B_6 vitamin C vitamin E
Skin cancer	alpha-linolenic acid betalains carotenoids coenzyme Q10	copper EPA and DHA vitamin B_3 vitamin D
Stomach cancer	conjugated linoleic acid iodine molybdenum	thiosulfinates (see page 160) vitamin B_6 vitamin C
Thyroid cancer	iodine	
Uterine cancer	glucosinolates (see page 160) polyphenols	
Cardiovascular disease		
Coronary heart disease	arginine carotenoids EPA and DHA ergothioneine glycine magnesium	selenium vitamin B_6 vitamin B_9 (folate) vitamin C vitamin D
Heart attack	conjugated linoleic acid coenzyme Q10 EPA and DHA gamma linolenic acid glycine	linoleic acid vitamin B_3 vitamin B_9 (folate) vitamin E
Heart failure	carnitine coenzyme Q10 EPA and DHA magnesium	pyrroloquinoline quinone short-chain fatty acids taurine vitamin D
Hypertension	alpha-linolenic acid arginine betalains carnitine calcium coenzyme Q10 fluoride gamma linolenic acid glutamic acid lysine magnesium	oleic acid (see page 95) polyphenols potassium (see page 115) short-chain fatty acids taurine thiosulfinates tyrosine vitamin B_2 vitamin C vitamin D

Disease/Symptom	Nutrients That Decrease Risk	
Hyperlipidemia (high cholesterol)	arginine betalains carnitine carotenoids chromium conjugated linoleic acid coenzyme Q10 copper EPA and DHA fiber gamma linolenic acid leucine linoleic acid medium-chain triglycerides	oleic acid (see page 95) phytosterols polyphenols pyrroloquinoline quinone short-chain fatty acids stearic acid taurine thiosulfinates valine vitamin B_3 vitamin B_5 vitamin C zinc
Stroke	alpha-linolenic acid carotenoids cysteine EPA and DHA gamma linolenic acid magnesium	polyphenols potassium (see page 115) vitamin B_3 vitamin B_9 (folate) vitamin C vitamin D
Thromboembolism	polyphenols thiosulfinates vitamin B_3	vitamin D vitamin E
Chronic pain	magnesium phenylalanine polyphenols (see page 151)	vitamin B_{12} vitamin C vitamin D
Dental problems	coenzyme Q10 fluoride molybdenum	
Eye problems		
Age-related macular degeneration	carotenoids (see page 157) polyphenols vitamin A	vitamin C vitamin E zinc
Blepharitis	biotin gamma linolenic acid vitamin B_2	vitamin B_6 zinc
Cataracts	carotenoids (see page 157) polyphenols vitamin B_1 vitamin B_2	vitamin C vitamin E zinc
Dry eye	alpha-linolenic acid vitamin A	
Retinitis pigmentosa	carotenoids (see page 157) vitamin A	

Disease/Symptom	Nutrients That Decrease Risk	
Retinopathy	vitamin E	
Fingernail problems	biotin vitamin B_{12} vitamin E	
Gout	fiber short-chain fatty acids vitamin C	
Gut problems		
Acid reflux/GERD	arginine glycine	vitamin B_2 vitamin B_9 (folate)
Constipation	fiber	
Diarrhea	glutamine lysine	
Diverticular disease	fiber (see page 90)	
Hemorrhoids	fiber	
Irritable bowel syndrome (IBS)	EPA and DHA fiber (see page 90)	glutamine short-chain fatty acids
Stomach Ulcers	alpha-linolenic acid fiber	glucosinolates glycine
Hair problems	biotin EPA and DHA iron lysine methionine polyphenols	vitamin A vitamin B_5 vitamin C vitamin D zinc
Immune problems		
Infection risk	alpha-linolenic acid glutamine leucine lysine selenium	vitamin B_1 vitamin A vitamin D vitamin E zinc (see page 122)

Disease/Symptom	Nutrients That Decrease Risk	
Inflammation	alpha-linolenic acid betalains biotin carnitine carotenoids conjugated linoleic acid coenzyme Q10 cysteine fiber glucosinolates glutamine glycine histidine magnesium	oleic acid phytosterols polyphenols pyrroloquinoline quinone selenium vitamin B_5 vitamin B_6 vitamin B_9 (folate) vitamin C vitamin D vitamin E vitamin K zinc (see page 122)
Kidney problems		
Chronic kidney disease	calcium carnitine fiber glucosinolates potassium vitamin B_1 vitamin B_2	vitamin B_3 vitamin B_5 vitamin B_6 vitamin B_9 (folate) vitamin C vitamin D
Kidney stones	calcium copper magnesium	potassium vitamin B_6
Liver problems		
Nonalcoholic fatty liver disease	carnitine carotenoids coenzyme Q10 glycine	oleic acid polyphenols vitamin B_5 vitamin E
Primary sclerosing cholangitis	EPA and DHA vitamin D	
Mental health challenges		
Anxiety	arginine EPA and DHA fiber lysine	taurine theanine tryptophan vitamin C (see page 139)
Depression	alpha-linolenic acid carnitine carnosine EPA and DHA fiber phenylalanine theanine	tryptophan vitamin B_6 (see page 133) vitamin B_9 (folate) vitamin B_{12} vitamin C (see page 139) zinc

Disease/Symptom	Nutrients That Decrease Risk	
Obsessive-compulsive disorder	glycine vitamin B_{12}	vitamin D zinc
Neurological and neurodegenerative disease		
Alzheimer's disease	betalains biotin carnitine carnosine EPA and DHA (see page 97) ergothioneine fiber glucosinolates medium-chain triglycerides polyphenols selenium short-chain fatty acids	stearic acid vitamin A vitamin B_1 vitamin B_2 vitamin B_3 vitamin B_6 vitamin B_9 (folate) vitamin B_{12} (see page 137) vitamin C vitamin D vitamin E zinc
Attention deficit and hyperactivity disorder (ADHD)	carnitine EPA and DHA magnesium	tryptophan vitamin B_{12} (see page 137) zinc
Autism spectrum disorder (ASD)	carnitine EPA and DHA fiber	short-chain fatty acids vitamin B_9 (folate) vitamin B_{12} (see page 137)
Chronic fatigue	carnitine coenzyme Q10 EPA and DHA magnesium tryptophan	vitamin B_9 (folate) vitamin B_{12} (see page 137) vitamin C zinc
Cognition issues	alanine carotenoids EPA and DHA (see page 97) ergothioneine histidine lysine medium-chain triglycerides phenylalanine	polyphenols short-chain fatty acids theanine threonine tyrosine vitamin B_{12} (see page 137) vitamin K
Epilepsy and other seizure disorders	carnosine EPA and DHA histidine magnesium manganese medium-chain triglycerides	serine taurine vitamin B_6 vitamin D vitamin E

Disease/Symptom	Nutrients That Decrease Risk	
Fatigue	biotin	vitamin B_3
	coenzyme Q10	vitamin B_5
	histidine	vitamin B_6
	iron	vitamin B_9 (folate)
	magnesium	vitamin B_{12} (see page 137)
	vitamin B_1	vitamin C
	vitamin B_2	zinc
Fibromyalgia	carnitine	magnesium
	coenzyme Q10	vitamin D
Memory issues	EPA and DHA (see page 97)	pyrroloquinoline quinone
	glycine	short-chain fatty acids
	histidine	theanine
	medium-chain triglycerides	tyrosine
	polyphenols	
Migraine headache	carnitine	vitamin B_2
	coenzyme Q10	vitamin B_6
	EPA and DHA	vitamin B_9 (folate)
	iron	vitamin B_{12}
	magnesium (see page 114)	vitamin D
	tryptophan	zinc
Parkinson's disease	betalains	pyrroloquinoline quinone
	carnitine	short-chain fatty acids
	coenzyme Q10	stearic acid
	glucosinolates	vitamin D
Schizophrenia	carnosine	serine
	EPA and DHA	theanine
	glycine	vitamin D
	lysine	
Obesity and overweight	arginine	medium-chain triglycerides
	betalains	oleic acid
	calcium	selenium
	carnitine	short-chain fatty acids
	carotenoids	theanine
	chromium	tryptophan
	conjugated linoleic acid	vitamin A
	fiber	vitamin B_1
	glucosinolates	vitamin B_2
	glycine	vitamin B_5
	histidine	vitamin B_6
	leucine	vitamin B_9 (folate)
	magnesium	vitamin D
Pregnancy-Related Concerns		
Fetal development problems	arginine	vitamin A
	biotin	vitamin B_9 (folate; see page 135)
	EPA and DHA	vitamin B_{12}
	iodine	vitamin E
	iron	

Disease/Symptom	Nutrients That Decrease Risk	
Gestational diabetes	chromium EPA and DHA serine	vitamin D zinc
Low birth weight	arginine biotin copper EPA and DHA	selenium vitamin B_9 (folate; see page 135)
Miscarriage	iodine vitamin B_9 (folate) vitamin E	
Morning sickness	vitamin B_6	
Placental abruption	iodine vitamin B_9 (folate) vitamin E	
Preeclampsia	arginine calcium coenzyme Q10 ergothioneine iodine	magnesium selenium vitamin B_2 vitamin B_9 (folate) vitamin D
Preterm birth	arginine biotin calcium EPA and DHA iodine	iron magnesium vitamin C vitamin E
Reproductive health		
Endometriosis	EPA and DHA magnesium vitamin C	vitamin E vitamin D
Erectile dysfunction	arginine copper magnesium	polyphenols selenium vitamin D
Female fertility issues	alpha-linolenic acid carnitine carotenoids coenzyme Q10 polyphenols	vitamin A vitamin B_9 (folate; see page 135) vitamin E
Male fertility issues	arginine calcium carnitine coenzyme Q10 copper magnesium selenium	vitamin A vitamin B_9 (folate) vitamin B_{12} vitamin C vitamin D zinc

Disease/Symptom	Nutrients That Decrease Risk	
Menopause symptoms	carotenoids calcium fiber magnesium protein selenium	vitamin B_6 (see page 133) vitamin B_{12} vitamin C vitamin D vitamin E vitamin K
Polycystic ovary syndrome (PCOS)	alpha-linolenic acid carnitine chromium (see page 118) coenzyme Q10	fiber selenium vitamin D vitamin E
Premenstrual syndrome (PMS)	calcium (see page 112) gamma linolenic acid	tryptophan vitamin B_6
Uterine fibroids	carotenoids polyphenols vitamin A	vitamin C vitamin D
Sarcopenia	calcium carnitine EPA and DHA isoleucine leucine	magnesium selenium tryptophan vitamin B_{12} vitamin D
Skin problems		
Acne	EPA and DHA vitamin A vitamin B_3	vitamin D zinc
Atopic dermatitis (eczema)	gamma linolenic acid histidine selenium	vitamin D vitamin E zinc
Hidradenitis suppurativa (acne inversus)	zinc	
Rosacea	EPA and DHA gamma linolenic acid zinc	
Visible signs of aging	carotenoids coenzyme Q10 EPA and DHA ergothioneine	linoleic acid vitamin A vitamin C vitamin E
Sleep issues		
Insomnia	glycine iron magnesium	tryptophan vitamin B_6 (see page 133) vitamin E

Disease/Symptom	Nutrients That Decrease Risk	
Restless leg syndrome	iron magnesium vitamin B_6	vitamin B_9 (folate) vitamin D
Thyroid health		
Goiter	iodine (see page 109) selenium (see page 121)	
Hyperthyroidism	carnitine iodine selenium (see page 121)	
Hypothyroidism	iodine iron magnesium selenium (see page 121)	vitamin A vitamin D zinc
Type 2 diabetes	alpha-linolenic acid alanine arginine betalains biotin carnitine carnosine carotenoids chromium (see page 118) conjugated linoleic acid coenzyme Q10 cysteine EPA and DHA ergothioneine fiber fluoride gamma linolenic acid glucosinolates glutamine glycine	histidine linoleic acid lysine magnesium manganese medium-chain triglycerides oleic acid phytosterols polyphenols serine short-chain fatty acids taurine tryptophan vitamin B_1 vitamin B_6 vitamin B_9 (folate) vitamin B_{12} vitamin C vitamin D (see page 24) zinc

Please note that while addressing nutrient shortfalls can often alleviate symptoms, and in many cases ameliorate chronic conditions, improving diet quality can only completely reverse disease in certain, specific circumstances. So focusing on nutrients related to your health complaints should be viewed as complementary to the advice and care of your health care provider, and never a substitute for medical intervention.

APPENDIX C

Food Family Average Nutrivore Scores

The following table shows the average nutrient density (Nutrivore Score) and energy density (calories per hundred grams) of all the food families. You can use this table as a rough guide when choosing foods, to narrow in on the most nutrient-dense option that makes sense with the meal you're preparing, and following the Nutrivore Meal Map from chapter 4.

	Average Nutrivore Score	Average Calories per 100 Grams
VEGETABLES	1,732	44
Crucifers	3,740	32
Leafy vegetables	3,476	25
Mushrooms	2,704	29
Alliums	2,142	56
Parsley family	1,422	40
Sea vegetables	1,036	36
Nightshades	812	40
Other vegetables	744	58
Root vegetables	701	74
Winter squash	503	36
Starchy vegetables	290	93

	Average Nutrivore Score	Average Calories per 100 Grams
FRUITS	457	61
Berries	489	53
Tropical and subtropical fruit	406	72
Citrus	391	51
Melons	307	34
Rosaceae Family	244	61
Stone fruits	294	48
Apple family	204	60
Fatty fruit	201	264
SEASONINGS	1,080	256
Fresh herbs	2,003	57
Spices	796	335
TEA and COFFEE	4,309	2
NUTS and SEEDS	276	575
Seeds	374	545
Nuts	294	594
LEGUMES	389	283
Fresh legumes	580	55
Pulses	358	307
Peanuts	219	568
GRAINS	156	307
Pseudograins	297	392
Whole grains	189	306
Refined grains	81	310
SEAFOOD	695	108
Shellfish	925	87
Fish	602	119

	Average Nutrivore Score	Average Calories per 100 Grams
OFFAL	680	170
Organ meat	903	133
Bone broth and stock	490	20
MEAT and EGGS	352	155
Eggs	373	168
Red meat	360	159
Poultry	343	149
DAIRY	149	257
Milk	218	66
Cheese	140	331
Milk alternatives	320	143
FATS and OILS	102	860
SUGARS	76	345

APPENDIX D

Alphabetical List of Nutrivore Scores

The following are Nutrivore Scores for more than seven hundred whole foods and common ingredients. The whole edible portion of the raw food is used in the calculation unless otherwise noted. You can also search the full Nutrivore Score database at Nutrivore.com.

Food	Nutrivore Score
Abalone	520
Acerola	7,877[1]
Acorn squash	297[1]
Adzuki beans	576[1]
Agar	456
Alaskan king crab	1,211
Alfalfa sprouts	902
Allspice, ground	408[1]
Almond butter	213
Almond flour	216
Almond milk, unsweetened	744
Almond oil	82
Almonds	234

Food	Nutrivore Score
Almonds, blanched	216
Amaranth	207
Anchovies	805
Anchovies (canned in oil)	736
Anise seed	285[1]
Aniseed	285[1]
Antelope	429[2]
Apple juice	69
Apples (with skin)	213
Apples, Fuji	131
Apples, Gala	141
Apples, Golden Delicious	141
Apples, Granny Smith	204

Food	Nutrivore Score
Apples, Red Delicious	140
Apricot	260
Apricots, dried	130
Arrowroot	361[1]
Arrowroot flour	14[2]
Artichokes	771
Arugula	2,019
Asparagus	1,385
Asparagus lettuce	957[2]
Atlantic salmon, wild	868
Aubergine	563
Avocado oil	71[1]
Avocados, California	251
Avocados, Florida	291
Baby Bella	2279
Bacon, pork	122
Baking powder, sodium aluminum sulfate	1,317
Baking powder, straight phosphate	2,815
Baking soda	N/A[4]
Balsamic vinegar	72[1]
Bamboo shoots, fresh	776
Bamboo shoots (canned)	420
Banana	185
Barley, pearled	158
Basil	3,381
Basil, dried	2,035
Bass, freshwater	555
Bass, striped	786

Food	Nutrivore Score
Bay leaf	572[1]
Beans, adzuki	576[1]
Beans, black	446
Beans, black-eyed peas	286[1]
Beans, broad	442
Beans, butter	340
Beans, chickpeas	454
Beans, cowpeas	286[1]
Beans, fava	442
Beans, garbanzo	454
Beans, great northern	419
Beans, green	605
Beans, green snap	605
Beans, kidney	413
Beans, lima	304
Beans, lima, green	340
Beans, mung	249
Beans, navy	269
Beans, pinto	390
Beans, red mung	576[1]
Beans, turtle	446
Beans, white	269
Beaver	431
Beef, arm pot roast	187
Beef, blade roast	189
Beef, brain	797
Beef, broth	336[1]
Beef, chuck eye roast	269

Food	Nutrivore Score
Beef, grass-fed, bottom round steak/roast	337
Beef, grass-fed, ground	208
Beef, grass-fed, rib eye steak/roast	283[1]
Beef, grass-fed, strip loin	371
Beef, grass-fed, top loin steak/roast	261
Beef, ground, 3% fat	360
Beef, ground, 5% fat	316
Beef, ground, 7% fat	284
Beef, ground, 10% fat	244
Beef, ground, 20% fat	165
Beef, ground, 25% fat	142
Beef, ground, 30% fat	125
Beef, heart	888
Beef, heart, New Zealand	1,001
Beef, kidney	2,543
Beef, liver	4,021
Beef, pancreas	429[1]
Beef, porterhouse steak	206
Beef, shoulder pot roast/ steak	446
Beef, spleen	867[1]
Beef, stock	336[1]
Beef, sweetbreads, pancreas	429[1]
Beef, sweetbreads, thymus	205[1]
Beef, tallow	38
Beef, T-bone steak	280
Beef, tenderloin roast	328

Food	Nutrivore Score
Beef, thymus	205[1]
Beef, tongue	215
Beef, tripe	259
Beef, tri-tip roast	250
Beer	70
Beet greens	3,259
Beets	2,013
Belgian endive	2,390
Bell peppers, green	1,094
Bell peppers, red	1,358
Bengal gram	454
Besan	454
Bibb lettuce	1,934
Bison, grass-fed, ground	322
Bison, ground	208
Bison, lean	394
Bison, rib eye, lean	370
Bison, top round, lean	417
Black beans	446
Black olives	164
Black tea	3,286
Blackberries	743
Black-eyed peas	286[1]
Blue cheese	130
Blue crab	1,073
Blueberries	396
Bluefin tuna	970
Bog blueberries	491
Bok choy	3,428

Food	Nutrivore Score
Bone marrow, caribou	56[1]
Boston lettuce	1,934
Brain, beef	797
Brain, lamb	767[1]
Brain, pork	469[1]
Brain, veal	682[1]
Brazil nuts	694
Bread, gluten-free, white, made with potato extract, rice starch, and rice flour	42[2]
Bread, gluten-free, white, made with rice flour, corn-starch, and/or tapioca	101
Bread, gluten-free, white, made with tapioca starch and brown rice flour	86[2]
Bread, gluten-free, whole grain, made with tapioca starch and brown rice flour	77[2]
Bread, multigrain	194
Bread, wheat	164[5]
Bread, white	128[5]
Bread, whole wheat	215
Brie cheese	130
Broad beans	442
Broccoli	2,833
Broccoli rabe	4,155
Broth, beef	336[1]
Broth, chicken	151[1]
Broth, fish	742[1]
Brown mushroom	2,279
Brussels sprouts	2,817
Buckwheat	303
Buffalo milk	159[1]
Bulgur	144
Bullock's heart	147[2]
Burdock root	182
Butter	57
Butter beans	340
Butter oil	33[1]
Butter, almond	213
Butter, cashew	182
Butter, cocoa	27
Butter, peanut, chunky	179
Butter, peanut, smooth	172
Butter, sesame seed	289
Butter, sunflower seed	308[1]
Butterhead lettuce	1,934
Butternut squash	670
Cabbage, green	2,034
Cabbage, kimchi	1,097
Cabbage, red	1,369
Canada goose, breast, skinless	556
Canola oil	176
Cantaloupe	457
Cape gooseberries	134[3]
Capers, canned	5,247
Carambola	378
Caraway seed	526
Cardamom	656[2]

Food	Nutrivore Score
Cardoon	1,039[2]
Caribou	750
Caribou, bone marrow	56[1]
Carp	480
Carrots	899
Casaba melon	304
Cashew butter	182
Cashews	203
Cassava	224
Cassava flour	224
Catfish, farmed	305
Catfish, wild	559
Catsup	253
Cauliflower	1,585
Caviar, black and red	1,582
Celeriac	345
Celery	767
Celery root	345
Celery seed	444
Celtuce	957[2]
Chamomile tea	988
Chanterelle mushroom	1,555
Chard, rainbow	6,573
Chard, Swiss	6,198
Chayote	871
Cheddar cheese	126
Cheese, blue	130
Cheese, brie	130
Cheese, cheddar	126
Cheese, cottage, 2%	201
Cheese, cream	78
Cheese, feta	189
Cheese, Gouda	136
Cheese, mozzarella	145
Cheese, Parmesan, grated	127
Cheese, Parmesan, hard	138
Cheese, ricotta	141
Cheese, Romano	129
Cheese, Roquefort	146
Cheese, sharp cheddar	121
Cheese, Swiss	157
Cherries, sweet	171
Chervil, dried	1,038[1]
Chestnuts	389
Chia seeds	450[1]
Chicken eggs	355
Chicken, breast, skinless	309
Chicken, broth	151[1]
Chicken, dark meat	281
Chicken, drumstick, meat and skin	230
Chicken, drumstick, meat only	297
Chicken, giblets	1,191[1]
Chicken, heart	689[1]
Chicken, light meat	306
Chicken, liver	2,502
Chicken, meat and skin	205
Chicken, meat only	341

Food	Nutrivore Score
Chicken, stock	151[1]
Chicken, thigh, meat and skin	167
Chicken, thigh, meat only	288
Chicken, wing, meat and skin	174
Chickpeas	454
Chickpea flour	454
Chicory greens	3,086
Chicory roots	207[1]
Chicory spear	2,390
Chicory, witloof	546[1]
Chinese broccoli	2,365[1]
Chinese cabbage	3,428
Chinese date	1,239[2]
Chinese kale	2,365[1]
Chinook salmon	775
Chitterlings, pork	133
Chives	3,531
Chocolate, 45-59%	169
Chocolate, 60-69%	192
Chocolate, 70-85%	235
Chocolate, ice cream	93
Chrysanthemum leaves	1,093[2]
Chum salmon	646
Cilantro	2,609
Cinnamon	1,146
Citronella	511[1]
Clams	1,046

Food	Nutrivore Score
Clarified butter	33[1]
Clementines	291
Cloudberries	646[1]
Cloves, ground	2,209
Cockles	457[3]
Cocoa butter	27
Cocoa, unsweetened	1,024
Coconut	179
Coconut butter	162
Coconut cream	165
Coconut flour	139[2]
Coconut milk	171
Coconut milk, canned	184
Coconut oil	112
Coconut water	271
Coconut, creamed	162
Cocoyam	178
Cod, Atlantic	431
Cod, Pacific	475
Coffee, brewed	7,036
Coffee, brewed, decaf	1,826
Coffee, espresso	2,304
Coffee, instant	6,633
Coffee, instant, chicory	2,412[1]
Coffee, instant, decaf	5,523
Coho salmon, wild	724
Collards	3,323
Coriander leaf, dried	1,460[1]

Food	Nutrivore Score
Coriander leaves	2,609
Coriander seed	353[2]
Corn oil	103
Corn, sweet, white	191
Corn, sweet, yellow	202
Cos lettuce	2,128
Cottage cheese, 2%	201
Cowpeas	286[1]
Crab apples	241[2]
Crab, Alaska king	1,211
Crab, blue	1,073
Crab, Dungeness	1,077
Crabapples	241[2]
Cranberries	288
Cranberries, dried, sweetened	40
Crayfish, farmed	578
Crayfish, wild	616
Cream cheese	78
Cremini mushroom	2,279
Cricket	1,071[1]
Cremini mushroom	2,279
Croaker	476
Crookneck squash	1,177
Cucumber	472
Cumin seed	641
Curly endive	3,086
Currants, black	811
Currants, red and white	393

Food	Nutrivore Score
Curry powder	544
Custard apple	147[2]
Cuttlefish	870[1]
Dandelion greens	2,815
Dates, deglet noor	70
Dates, medjool	81
Deer, ground	437
Deer, meat	683
Dill seed	333[1]
Dill weed	1,940
Dill weed, dried	557[2]
Dragon fruit, red	800[1]
Dragon fruit, white	357[1]
Drum, freshwater	494[1]
Duck eggs	396
Duck, meat and skin	201
Dungeness crab	1,077
Durian	148[2]
Edamame	362[1]
Edible podded peas	669
Eel	385
Egg, white	272
Egg, yolk	342
Eggplant	563
Eggs, chicken	355
Eggs, duck	396
Eggs, goose	398
Eggs, quail	341

Food	Nutrivore Score
Elderberries	546[1]
Elk	718
Emu	733[1]
Endive	2,390
Enoki mushroom	4,434
Enokitake	4,434
Epazote	1,270[2]
Fat, goose	43[1]
Fava beans	442
Feet, pork	112
Fennel	663
Fennel seed	373[2]
Fenugreek seed	264[2]
Feta cheese	189
Fiddlehead ferns	1,721[2]
Figs	158
Figs, dried	141
Filberts	292
Filberts, blanched	323
Fish sauce	523
Fish, anchovies	805
Fish, anchovies (canned in oil)	736
Fish, bass, freshwater	555
Fish, bass, striped	786
Fish, broth	742[1]
Fish, carp	480
Fish, catfish, farmed	305
Fish, catfish, wild	559

Food	Nutrivore Score
Fish, caviar	1,582
Fish, cod, Atlantic	431
Fish, cod, Pacific	475
Fish, croaker	476
Fish, drum, freshwater	494[1]
Fish, eel	385
Fish, flatfish	749
Fish, flounder	749
Fish, grouper	400[1]
Fish, haddock	464
Fish, halibut	523
Fish, herring, Atlantic	996
Fish, mackerel, Atlantic	922
Fish, mackerel, king	1,242
Fish, mahimahi	416[1]
Fish, milkfish	266[1]
Fish, monkfish	338[1]
Fish, mullet, striped	396
Fish, orange roughy	392
Fish, perch	508
Fish, perch, ocean	464
Fish, pike, walleye	560
Fish, pollock, Alaskan	528
Fish, pollock, Atlantic	650
Fish, roe	1,349
Fish, salmon, chinook	775
Fish, salmon, chum	646
Fish, salmon, pink	625

Food	Nutrivore Score
Fish, salmon, sockeye	750
Fish, salmon, wild Atlantic	868
Fish, salmon, wild coho	724
Fish, sardines (canned in oil)	654
Fish, sea bass	575
Fish, shad	701
Fish, shark	524
Fish, sheepshead	416[1]
Fish, smelt, rainbow	834
Fish, snapper	548
Fish, sole	749
Fish, stock	732
Fish, sturgeon	528
Fish, swordfish	557
Fish, tilapia	409
Fish, tilefish	553[1]
Fish, trout	710
Fish, trout, rainbow	645
Fish, tuna, bluefin	970
Fish, tuna, skipjack	645
Fish, tuna, yellowfin	642
Fish, whitefish	663
Fish, whiting	455
Flatfish	749
Flaxseed	515
Flaxseed oil	428
Flounder	749
Flour, arrowroot	14[2]

Food	Nutrivore Score
Flour, cassava	224
Flour, coconut	139[2]
Flour, manioc	224
Flour, wheat, soft-grain	185
Flour, wheat, white, all-purpose	70
Flour, wheat, whole-grain	227
Fuyu, tofu	295
Gai lan	2,365[1]
Garbanzo	454
Garbanzo flour	454
Garden cress	11,265
Garden pepper cress	11,265
Garlic	5,622
Garlic powder	5,529
Ghee	33[1]
Giblets, chicken	1,191[1]
Giblets, turkey	1,567
Ginger, ground	668
Ginger, root	192
Goat	525
Goat milk (added vitamin D)	178[5]
Goji berries, dried	780[3]
Goose eggs	398
Goose, liver	4,529[1]
Goose, meat and skin	149
Goose, meat only	311
Gooseberries	459

Food	Nutrivore Score
Gouda cheese	136
Granadilla	261[1]
Grape juice	110
Grape leaves	1,197
Grapefruit juice, pink	293
Grapefruit juice, white	287
Grapefruit, pink and red	361
Grapes, American (slip skin)	365
Grapes, European (red or green)	271
Grapes, muscadine	644
Grapeseed oil	82[1]
Graviola	255[1]
Great northern beans	419
Green beans	605
Green leaf lettuce	2,245
Green olives	160
Green onions	2,097
Green peas	431
Green snap beans	605
Green tea	3,055
Groundcherries	134[3]
Grouper	400[1]
Guanabana	255[1]
Guavas, common	761
Guavas, strawberry	410
Guinea hen, meat	349[1]
Guinea hen, meat and skin	257[1]

Food	Nutrivore Score
Haddock	464
Halibut	523
Ham, pork	214
Hazelnut oil	87[1]
Hazelnuts	292
Hazelnuts, blanched	323
Heart, beef	888
Heart, beef, New Zealand	1,001
Heart, chicken	689[1]
Heart, lamb	916[1]
Heart, pork	977
Hearts of palm	545
Hemp seeds	415[1]
Herring, Atlantic	996
Honey	20
Honeydew	228
Horned melon	139[2]
Horse	507
Horseradish, prepared	850
Hot chili sauce	262[2]
Hubbard squash	358
Huckleberries	317[3]
Hummus	139
Ice cream, chocolate	93
Ice cream, strawberry	99
Ice cream, vanilla	86
Iceberg lettuce	773
Indian date	77[1]

Food	Nutrivore Score
Indian fig	881[1]
Inkberry	2,330
Intestines, pork	133
Irish moss	602
Italian brown mushroom	2,279
Jackfruit	132[1]
Jam	30
Japanese horseradish	710
Jerusalem artichokes	195
Jicama	234
Jowl, pork	64[1]
Juice, apple	69
Juice, grape	110
Juice, grapefruit, pink	293
Juice, grapefruit, white	287
Juice, orange	301
Juice, pomegranate	148
Juice, tomato	1,568
Jujube	1,239[2]
Kaki fruit	537
Kale	4,233
Kefir	296
Kelp	700
Ketchup	253
Kidney beans	413
Kidney, beef	2,543
Kidney, lamb	3,481[1]
Kidney, pork	1,650

Food	Nutrivore Score
Kimchi (cabbage)	1,097
Kiwano	139[2]
Kiwi, golden	500
Kiwi, green	453
Knob celery	345
Kohlrabi	2,497
Komatsuna	5,784[1]
Koyadofu, tofu	254[1]
Kumquat	381
Lamb, brain	767[1]
Lamb, ground	186
Lamb, heart	916[1]
Lamb, kidney	3,481[1]
Lamb, lean and fat	215
Lamb, leg, lean and fat	191
Lamb, liver	4,925[1]
Lamb, pancreas	376[1]
Lamb, shoulder	360
Lamb, spleen	765[1]
Lamb, sweetbreads, pancreas	376[1]
Lamb, tongue	298[1]
Lard	43
Laver	1,520
Leeks	1,128
Lemongrass	511[1]
Lemon peel	618
Lemons	477
Lentils	489

Food	Nutrivore Score
Lettuce, Bibb	1,934
Lettuce, Boston	1,934
Lettuce, butterhead	1,934
Lettuce, cos	2,128
Lettuce, green leaf	2,245
Lettuce, iceberg	773
Lettuce, red leaf	2,684
Lettuce, romaine	2,128
Lichee	319
Lima beans	304
Lima beans, green	340
Limes	344
Linseed	515
Linseed oil	428
Litchi	319
Liver, beef	4,021
Liver, chicken	2,502
Liver, goose	4,529[1]
Liver, lamb	4,925[1]
Liver, pork	2,483
Lobster, northern	839
Lobster, spiny	637
Longan	264[2]
Loquat	170[1]
Lotus root	344[1]
Lychee	319
Macadamia nuts	167
Mace, ground	210[1]
Mackerel, Atlantic	922

Food	Nutrivore Score
Mackerel, king	1,242
Mahimahi	416[1]
Maitake mushroom	3,551
Malay apple	210[2]
Mamey sapote	488[1]
Mandarin orange	238
Mango	342
Mango, dried, sweetened	247
Manioc	224
Manioc flour	224
Maple syrup	103
Margarine	78[1]
Marjoram, dried	1,278[1]
Marmalade, orange	77
Matai	257
Mayonnaise	90
Melon, cantaloupe	457
Melon, casaba	304
Melon, horned	139[2]
Melon, watermelon	405
Milk, 1%	251
Milk, 2%	224
Milk, almond, unsweetened	744
Milk, buffalo	159[1]
Milk, coconut	171
Milk, coconut, canned	184
Milk, goat (added vitamin D)	178[5]
Milk, rice, unsweetened	234

Food	Nutrivore Score
Milk, sheep	210[1]
Milk, skim	305
Milk, soy, unsweetened	425[1]
Milk, whole	202
Milkfish	266[1]
Millet	132
Molasses	367
Monkfish	338[1]
Moose	691
Morel mushroom	2,271[1]
Mountain apple	210[2]
Mountain yam, Hawaii	783[1]
Mozzarella cheese	145
Mulberries	719[1]
Mullet, striped	396
Mung bean sprouts	711
Mung beans	249
Mushroom, brown	2,279
Mushroom, chanterelle	1,555
Mushroom, cremini	2,279
Mushroom, enoki	4,434
Mushroom, maitake	3,551
Mushroom, morel	2,271[1]
Mushroom, oyster	2,550
Mushroom, portobello	1,483
Mushroom, shiitake	4,343
Mushroom, white button	1,872
Mussels	1,564

Food	Nutrivore Score
Mustard and cress	11,265
Mustard greens	5,391
Mustard oil	221[1]
Mustard seed, ground	1,904
Mustard spinach	5,784[1]
Mustard, yellow	718
Navy beans	269
Nectarines	222
New Zealand spinach	5,541[1]
Nigari, tofu, hard	282
Nori	1,520
Nutmeg, ground	157
Nuts, almonds	234
Nuts, almonds, blanched	216
Nuts, Brazil	694
Nuts, cashews	203
Nuts, chestnuts	389
Nuts, filbert	292
Nuts, filbert, blanched	323
Nuts, hazelnuts	292
Nuts, hazelnuts, blanched	323
Nuts, macadamia	167
Nuts, peanuts	219
Nuts, peanuts, Spanish	223
Nuts, peanuts, Valencia	217
Nuts, peanuts, Virginia	217
Nuts, pecans	221
Nuts, pine	222
Nuts, pistachios	265

Food	Nutrivore Score
Nuts, tigernut	192[2]
Nuts, walnuts	303
Oats	208
Octopus	1,618
Oil, almond	82
Oil, avocado	71[1]
Oil, canola	176
Oil, coconut	112
Oil, corn	103
Oil, flaxseed	428
Oil, grapeseed	82[1]
Oil, hazelnut	87[1]
Oil, linseed	428
Oil, mustard	221[1]
Oil, olive, extra-virgin	139
Oil, olive, virgin	106
Oil, palm	42
Oil, peanut	90
Oil, poppyseed	86[1]
Oil, safflower, high oleic	82
Oil, safflower, linoleic	88
Oil, sesame	127
Oil, soybean	160
Oil, sunflower, high-oleic	105
Oil, sunflower, linoleic	104
Oil, sunflower, mid-oleic	104
Oil, walnut	126
Okra	859

Food	Nutrivore Score
Olive oil, extra-virgin	139
Olive oil, virgin	106
Olives, black	164
Olives, green	160
Onion powder	348
Onions	380
Onions, dehydrated flakes	392
Onions, green	2,097
Onions, spring	1,932
Onions, Welsh	1,704
Oolong tea	4,821
Orange juice	301
Orange peel	353[1]
Orange roughy	392
Oranges	418
Oranges, California, Valencia	397
Oranges, Florida	401
Oranges, navels	408
Oregano, dried	1,075
Ostrich, ground	357
Ostrich, inside leg	546[1]
Ostrich, outside leg	536[1]
Ostrich, tenderloin	505[1]
Ostrich, top loin	504[1]
Oyster mushroom	2,550
Oyster sauce	162
Oysters, eastern, wild	3,049
Oysters, Pacific	2,255

Food	Nutrivore Score
Pak choy	3,428
Palm oil	42
Pancreas, beef	429[1]
Pancreas, lamb	376[1]
Pancreas, pork	570[1]
Pancreas, veal	467[1]
Papaya	636
Paprika	847
Parmesan cheese, grated	127
Parmesan cheese, hard	138
Parsley	5,491
Parsley, dried	1,297
Parsnip	372
Passion fruit, purple	261[1]
Pea sprouts	310[1]
Peaches, yellow	295
Peanut butter, chunky	179
Peanut butter, smooth	172
Peanut oil	90
Peanuts	219
Peanuts, Spanish	223
Peanuts, Valencia	217
Peanuts, Virginia	217
Pears	145
Pears, Asian	621
Pears, Bartlett	132
Pears, Bosc	147
Pears, green Anjou	125

Food	Nutrivore Score
Pears, red Anjou	135
Peas, edible podded	669
Peas, green	431
Peas, split	274
Pecans	221
Pepitas	271
Pepper grass	11,265
Pepper, black	635
Pepper, red or cayenne	689
Pepper, white	246[1]
Peppermint	1,011[2]
Peppers, hot chili, green	1,234
Peppers, hot chili, red	987
Peppers, sweet, green	1,094
Peppers, sweet, red	1,358
Pepperwort	11,265
Perch	508
Perch, ocean	464
Persimmons, Japanese	537
Persimmons, native	292
Pheasant, breast, skinless	266
Pheasant, leg, skinless	279
Pheasant, meat and skin	246
Pheasant, meat only	318
Pickle relish, hamburger	42[1]
Pickle relish, hot dog	60[1]
Pickle relish, sweet	101
Pickles, dill or kosher dill	593

Food	Nutrivore Score
Pickles, sour	702
Pickles, sweet	107
Pigeon, light meat, skinless	308[1]
Pigeon, meat and skin	180[1]
Pigeon, meat only	368[1]
Pike, walleye	560
Pine nuts	222
Pineapple	358
Pink salmon	625
Pinto beans	390
Pistachios	265
Pitahaya, red	800[1]
Pitahaya, white	357[1]
Pitaya, red	800[1]
Pitaya, white	357[1]
Plantains, green	173
Plantains, yellow	186
Plum, dried	176
Plums	521
Poha	134[3]
Poke	2,330
Pokeberry shoots	2,330
Pokeweed	2,330
Pollack, Alaskan	528
Pollack, Atlantic	650
Pomegranate juice	148
Pomegranates	256
Poor man's pepper	11,265

Food	Nutrivore Score
Popcorn, air-popped	118
Popcorn, microwave	95
Popcorn, oil-popped	104
Poppy seed	333
Poppyseed oil	86[1]
Pork, bacon	122
Pork, brain	469[1]
Pork, chitterlings	133
Pork, feet	112
Pork, ground	186
Pork, ham	214
Pork, heart	977
Pork, intestine	133
Pork, jowl	64[1]
Pork, kidney	1,650
Pork, liver	2,483
Pork, loin, lean	315
Pork, loin, lean and fat	222
Pork, pancreas	570[1]
Pork, spleen	591[1]
Pork, sweetbreads, pancreas	570[1]
Pork, tail	91[1]
Pork, tongue	211
Portobello mushroom	1,483
Potato	272
Potato chips, plain	105
Potatoes, red	278
Potatoes, russet	248

Food	Nutrivore Score
Potatoes, white	273
Prairie turnips	118[2]
Prickly pears	881[1]
Prunes	176
Pumpkin	1,036
Pumpkin flowers	1,564[1]
Pumpkin leaves	1,840
Pumpkin seeds, shelled	271
Quail eggs	341
Quail, breast, skinless	337[1]
Quail, meat and skin	297[1]
Quail, meat only	393[1]
Quince	336[1]
Quinoa	227
Rabbit	378
Radicchio	2,471
Radish sprouts	3,429[1]
Radishes	5,863
Rainbow trout	645
Raisins, dark, seedless	106
Raisins, golden, seedless	103
Raisins, seeded	114
Rapeseed oil	176
Rapini	4,155
Raspberries	491
Red leaf lettuce	2,684
Red mung beans	576[1]
Rhubarb	598

Food	Nutrivore Score
Rice milk, unsweetened	234
Rice, brown	154
Rice, white	66
Rice, wild	154
Ricotta cheese	141
Rocket	2,019
Roe	1,349
Romaine lettuce	2,128
Romano cheese	129
Roquefort cheese	146
Rose apple	210[2]
Rose haw	640
Rose hip	640
Roselle	191[3]
Rosemary	438[1]
Rosemary, dried	459[1]
Ruffed grouse, breast, skinless	397[1]
Rutabaga	766
Safflower oil, high oleic	82
Safflower oil, linoleic	88
Saffron	609[1]
Sage, ground	1,121
Salmon, Chinook	775
Salmon, chum	646
Salmon, pink	625
Salmon, sockeye	750
Salmon, wild Atlantic	868
Salmon, wild coho	724

Food	Nutrivore Score
Salmonberries	327[2]
Salsify	182
Salt, table	N/A[4]
Sapote	488[1]
Sardines (canned in oil)	654
Sauce, fish	523
Sauce, hot chili	262[2]
Sauce, oyster	162
Sauce, soy, made from hydrolyzed vegetable protein	259
Sauce, soy, made from soy (tamari)	373
Sauce, soy, made from soy and wheat (shoyu)	433
Sauerkraut	710
Savory, ground	635[2]
Scallions	1,932
Scallop squash	1,394
Scallops	645
Sea bass	575
Sea cucumber, yane	283[3]
Seaweed, agar	456
Seaweed, Irish moss	602
Seaweed, kelp	700
Seaweed, laver	1,520
Seaweed, nori	1,520
Seaweed, spirulina	1,903
Seaweed, wakame	841
Seed, chia	450[1]

Food	Nutrivore Score
Seeds, flax	515
Seeds, hemp	415[1]
Seeds, pumpkin	271
Seeds, sesame	299
Seeds, sunflower	340
Sesame oil	127
Sesame seed butter	212
Sesame seed butter, paste	289
Sesame seeds	299
Shad	701
Shallots	740
Shark	524
Sharp cheddar cheese	121
Sheep milk	210[1]
Sheepshead	416[1]
Shiitake mushroom	4,343
Shortening	42
Shoyu	433
Shrimp	535
Skipjack tuna	645
Smelt, rainbow	834
Snail	435
Snapper	548
Sockeye salmon	750
Sole	749
Sour cream	82
Soursop	255[1]
Soy milk, unsweetened	425[1]

Food	Nutrivore Score
Soy sauce made from hydrolyzed vegetable protein	259
Soy sauce made from soy (tamari)	373
Soy sauce made from soy and wheat (shoyu)	433
Soybean oil	160
Soybeans	326
Soybeans, green	362[1]
Spaghetti squash	286
Spearmint	914[2]
Spearmint, dried	1,336[2]
Spinach	4,548
Spirulina	1,903
Spleen, beef	867[1]
Spleen, lamb	765[1]
Spleen, pork	591[1]
Spleen, veal	674[1]
Split peas	274
Spring onion	1,932
Sprouts, alfalfa	902
Sprouts, mung bean	711
Sprouts, pea	310[1]
Sprouts, radish	3,429[1]
Squab, light meat, skinless	308[1]
Squab, meat and skin	180[1]
Squab, meat only	368[1]
Squash, acorn	297[1]
Squash, butternut	670

Food	Nutrivore Score
Squash, crookneck	1,177
Squash, Hubbard	358
Squash, scallop	1,394
Squash, spaghetti	286
Squash, straightneck	1,177
Squash, summer	1,596
Squash, winter	370
Squash, zucchini	1,477
Squid	890
Sriracha	262[2]
Starfruit	378
Stock, beef	336[1]
Stock, chicken	151[1]
Stock, fish	732
Straightneck squash	1,177
Strawberries	762
Sturgeon	528
Sugar apple	204[1]
Sugar, brown	22
Sugar, granulated	1
Sugar, maple	82[1]
Sugar, powdered	1[1]
Sugar, turbinado	14[2]
Summer squash	1,596
Sun-dried tomatoes	655
Sunflower oil, high oleic	105
Sunflower oil, linoleic	104
Sunflower oil, mid-oleic	104

Food	Nutrivore Score
Sunflower seed butter	308[1]
Sunflower seeds	340
Swede	766
Sweet potato	379
Sweet potato leaves	1,775
Sweetbreads, beef, pancreas	429[1]
Sweetbreads, beef, thymus	205[1]
Sweetbreads, lamb, pancreas	376[1]
Sweetbreads, pork, pancreas	570[1]
Sweetbreads, veal, pancreas	467[1]
Sweetbreads, veal, thymus	475
Sweetsop	204[1]
Swiss cheese	157
Swordfish	557
Tahini	212
Tail, pork	91[1]
Tallow, beef	38
Tamari	373
Tamarind	77[1]
Tangerine	238
Tapioca, pearl	8[1]
Taro	178
Tarragon, dried	642[1]
Tea, black	3,286
Tea, chamomile	988
Tea, green	3,055

Food	Nutrivore Score
Tea, oolong	4,821
Tempeh	438[1]
Thyme	942[1]
Thyme, dried	1,335
Thymus, beef	205[1]
Thymus, veal	475
Tigernut	192[2]
Tilapia	409
Tilefish	553[1]
Tofu, fuyu	295
Tofu, hard, nigari	282
Tofu, koyadofu	254[1]
Tomatillos	621
Tomato juice	1,568
Tomato puree	1,248
Tomatoes, green	611
Tomatoes, orange	1,780
Tomatoes, red	983
Tomatoes, sun-dried	655
Tomatoes, yellow	1,738
Tongue, beef	215
Tongue, lamb	298[1]
Tongue, pork	211
Tongue, veal	402
Tripe, beef	259
Trotters	112
Trout	710
Trout, rainbow	645

Food	Nutrivore Score
Tuna, bluefin	970
Tuna, skipjack	645
Tuna, yellowfin	642
Turkey, breast, meat only	317
Turkey, dark meat	418
Turkey, giblets	1,567
Turkey, ground	295
Turkey, light meat	315
Turkey, light meat with skin	228
Turkey, whole, meat and skin	299
Turmeric	637
Turnip	1,954
Turnip greens	6,370
Turnip-rooted celery	345
Turtle beans	446
Vanilla extract	65[1]
Vanilla, ice cream	86
Veal, brain	682[1]
Veal, ground	230
Veal, leg (top round), lean	369
Veal, leg, top round, cap off, cutlet, boneless	425
Veal, loin, lean and fat	266
Veal, pancreas	467[1]
Veal, rib, lean	329
Veal, shank, lean and fat	385
Veal, shank, separable lean and fat	338[1]
Veal, shoulder, arm, lean and fat	314

Food	Nutrivore Score
Veal, shoulder, blade chop, lean	435
Veal, shoulder, whole, lean	358[1]
Veal, sirloin, lean	365[1]
Veal, spleen	674[1]
Veal, sweetbreads, pancreas	467[1]
Veal, sweetbreads, thymus	475
Veal, thymus	475
Veal, tongue	402
Vegetable oyster	182
Vinegar, balsamic	72[1]
Vinegar, cider	131
Vinegar, distilled	33
Wakame	841
Walnut oil	126
Walnuts	303
Wasabi	523
Wasabi, root	710
Water convolvulus	1,271[2]
Water spinach	1,271[2]
Water chestnuts	257
Watercress	6,929
Watermelon	405
Wax apple	210[2]
Welsh onions	1,704
West Indian cherries	7,877[1]
Wheat flour, soft grain	185
Wheat flour, white, all-purpose	70

Food	Nutrivore Score
Wheat flour, whole-grain	227
Whelk	730
White beans	269
White button mushroom	1,872
Whitefish	663
Whiting	455
Wild rice	154
Wine, red	104
Wine, white	42
Winter mushroom	4,434

Food	Nutrivore Score
Winter squash	370
Yam	167
Yam bean	234
Yeast, baker's, active dry	1,202
Yellowfin tuna	642
Yogurt, Greek, whole	178
Yogurt, plain, skim	263
Yogurt, plain, whole	184
Yuca	224
Zucchini	1,477

1. Nutrivore Score may be higher since 10 to 25 percent of data is missing.
2. Nutrivore Score is likely higher since 25 to 50 percent of data is missing.
3. Nutrivore Score is unreliable as more than 50 percent of data is missing.
4. Nutrivore Score can't be calculated for noncaloric foods or ingredients.
5. Nutrivore Score is artificially high due to fortification.

Acknowledgments

While my name may be listed as the author, a book is never the work of one sole person—a huge team of experts helped make this book a reality. To Leah Miller, my amazing editor, and the entire team at Simon Element, thank you for encouraging me to tell a story, for honing my words, for making this dream become a reality, and for believing in me. To Jaidree Braddix, my phenomenal agent, and the entire team at Park & Fine Literary and Media, thank you for being my advocate, my sounding board, my cheerleader, and for helping to create the vision that is realized with this book. To my amazing team, past and present, but most notably Charissa Joy, Denise Minger, Lisa Hunter, Jacqueline Leeflang, Kiersten Peterson, and Nicole Anouar, thank you for always having my back; for the million ways your hard work, expertise, and creativity is reflected in this book; and for being as passionate about everything Nutrivore as I am.

This book also wouldn't exist with the support of many people in my personal life. To my husband, David, always quick to ask, "What can I do to help," Nutrivore as a concept, website, or book would not exist without your love, patience, and support. To my daughters, Adele and Mira, being your mom makes me a better person and is my motivation to help make the world a better place for you—no words can ever fully express how much I love and am proud of both of you. To my mom, Patsy, so much of who I am is thanks to who you helped me become—thank you for always being my biggest fan. To my coach, Anne Marie, thank you for always being flexible and helping me stay physically and mentally healthy during the craziness of writing yet another book. And to my dog, Soka, who can't read and will never understand how much you have enriched my life with your antics and our morning hikes in the woods.

I also want to thank you, dear reader, and the audience I have amassed online. Without your support and enthusiasm for my work, none of this ever would have been possible. Thank you for so many thoughtful questions, your heartwarming stories, your encouraging comments, and for making my social media pages a welcoming community for everyone who wants to nerd out about nutrients.

Notes

Introduction

1. Stephen D. Anton et al., "Effects of Popular Diets without Specific Calorie Targets on Weight Loss Outcomes: Systematic Review of Findings from Clinical Trials," *Nutrients* 9, no. 8 (July 2017): 822, doi: 10.3390/nu9080822.

Part I: Why Nutrivore?

1. Jomana Khawandanah and Ihab Tewfik, "Fad Diets: Lifestyle Promises and Health Challenges," *Journal of Food Research* 5, no. 6 (2016): 80–94, doi: 10.5539/jfr.v5n6p80.
2. E. B. Krumbhaar, "The Post-Mortem Examination of Lord Byron's Body," *Annals of Medical History* 5, no. 3 (September 1923): 283–84, https://pubmed.ncbi.nlm.nih.gov/33943256/.
3. I. Santos et al., "Prevalence of Personal Weight Control Attempts in Adults: A Systematic Review and Meta-Analysis," *Obesity Reviews* 18, no. 1 (January 2017): 32–50, doi: 10.1111/obr.12466.
4. Crescent B. Martin et al., "Attempts to Lose Weight among Adults in the United States, 2013–2016," *NCHS Data Brief* no. 313 (July 2018): 1–8, https://pubmed.ncbi.nlm.nih.gov/30044214/.
5. A. Janet Tomiyama et al., "Low Calorie Dieting Increases Cortisol," *Psychosomatic Medicine* 72, no. 4 (May 2010): 357–64, doi: 10.1097/PSY.0b013e3181d9523c.
6. C. M. Shisslak, M. Crago, and L. S. Estes, "The Spectrum of Eating Disturbances," *International Journal of Eating Disorders* 18, no. 3 (November 1995): 209–19, https://pubmed.ncbi.nlm.nih.gov/8556017/.

Chapter 1: You're Not Getting Enough Nutrients

1. Victor L. Fulgoni III et al., "Foods, Fortificants, and Supplements: Where Do Americans Get Their Nutrients?" *Journal of Nutrition* 141, no. 10 (October 2011): 1,847–54, doi: 10.3945/jn.111.142257.
2. Bill Misner, "Food Alone May Not Provide Sufficient Micronutrients for

Preventing Deficiency," *Journal of the International Society of Sports Nutrition* 3, no. 1 (2006): 51–55, doi: 10.1186/1550-2783-3-1-51.

3. Biji T. Kurien, "Just a Minute: Incredible Numbers at Play at the Macro and Micro Level," *CMAJ: Canadian Medical Association Journal* 171, no. 12 (December 2004): 1497, doi: 10.1503/cmaj.1040579.
4. Julia K. Bird et al., "Risk of Deficiency in Multiple Concurrent Micronutrients in Children and Adults in the United States," *Nutrients* 9, no. 7 (2017): 655, doi: 10.3390/nu9070655.
5. Ross M. Welch and Robin D. Graham, "Breeding for Micronutrients in Staple Food Crops from a Human Nutrition Perspective," *Journal of Experimental Botany* 55, no. 396 (February 2004): 353–64, doi: 10.1093/jxb/erh064.
6. Centers for Disease Control and Prevention, *Second National Report on Biochemical Indicators of Diet and Nutrition in the U.S. Population* (Atlanta: National Center for Environmental Health, 2012), http://www.cdc.gov/nutritionreport.
7. Fulgoni III et al., "Foods, Fortificants, and Supplements."
8. Alexandra E. Cowan et al., "Total Usual Micronutrient Intakes Compared to the Dietary Reference Intakes among U.S. Adults by Food Security Status," *Nutrients* 12, no. 1 (December 2019): 38, doi: 10.3390/nu12010038.
9. Eurídice Martínez Steele et al., "Ultra-Processed Foods and Added Sugars in the US Diet: Evidence from a Nationally Representative Cross-Sectional Study," *BMJ Open* 6, no. 3 (March 2016): e009892, doi: 10.1136/bmjopen-2015-009892.
10. Ashley N. Gearhardt et al., "Can Food Be Addictive? Public Health and Policy Implications," *Addiction (Abingdon, England)* 106, no. 7 (July 2011): 1,208–12, doi: 10.1111/j.1360-0443.2010.03301.x.
11. Daniela Martini et al., "Ultra-Processed Foods and Nutritional Dietary Profile: A Meta-Analysis of Nationally Representative Samples," *Nutrients* 13, no. 10 (September 2021): 3,390, doi: 10.3390/nu13103390.
12. Isabel Cristina de Macedo, Joice Soares de Freitas, and Iraci Lucena da Silva Torres, "The Influence of Palatable Diets in Reward System Activation: A Mini Review," *Advances in Pharmacological Sciences* 2016 (2016): 7238679, doi: 10.1155/2016/7238679.
13. Kevin D. Hall et al., "Ultra-Processed Diets Cause Excess Calorie Intake and Weight Gain: An Inpatient Randomized Controlled Trial of Ad Libitum Food Intake," *Cell Metabolism* 30, no. 1 (July 2019): 67–77.e3, doi: 10.1016/j.cmet.2019.05.008.
14. Paul R. Marantz, Elizabeth D. Bird, and Michael H. Alderman, "A Call for Higher Standards of Evidence for Dietary Guidelines," *American Journal of Preventive Medicine* 34, no. 3 (March 2008): 234–40, doi: 10.1016/j.amepre.2007.11.017; and Nina Teicholz, "The Scientific Report Guiding the US Dietary Guidelines: Is It Scientific?" *BMJ (Clinical Research Ed.)* 351 (September 2015): h4962, doi: 10.1136/bmj.h4962.
15. USDA Food and Nutrition Service, US Department of Agriculture, "HEI Scores for Americans," FNS.USDA.gov, April 2022, https://www.fns.usda.gov/cnpp/hei-scores-americans.

16. Edwina Wambogo et al., "Awareness of the MyPlate Plan: United States, 2017–March 2020," *National Health Statistics Reports* no. 178 (November 2022): 1–14, https://pubmed.ncbi.nlm.nih.gov/36454172/.
17. Dagfinn Aune et al., "Fruit and Vegetable Intake and the Risk of Cardiovascular Disease, Total Cancer and All-Cause Mortality—A Systematic Review and Dose-Response Meta-Analysis of Prospective Studies," *International Journal of Epidemiology* 46, no. 3 (June 2017): 1,029–56, doi: 10.1093/ije/dyw319.
18. Seung Hee Lee, PhD, et al., "Adults Meeting Fruit and Vegetable Intake Recommendations—United States, 2019," *Morbidity and Mortality Weekly Report (MMWR)* 71, no. 1 (January 2022): 1–9, doi: 10.15585/mmwr.mm7101a1.
19. US Department of Health and Human Services and US Department of Agriculture, *2015–2020 Dietary Guidelines for Americans*, 8th edition (December 2015), https://www.dietaryguidelines.gov/about-dietary-guidelines/previous-editions/2015-dietary-guidelines.
20. US Department of Agriculture and US Department of Health and Human Services, *Dietary Guidelines for Americans, 2020–2025*, 9th edition (December 2020), https://www.dietaryguidelines.gov/resources/2020-2025-dietary-guidelines-online-materials.
21. Laural K. English, PhD, et al., "Evaluation of Dietary Patterns and All-Cause Mortality: A Systematic Review," *JAMA Network Open* 4, no. 8 (2021): e2122277, doi: 10.1001/jamanetworkopen.2021.22277.
22. Josefine Nebl et al., "Micronutrient Status of Recreational Runners with Vegetarian or Non-Vegetarian Dietary Patterns," *Nutrients* 11, no. 5 (2019): 1146, doi: 10.3390/nu11051146; and R. Schüpbach et al., "Micronutrient Status and Intake in Omnivores, Vegetarians and Vegans in Switzerland," *European Journal of Nutrition* 56, no. 1 (February 2017): 283–93, doi: 10.1007/s00394-015-1079-7.
23. Jayson B. Calton, "Prevalence of Micronutrient Deficiency in Popular Diet Plans," *Journal of the International Society of Sports Nutrition* 7 (June 2010): 24, doi: 10.1186/1550-2783-7-24; Matthew G. Engel et al., "Micronutrient Gaps in Three Commercial Weight-Loss Diet Plans," *Nutrients* 10, no. 1 (January 2018): 108, doi: 10.3390/nu10010108; and Maximilian Andreas Storz and Alvaro Luis Ronco, "Nutrient Intake in Low-Carbohydrate Diets in Comparison to the 2020–2025 Dietary Guidelines for Americans: A Cross-Sectional Study," *British Journal of Nutrition* 129, no. 6 (June 2022): 1–14, doi: 10.1017/S0007114522001908.
24. Christopher D. Gardner et al., "Micronutrient Quality of Weight-Loss Diets That Focus on Macronutrients: Results from the A TO Z Study," *American Journal of Clinical Nutrition* 92, no. 2 (August 2010): 304–12, doi: 10.3945/ajcn.2010.29468; and Catherine A. Chenard et al., "Nutrient Composition Comparison between the Low Saturated Fat Swank Diet for Multiple Sclerosis and Healthy U.S.–Style Eating Pattern," *Nutrients* 11, no. 3 (March 2019): 616, doi: 10.3390/nu11030616.
25. Antje Damms-Machado, Gesine Weser, and Stephan C. Bischoff, "Micronutrient Deficiency in Obese Subjects Undergoing Low Calorie Diet," *Nutrition Journal* 11 (2012): 34, doi: 10.1186/1475-2891-11-34.

26. Anna Szaflarska-Popławska, Aleksandra Dolińska, and Magdalena Kuśmierek, "Nutritional Imbalances in Polish Children with Coeliac Disease on a Strict Gluten-Free Diet," *Nutrients* 14, no. 19 (September 2022): 3969, doi: 10.3390/nu14193969; Aynur Unalp-Arida, Rui Liu, and Constance E. Ruhl, "Nutrient Intake Differs among Persons with Celiac Disease and Gluten-Related Disorders in the United States," *Scientific Reports* 12, no. 1 (April 2022): 5566, doi: 10.1038/s41598-022-09346-y; and Teba González et al., "Celiac Male's Gluten-Free Diet Profile: Comparison to That of the Control Population and Celiac Women," *Nutrients* 10, no. 11 (November 2018): 1713, doi: 10.3390/nu10111713.
27. Chaitong Churuangsuk et al., "Impacts of Carbohydrate-Restricted Diets on Micronutrient Intakes and Status: A Systematic Review," *Obesity Reviews* 20, no. 8 (August 2019): 1,132–47, doi: 10.1111/obr.12857.
28. Mariana Baldini Prudencio et al., "Micronutrient Supplementation Needs More Attention in Patients with Refractory Epilepsy under Ketogenic Diet Treatment," *Nutrition (Burbank, Los Angeles County, Calif.)* 86 (June 2021): 111158, doi: 10.1016/j.nut.2021.111158.
29. Research and Markets, "Global Weight Loss Products and Services Market Report 2023: Rising Ageing Population Drives Growth," press release, PR Newswire, May 2, 2023, https://www.prnewswire.com/news-releases/global-weight-loss-products-and-services-market-report-2023-rising-ageing-population-drives-growth-301813238.html.
30. Steven N. Blair and Tim S. Church, "The Fitness, Obesity, and Health Equation: Is Physical Activity the Common Denominator?" *JAMA* 292, no. 10 (September 2004): 1,232–34, doi: 10.1001/jama.292.10.1232.
31. Rachel P. Wildman et al., "The Obese without Cardiometabolic Risk Factor Clustering and the Normal Weight with Cardiometabolic Risk Factor Clustering: Prevalence and Correlates of 2 Phenotypes among the US Population (NHANES 1999–2004)," *Archives of Internal Medicine* 168, no. 15 (August 2008): 1,617–24, doi: 10.1001/archinte.168.15.1617.
32. Katherine M. Flegal et al., "Association of All-Cause Mortality with Overweight and Obesity Using Standard Body Mass Index Categories: A Systematic Review and Meta-Analysis," *JAMA* 309, no. 1 (2013): 71–82, doi: 10.1001/jama.2012.113905.
33. Eun-Jung Rhee, "Weight Cycling and Its Cardiometabolic Impact," *Journal of Obesity & Metabolic Syndrome* 26, no. 4 (2017): 237–42, doi: 10.7570/jomes.2017.26.4.237.
34. Mee Kyoung Kim et al., "Associations of Variability in Blood Pressure, Glucose and Cholesterol Concentrations, and Body Mass Index with Mortality and Cardiovascular Outcomes in the General Population," *Circulation* 138, no. 23 (October 2018): 2,627–37, doi: 10.1161/CIRCULATIONAHA.118.034978.
35. Olga P. García, Kurt Z. Long, and Jorge L. Rosado, "Impact of Micronutrient Deficiencies on Obesity," *Nutrition Reviews* 67, no. 10 (October 2009): 559–72, doi: 10.1111/j.1753-4887.2009.00228.x.
36. Helen Macpherson, Andrew Pipingas, and Matthew P. Pase, "Multivitamin-Multimineral Supplementation and Mortality: A Meta-Analysis of Randomized

Controlled Trials," *American Journal of Clinical Nutrition* 97, no. 2 (February 2013): 437–44, doi: 10.3945/ajcn.112.049304.

37. Joonseok Kim et al., "Association of Multivitamin and Mineral Supplementation and Risk of Cardiovascular Disease: A Systematic Review and Meta-Analysis," *Circulation. Cardiovascular Quality and Outcomes* 11, no. 7 (July 2018): e004224, doi: 10.1161/CIRCOUTCOMES.117.004224.
38. Stephen P. Fortmann et al., "Vitamin and Mineral Supplements in the Primary Prevention of Cardiovascular Disease and Cancer: An Updated Systematic Evidence Review for the U.S. Preventive Services Task Force," *Annals of Internal Medicine* 159, no. 12 (December 2013): 824–34, doi: 10.7326/0003-4819-159-12-201312170-00729.
39. Fan Chen et al., "Association among Dietary Supplement Use, Nutrient Intake, and Mortality among U.S. Adults: A Cohort Study," *Annals of Internal Medicine* 170, no. 9 (May 2019): 604–13, doi: 10.7326/M18-2478.
40. Elizabeth A. O'Connor et al., "Vitamin and Mineral Supplements for the Primary Prevention of Cardiovascular Disease and Cancer: Updated Evidence Report and Systematic Review for the US Preventive Services Task Force," *JAMA* 327, no. 23 (June 2022): 2,334–47, doi: 10.1001/jama.2021.15650.
41. V. S. Srinivasan, "Bioavailability of Nutrients: A Practical Approach to In Vitro Demonstration of the Availability of Nutrients in Multivitamin-Mineral Combination Products," *Journal of Nutrition* 131, Supplement 4 (April 2001): 1,349S–50S, doi: 10.1093/jn/131.4.1349S.
42. Cristina Palacios et al., "Current Calcium Fortification Experiences: A Review," *Annals of the New York Academy of Sciences* 1484, no. 1 (January 2021): 55–73, doi: 10.1111/nyas.14481.
43. Penjani Mkambula et al., "The Unfinished Agenda for Food Fortification in Low- and Middle-Income Countries: Quantifying Progress, Gaps and Potential Opportunities," *Nutrients* 12, no. 2 (2020): 354, doi: 10.3390/nu12020354.

Chapter 2: Fix Your Diet (and Health) with Nutrivore

1. GBD 2017 Diet Collaborators, "Health Effects of Dietary Risks in 195 Countries, 1990–2017: A Systematic Analysis for the Global Burden of Disease Study 2017," *Lancet* 393, no. 10,184 (May 2019): 1,958–72, doi: 10.1016/S0140-6736(19)30041-8.
2. Stephanie M. Fanelli et al., "Poorer Diet Quality Observed among US Adults with a Greater Number of Clinical Chronic Disease Risk Factors," *Journal of Primary Care & Community Health* 11 (January–December 2020): 2150132720945898, doi: 10.1177/2150132720945898.
3. "Diabetes," World Health Organization, September 16, 2022, https://www.who.int/news-room/fact-sheets/detail/diabetes.
4. "National Diabetes Statistics Report," Centers for Disease Control and Prevention, June 29, 2022, https://www.cdc.gov/diabetes/data/statistics-report/index.html.
5. Izabela Szymczak-Pajor and Agnieszka Śliwińska, "Analysis of Association between Vitamin D Deficiency and Insulin Resistance," *Nutrients* 11, no. 4 (2019): 794, doi: 10.3390/nu11040794.

6. Rathish Nair and Arun Maseeh, "Vitamin D: The 'Sunshine' Vitamin," *Journal of Pharmacology & Pharmacotherapeutics* 3, no. 2 (April 2012): 118–26, doi: 10.4103/0976-500X.95506.
7. Xuefeng Liu, Ana Baylin, and Phillip D. Levy, "Vitamin D Deficiency and Insufficiency among US Adults: Prevalence, Predictors and Clinical Implications," *British Journal of Nutrition* 119, no. 8 (April 2018): 928–36, doi: 10.1017/S0007114518000491.
8. Andrius Bleizgys, "Vitamin D Dosing: Basic Principles and a Brief Algorithm (2021 Update)," *Nutrients* 13, no. 12 (2021): 4415, doi: 10.3390/nu13124415.
9. Cem Ekmekcioglu, Daniela Haluza, and Michael Kundi, "25-Hydroxyvitamin D Status and Risk for Colorectal Cancer and Type 2 Diabetes Mellitus: A Systematic Review and Meta-Analysis of Epidemiological Studies," *International Journal of Environmental Research and Public Health* 14, no. 2 (2017): 127, doi: 10.3390/ijerph14020127.
10. Zahra Sadat Khosravi et al., "Effect of Vitamin D Supplementation on Weight Loss, Glycemic Indices, and Lipid Profile in Obese and Overweight Women: A Clinical Trial Study," *International Journal of Preventive Medicine* 9 (July 2018): 63, doi: 10.4103/ijpvm.IJPVM_329_15.
11. Ken C. Chiu et al., "Hypovitaminosis D Is Associated with Insulin Resistance and Beta Cell Dysfunction," *American Journal of Clinical Nutrition* 79, no. 5 (May 2004): 820–25, doi: 10.1093/ajcn/79.5.820.
12. Paola Lucato et al., "Low Vitamin D Levels Increase the Risk of Type 2 Diabetes in Older Adults: A Systematic Review and Meta-Analysis," *Maturitas* 100 (June 2017): 8–15, doi: 10.1016/j.maturitas.2017.02.016.
13. A. Deleskog et al., "Low Serum 25-Hydroxyvitamin D Level Predicts Progression to Type 2 Diabetes in Individuals with Prediabetes but Not with Normal Glucose Tolerance," *Diabetologia* 55, no. 6 (June 2012): 1,668–78, doi: 10.1007/s00125-012-2529-x.
14. J. Michael McGinnis, Pamela Williams-Russo, and James R. Knickman, "The Case for More Active Policy Attention to Health Promotion," *Health Affairs* 21, no. 2 (March/April 2002): 78–93, doi: 10.1377/hlthaff.21.2.78.
15. Karen Hacker et al., "Social Determinants of Health—An Approach Taken at CDC," *Journal of Public Health Management and Practice* 28, no. 6 (November–December 2022): 589–94, doi: 10.1097/PHH.0000000000001626.
16. Paula Braveman and Laura Gottlieb, "The Social Determinants of Health: It's Time to Consider the Causes of the Causes," *Public Health Reports* 129, Supplement 2 (January–February 2014): 19–31, doi: 10.1177/00333549141291S206.
17. Shan Pou Tsai et al., "Converting Health Risks into Loss of Life Years—A Paradigm Shift in Clinical Risk Communication," *Aging (Albany, NY)* 13, no. 17 (September 2021): 21,513–25, doi: 10.18632/aging.203491.
18. Lars T. Fadnes et al., "Estimating Impact of Food Choices on Life Expectancy: A Modeling Study," *PLoS Medicine* 19, no. 3 (March 2022): e1003889, doi: 10.1371/journal.pmed.1003889.
19. Aikaterini Palascha, Ellen van Kleef, and Hans C. M. van Trijp, "How Does Thinking in Black and White Terms Relate to Eating Behavior and Weight

Regain?" *Journal of Health Psychology* 20, no. 5 (May 2015): 638–48, doi: 10.1177/1359105315573440; and Atsushi Oshio, "Development and Validation of the Dichotomous Thinking Inventory," *Social Behavior and Personality* 37, no. 6 (2009): 729–41, doi: 10.2224/sbp.2009.37.6.729.

20. Esther Jansen, Sandra Mulkens, and Anita Jansen, "Do Not Eat the Red Food!: Prohibition of Snacks Leads to Their Relatively Higher Consumption in Children," *Appetite* 49, no. 3 (November 2007): 572–77, doi: 10.1016/j.appet.2007.03.229.
21. J. W. Anderson et al., "Long-Term Weight-Loss Maintenance: A Meta-Analysis of US Studies," *American Journal of Clinical Nutrition* 74, no. 5 (November 2001): 579–84, doi: 10.1093/ajcn/74.5.579.
22. Cecilie Thøgersen-Ntoumani et al., "Does Self-Compassion Help to Deal with Dietary Lapses among Overweight and Obese Adults Who Pursue Weight-Loss Goals?" *British Journal of Health Psychology* 26, no. 3 (September 2021): 767–88, doi: 10.1111/bjhp.12499.
23. Ehab S. Eshak et al., "Rice Intake Is Associated with Reduced Risk of Mortality from Cardiovascular Disease in Japanese Men but Not Women," *Journal of Nutrition* 141, no. 4 (April 2011): 595–602, doi: 10.3945/jn.110.132167.

Chapter 3: The Nutrivore Score

1. Adam Drewnowski, "Defining Nutrient Density: Development and Validation of the Nutrient Rich Foods Index," *Journal of the American College of Nutrition* 28, no. 4 (August 2009): 421S–26S, doi: 10.1080/07315724.2009.10718106.
2. Adam Drewnowski, "Concept of a Nutritious Food: Toward a Nutrient Density Score," *American Journal of Clinical Nutrition* 82, no. 4 (October 2005): 721–32, doi: 10.1093/ajcn/82.4.721.
3. Gregory D. Miller et al., "It Is Time for a Positive Approach to Dietary Guidance Using Nutrient Density as a Basic Principle," *Journal of Nutrition* 139, no. 6 (June 2009): 1,198–202, doi: 10.3945/jn.108.100842.
4. Theresa A. Nicklas, Adam Drewnowski, and Carol E. O'Neil, "The Nutrient Density Approach to Healthy Eating: Challenges and Opportunities," *Public Health Nutrition* 17, no. 12 (December 2014): 2,626–36, doi: 10.1017/S136898001400158X.
5. Peter Scarborough et al., "Testing Nutrient Profile Models Using Data from a Survey of Nutrition Professionals," *Public Health Nutrition* 10, no. 4 (April 2007): 337–45, doi: 10.1017/S1368980007666671.
6. Adam Drewnowski and Victor L. Fulgoni III, "Nutrient Density: Principles and Evaluation Tools," *American Journal of Clinical Nutrition* 99, Supplement 5 (May 2014): 1,223S–28S, doi: 10.3945/ajcn.113.073395.
7. Flaminia Ortenzi et al., "Limitations of the Food Compass Nutrient Profiling System," *Journal of Nutrition* 153, no. 3 (March 2023): 610–14, doi: 10.1016/j.tjnut.2023.01.027.

Chapter 4: Easy Steps to Nutrivore

1. Yin Zhang and Edward L. Giovannucci, "Ultra-Processed Foods and Health: A Comprehensive Review," *Critical Reviews in Food Science and Nutrition* 63, no. 31 (2023): 10,836–48, doi: 10.1080/10408398.2022.2084359.

2. Anaïs Rico-Campà et al., "Association between Consumption of Ultra-Processed Foods and All-Cause Mortality: SUN Prospective Cohort Study," *BMJ (Clinical Research Ed.)* 365 (May 2019): I1949, doi: 10.1136/bmj.l1949.
3. Xuanli Chen et al., "Associations of Ultra-Processed Food Consumption with Cardiovascular Disease and All-Cause Mortality: UK Biobank," *European Journal of Public Health* 32, no. 5 (October 2022): 779–85, doi: 10.1093/eurpub/ckac104.
4. Wanich Suksatan et al., "Ultra-Processed Food Consumption and Adult Mortality Risk: A Systematic Review and Dose-Response Meta-Analysis of 207,291 Participants," *Nutrients* 14, no. 1 (December 2021): 174, doi: 10.3390/nu14010174.
5. Petek Eylul Taneri et al., "Association between Ultra-Processed Food Intake and All-Cause Mortality: A Systematic Review and Meta-Analysis," *American Journal of Epidemiology* 191, no. 7 (July 2022): 1,323–35, doi: 10.1093/aje/kwac039.
6. David Wiss, "Clinical Considerations of Ultra-Processed Food Addiction across Weight Classes: An Eating Disorder Treatment and Care Perspective," *Current Addiction Reports* 9, no. 4 (2022): 255–67, doi: 10.1007/s40429-022-00411-0.
7. Quanhe Yang et al., "Added Sugar Intake and Cardiovascular Diseases Mortality among US Adults," *JAMA Internal Medicine* 174, no. 4 (2014): 516–24, doi: 10.1001/jamainternmed.2013.13563.
8. Sigrid Gibson et al., "The Effects of Sucrose on Metabolic Health: A Systematic Review of Human Intervention Studies in Healthy Adults," *Critical Reviews in Food Science and Nutrition* 53, no. 6 (2013): 591–614, doi: 10.1080/10408398.2012.691574.
9. Charlotte Debras et al., "Artificial Sweeteners and Risk of Cardiovascular Diseases: Results from the Prospective NutriNet-Santé Cohort," *BMJ (Clinical Research Ed.)* 378 (September 2022): e071204, doi: 10.1136/bmj-2022-071204.
10. Charlotte Debras et al., "Artificial Sweeteners and Cancer Risk: Results from the NutriNet-Santé Population-Based Cohort Study," *PLoS Medicine* 19, no. 3 (March 2022): e1003950, doi: 10.1371/journal.pmed.1003950.
11. Victor L. Fulgoni III and Adam Drewnowski, "No Association between Low-Calorie Sweetener (LCS) Use and Overall Cancer Risk in the Nationally Representative Database in the US: Analyses of NHANES 1988–2018 Data and 2019 Public-Use Linked Mortality Files," *Nutrients* 14, no. 23 (November 2022): 4957, doi: 10.3390/nu14234957.
12. Bo Yang et al., "Added Sugar, Sugar-Sweetened Beverages, and Artificially Sweetened Beverages and Risk of Cardiovascular Disease: Findings from the Women's Health Initiative and a Network Meta-Analysis of Prospective Studies," *Nutrients* 14, no. 20 (October 2022): 4226, doi: 10.3390/nu14204226.
13. Yan-Bo Zhang et al., "Association of Sugar-Sweetened Beverage and Artificially Sweetened Beverage Intakes with Mortality: An Analysis of US National Health and Nutrition Examination Survey," *European Journal of Nutrition* 60, no. 4 (June 2021): 1,945–55, doi: 10.1007/s00394-020-02387-x.
14. Lisa J. Harnack et al., "Sources of Sodium in US Adults from 3 Geographic Regions," *Circulation* 135, no. 19 (May 2017): 1,775–83, doi: 10.1161/CIRCULATIONAHA.116.024446.

15. Giles T. Hanley-Cook et al., "Food Biodiversity and Total and Cause-Specific Mortality in 9 European Countries: An Analysis of a Prospective Cohort Study," *PLoS Medicine* 18, no. 10 (October 2021): e1003834, doi: 10.1371/journal.pmed.1003834.
16. Hadis Mozaffari et al., "Is Eating a Mixed Diet Better for Health and Survival?: A Systematic Review and Meta-Analysis of Longitudinal Observational Studies," *Critical Reviews in Food Science and Nutrition* 62, no. 29 (2022): 8,120–36, doi: 10.1080/10408398.2021.1925630.
17. S. M. Krebs-Smith et al., "The Effects of Variety in Food Choices on Dietary Quality," *Journal of the American Dietetic Association* 87, no. 7 (July 1987): 897–903, https://pubmed.ncbi.nlm.nih.gov/3598038/.
18. Kumari Malkanthi Rathnayake, Pae Madushani, and Kdrr Silva, "Use of Dietary Diversity Score as a Proxy Indicator of Nutrient Adequacy of Rural Elderly People in Sri Lanka," *BMC Research Notes* 5 (August 2012): 469, doi: 10.1186/1756-0500-5-469.
19. Taylor C. Wallace et al., "Fruits, Vegetables, and Health: A Comprehensive Narrative, Umbrella Review of the Science and Recommendations for Enhanced Public Policy to Improve Intake," *Critical Reviews in Food Science and Nutrition* 60, no. 13 (2020): 2,174–211, doi: 10.1080/10408398.2019.1632258.
20. Dagfinn Aune et al., "Fruit and Vegetable Intake and the Risk of Cardiovascular Disease, Total Cancer and All-Cause Mortality—A Systematic Review and Dose-Response Meta-Analysis of Prospective Studies," *International Journal of Epidemiology* 46, no. 3 (June 2017): 1,029–56, doi: 10.1093/ije/dyw319.
21. Michelle Blumfield et al., "Should We 'Eat a Rainbow'? An Umbrella Review of the Health Effects of Colorful Bioactive Pigments in Fruits and Vegetables," *Molecules (Basel, Switzerland)* 27, no. 13 (June 2022): 4061, doi: 10.3390/molecules27134061.
22. Redzo Mujcic and Andrew J. Oswald, "Evolution of Well-Being and Happiness after Increases in Consumption of Fruit and Vegetables," *American Journal of Public Health* 106, no. 8 (August 2016): 1,504–10, doi: 10.2105/AJPH.2016.303260.
23. Yu Zhang et al., "Cooking Oil/Fat Consumption and Deaths from Cardiometabolic Diseases and Other Causes: Prospective Analysis of 521,120 Individuals," *BMC Medicine* 19, no. 1 (April 2021): 92, doi: 10.1186/s12916-021-01961-2.
24. Tauseef A. Khan et al., "A Lack of Consideration of a Dose-Response Relationship Can Lead to Erroneous Conclusions Regarding 100% Fruit Juice and the Risk of Cardiometabolic Disease," *European Journal of Clinical Nutrition* 73, no. 12 (December 2019): 1,556–60, doi: 10.1038/s41430-019-0514-x.
25. Janette de Goede et al., "Dairy Consumption and Risk of Stroke: A Systematic Review and Updated Dose-Response Meta-Analysis of Prospective Cohort Studies," *Journal of the American Heart Association* 5, no. 5 (May 2016): e002787, doi: 10.1161/JAHA.115.002787.
26. Jinhui Zhao et al., "Association between Daily Alcohol Intake and Risk of All-Cause Mortality: A Systematic Review and Meta-Analyses," *JAMA Network Open* 6, no. 3 (March 2023): e236185, doi: 10.1001/jamanetworkopen.2023.6185.

27. Kiran J. Biddinger et al., "Association of Habitual Alcohol Intake with Risk of Cardiovascular Disease," *JAMA Network Open* 5, no. 3 (March 2022): e223849, doi: 10.1001/jamanetworkopen.2022.3849.
28. V. Bagnardi et al., "Alcohol Consumption and Site-Specific Cancer Risk: A Comprehensive Dose-Response Meta-Analysis," *British Journal of Cancer* 112, no. 3 (February 2015): 580–93, doi: 10.1038/bjc.2014.579; and David E. Nelson et al., "Alcohol-Attributable Cancer Deaths and Years of Potential Life Lost in the United States," *American Journal of Public Health* 103, no. 4 (April 2013): 641–48, doi: 10.2105/AJPH.2012.301199.
29. GBD 2016 Alcohol Collaborators, "Alcohol Use and Burden for 195 Countries and Territories, 1990–2016: A Systematic Analysis for the Global Burden of Disease Study 2016," *Lancet* 392, no. 10,152 (September 2018): 1,015–35, doi: 10.1016/S0140-6736(18)31310-2.
30. Laura C. Ortinau et al., "Effects of High-Protein vs. High-Fat Snacks on Appetite Control, Satiety, and Eating Initiation in Healthy Women," *Nutrition Journal* 13 (September 2014): 97, doi: 10.1186/1475-2891-13-97.
31. Santiago Navas-Carretero et al., "Chronologically Scheduled Snacking with High-Protein Products within the Habitual Diet in Type-2 Diabetes Patients Leads to a Fat Mass Loss: A Longitudinal Study," *Nutrition Journal* 10 (July 2011): 74, doi: 10.1186/1475-2891-10-74.
32. Gemma Williams et al., "High Protein High Fibre Snack Bars Reduce Food Intake and Improve Short Term Glucose and Insulin Profiles Compared with High Fat Snack Bars," *Asia Pacific Journal of Clinical Nutrition* 15, no. 4 (2006): 443–50, https://pubmed.ncbi.nlm.nih.gov/17077058/.
33. Wei Wei et al., "Association of Meal and Snack Patterns with Mortality of All-Cause, Cardiovascular Disease, and Cancer: The US National Health and Nutrition Examination Survey, 2003 to 2014," *Journal of the American Heart Association* 10, no. 13 (June 2021): e020254, doi: 10.1161/JAHA.120.020254.

Part 2: Nutrients and Your Health

1. Emma Seifrit Weigley, PhD, "Sarah Tyson Rorer: First American Dietitian?" *Journal of the American Dietetic Association* 77, no. 1 (July 1980): 11–15, https://www.sciencedirect.com/science/article/abs/pii/S0002822321049130.

Chapter 5: Mighty Macronutrients: Protein, Carbs, and Fat

1. Kenneth J. Carpenter, "A Short History of Nutritional Science: Part 1 (1785–1885)," *Journal of Nutrition* 133, no. 3 (March 2003): 638–45, doi: 10.1093/jn/133.3.638.
2. James L. Hargrove, "History of the Calorie in Nutrition," *Journal of Nutrition* 136, no. 12 (December 2006): 2,957–61, doi: 10.1093/jn/136.12.2957.
3. F. W. Leigh, "Sir Hans Adolf Krebs (1900–81), Pioneer of Modern Medicine, Architect of Intermediary Metabolism," *Journal of Medical Biography* 17, no. 3 (August 2009): 149–54, doi: 10.1258/jmb.2009.009032.
4. Kenneth J. Carpenter, "The History of Enthusiasm for Protein," *Journal of Nutrition* 116, no. 7 (July 1986): 1,364–70, doi: 10.1093/jn/116.7.1364.

5. Kenneth J. Carpenter, "A Short History of Nutritional Science: Part 2 (1885–1912)," *Journal of Nutrition* 133, no. 4 (April 2003): 975–84, doi: 10.1093/jn/133.4.975.
6. M. R. Finlay, "Quackery and Cookery: Justus von Liebig's Extract of Meat and the Theory of Nutrition in the Victorian Age," *Bulletin of the History of Medicine* 66, no. 3 (Fall 1992): 404–18, https://pubmed.ncbi.nlm.nih.gov/1392506/.
7. W. O. Atwater, PhD, *Farmers' Bulletin no. 23: Foods: Nutritive Value and Cost* (Washington, DC: Government Printing Office, 1894), https://www.ars.usda.gov/ARSUserFiles/80400530/pdf/hist/oes_1894_farm_bul_23.pdf.
8. Stephan Rössner, "Anthelme Brillat-Savarin (1755–1826)," *Obesity Reviews* 8, no. 6 (November 2007): 531–32, doi: 10.1111/j.1467-789X.2007.00380.x.
9. R. E. Olson, "Evolution of Ideas about the Nutritional Value of Dietary Fat: Introduction," *Journal of Nutrition* 128, Supplement 2 (February 1998): 421S–22S, doi: 10.1093/jn/128.2.421S.
10. Germain Honvo et al., "Role of Collagen Derivatives in Osteoarthritis and Cartilage Repair: A Systematic Scoping Review with Evidence Mapping," *Rheumatology and Therapy* 7, no. 4 (December 2020): 703–40, doi: 10.1007/s40744-020-00240-5.
11. T. E. McAlindon et al., "Change in Knee Osteoarthritis Cartilage Detected by Delayed Gadolinium Enhanced Magnetic Resonance Imaging Following Treatment with Collagen Hydrolysate: A Pilot Randomized Controlled Trial," *Osteoarthritis and Cartilage* 19, no. 4 (April 2011): 399–405, doi: 10.1016/j.joca.2011.01.001.
12. P. Benito-Ruiz et al., "A Randomized Controlled Trial on the Efficacy and Safety of a Food Ingredient, Collagen Hydrolysate, for Improving Joint Comfort," *International Journal of Food Sciences and Nutrition* 60, Supplement 2 (2009): 99–113, doi: 10.1080/09637480802498820.
13. Kristine L. Clark et al., "24-Week Study on the Use of Collagen Hydrolysate as a Dietary Supplement in Athletes with Activity-Related Joint Pain," *Current Medical Research and Opinion* 24, no. 5 (May 2008): 1,485–96, doi: 10.1185/030079908x291967.
14. Anita Laser Reutersward and Stefan Fabiansson, "In Vivo Digestibility of Insoluble Collagen from Bovine Tendon as Influenced by the Inhibition of Gastric Acid Secretion," *Journal of Food Science* 50, no. 6 (November 1985): 1,523–25, doi: 10.1111/j.1365-2621.1985.tb10524.x.
15. Rebekah D. Alcock, Gregory C. Shaw, and Louise M. Burke, "Bone Broth Unlikely to Provide Reliable Concentrations of Collagen Precursors Compared with Supplemental Sources of Collagen Used in Collagen Research," *International Journal of Sport Nutrition and Exercise Metabolism* 29, no. 3 (May 2019): 265–72, doi: 10.1123/ijsnem.2018-0139.
16. Irwin K. Cheah and Barry Halliwell, "Ergothioneine, Recent Developments," *Redox Biology* 42 (June 2021): 101868, doi: 10.1016/j.redox.2021.101868.
17. Irina Borodina et al., "The Biology of Ergothioneine, an Antioxidant Nutraceutical," *Nutrition Research Reviews* 33, no. 2 (December 2020): 190–217, doi: 10.1017/S0954422419000301.

18. Einar Smith et al., "Ergothioneine Is Associated with Reduced Mortality and Decreased Risk of Cardiovascular Disease," *Heart (British Cardiac Society)* 106, no. 9 (May 2020): 691–97, doi: 10.1136/heartjnl-2019-315485.
19. Masahiro Kameda et al., "Frailty Markers Comprise Blood Metabolites Involved in Antioxidation, Cognition, and Mobility," *Proceedings of the National Academy of Sciences of the United States of America* 117, no. 17 (April 2020): 9,483–89, doi: 10.1073/pnas.1920795117.
20. Robert B. Beelman et al., "Is Ergothioneine a 'Longevity Vitamin' Limited in the American Diet?" *Journal of Nutritional Science* 9 (November 2020): e52, doi: 10.1017/jns.2020.44.
21. P. C. Barko et al., "The Gastrointestinal Microbiome: A Review," *Journal of Veterinary Internal Medicine* 32, no. 1 (January 2018): 9–25, doi: 10.1111/jvim.14875.
22. Eman Zakaria Gomaa, "Human Gut Microbiota/Microbiome in Health and Diseases: A Review," *Antonie van Leeuwenhoek* 113, no. 12 (December 2020): 2,019–40, doi: 10.1007/s10482-020-01474-7.
23. Gary D. Wu, "The Gut Microbiome, Its Metabolome, and Their Relationship to Health and Disease," *Nestle Nutrition Institute Workshop Series* 84 (2016): 103–10, doi: 10.1159/000436993.
24. Daniel So et al., "Dietary Fiber Intervention on Gut Microbiota Composition in Healthy Adults: A Systematic Review and Meta-Analysis," *American Journal of Clinical Nutrition* 107, no. 6 (June 2018): 965–83, doi: 10.1093/ajcn/nqy041.
25. H. L. Simpson and B. J. Campbell, "Review Article: Dietary Fibre–Microbiota Interactions," *Alimentary Pharmacology & Therapeutics* 42, no. 2 (July 2015): 158–79, doi: 10.1111/apt.13248.
26. Daniel McDonald et al., "American Gut: An Open Platform for Citizen Science Microbiome Research," *mSystems* 3, no. 3 (May 2018): e00031-18, doi: 10.1128/mSystems.00031-18.
27. Adam V. Weizman and Geoffrey Christopher Nguyen, "Diverticular Disease: Epidemiology and Management," *Canadian Journal of Gastroenterology* 25, no. 7 (July 2011): 385–89, doi: 10.1155/2011/795241.
28. Juozas Kupcinskas et al., "Pathogenesis of Diverticulosis and Diverticular Disease," *Journal of Gastrointestinal and Liver Diseases* 28, Supplement 4 (December 2019): 7–10, doi: 10.15403/jgld-551.
29. Mona Rezapour, Saima Ali, and Neil Stollman, "Diverticular Disease: An Update on Pathogenesis and Management," *Gut and Liver* 12, no. 2 (March 2018): 125–32, doi: 10.5009/gnl16552.
30. Marilia Carabotti et al., "Role of Fiber in Symptomatic Uncomplicated Diverticular Disease: A Systematic Review," *Nutrients* 9, no. 2 (February 2017): 161, doi: 10.3390/nu9020161.
31. James M. Dahlhamer, PhD, et al., "Prevalence of Inflammatory Bowel Disease among Adults Aged ≥18 Years—United States, 2015," *Morbidity and Mortality Weekly Report* 65, no. 42 (October 2016): 1,166–69, doi: 10.15585/mmwr.mm6542a3.
32. Jason K. Hou, Bincy Abraham, and Hashem El-Serag, "Dietary Intake and

Risk of Developing Inflammatory Bowel Disease: A Systematic Review of the Literature," *American Journal of Gastroenterology* 106, no. 4 (April 2011): 563–73, doi: 10.1038/ajg.2011.44.

33. Donald Goens and Dejan Micic, "Role of Diet in the Development and Management of Crohn's Disease," *Current Gastroenterology Reports* 22, no. 4 (March 2020): 19, doi: 10.1007/s11894-020-0755-9.
34. Caroline Canavan, Joe West, and Timothy Card, "The Epidemiology of Irritable Bowel Syndrome," *Clinical Epidemiology* 6 (February 2014): 71–80, doi: 10.2147/CLEP.S40245.
35. Magdy El-Salhy et al., "Dietary Fiber in Irritable Bowel Syndrome (Review)," *International Journal of Molecular Medicine* 40, no. 3 (September 2017): 607–13, doi: 10.3892/ijmm.2017.3072.
36. Tao Zhang et al., "Efficacy of Probiotics for Irritable Bowel Syndrome: A Systematic Review and Network Meta-Analysis," *Frontiers in Cellular and Infection Microbiology* 12 (April 2022): 859967, doi: 10.3389/fcimb.2022.859967.
37. Adelina Nicoleta Galica, Reitano Galica, and Dan Lucian Dumitraşcu, "Diet, Fibers, and Probiotics for Irritable Bowel Syndrome," *Journal of Medicine and Life* 15, no. 2 (February 2022): 174–79, doi: 10.25122/jml-2022-0028.
38. Yang Yang et al., "Association between Dietary Fiber and Lower Risk of All-Cause Mortality: A Meta-Analysis of Cohort Studies," *American Journal of Epidemiology* 181, no. 2 (January 2015): 83–91, doi: 10.1093/aje/kwu257.
39. Robynne Chutkan et al., "Viscous versus Nonviscous Soluble Fiber Supplements: Mechanisms and Evidence for Fiber-Specific Health Benefits," *Journal of the American Academy of Nurse Practitioners* 24, no. 8 (August 2012): 476–87, doi: 10.1111/j.1745-7599.2012.00758.x.
40. Maria L. Marco et al., "Health Benefits of Fermented Foods: Microbiota and Beyond," *Current Opinion in Biotechnology* 44 (April 2017): 94–102, doi: 10.1016/j.copbio.2016.11.010; and Nevin Şanlier, Büsra Basar Gökcen, and Aybüke Ceyhun Sezgin, "Health Benefits of Fermented Foods," *Critical Reviews in Food Science and Nutrition* 59, no. 3 (2019): 506–27, doi: 10.1080/10408398.2017.1383355.
41. Hannah C. Wastyk et al., "Gut-Microbiota-Targeted Diets Modulate Human Immune Status," *Cell* 184, no. 16 (August 2021): 4,137–53.e14, doi: 10.1016/j.cell.2021.06.019.
42. In Hwa Choi et al., "Kimchi, a Fermented Vegetable, Improves Serum Lipid Profiles in Healthy Young Adults: Randomized Clinical Trial," *Journal of Medicinal Food* 16, no. 3 (March 2013): 223–29, doi: 10.1089/jmf.2012.2563.
43. Connie W. Tsao et al., "Heart Disease and Stroke Statistics—2022 Update: A Report from the American Heart Association," *Circulation* 145, no. 8 (February 2022): e153–e639, doi: 10.1161/CIR.0000000000001052.
44. Ghada A. Soliman, "Dietary Cholesterol and the Lack of Evidence in Cardiovascular Disease," *Nutrients* 10, no. 6 (June 2018): 780, doi: 10.3390/nu10060780.
45. Lukas Schwingshackl and Georg Hoffmann, "Monounsaturated Fatty Acids, Olive Oil and Health Status: A Systematic Review and Meta-Analysis of Cohort

Studies," *Lipids in Health and Disease* 13 (October 2014): 154, doi: 10.1186/1476-511X-13-154.

46. Marta Guasch-Ferré et al., "Olive Oil Intake and Risk of Cardiovascular Disease and Mortality in the PREDIMED Study," *BMC Medicine* 12 (May 2014): 78, doi: 10.1186/1741-7015-12-78.
47. Saeed Ghobadi et al., "Comparison of Blood Lipid–Lowering Effects of Olive Oil and Other Plant Oils: A Systematic Review and Meta-Analysis of 27 Randomized Placebo-Controlled Clinical Trials," *Critical Reviews in Food Science and Nutrition* 59, no. 13 (2019): 2,110–24, doi: 10.1080/10408398.2018.1438349.
48. Marta Guasch-Ferré et al., "Consumption of Olive Oil and Risk of Total and Cause-Specific Mortality among U.S. Adults," *Journal of the American College of Cardiology* 79, no. 2 (January 2022): 101–12, doi: 10.1016/j.jacc.2021.10.041.
49. Helioswilton Sales-Campos et al., "An Overview of the Modulatory Effects of Oleic Acid in Health and Disease," *Mini Reviews in Medicinal Chemistry* 13, no. 2 (February 2013): 201–10, https://pubmed.ncbi.nlm.nih.gov/23278117/.
50. P. M. Kris-Etherton et al., "High-Monounsaturated Fatty Acid Diets Lower Both Plasma Cholesterol and Triacylglycerol Concentrations," *American Journal of Clinical Nutrition* 70, no. 6 (December 1999): 1,009–15, doi: 10.1093/ajcn/70.6.1009.
51. Keyhan Lotfi et al., "Dietary Intakes of Monounsaturated Fatty Acids and Risk of Mortality from All Causes, Cardiovascular Disease and Cancer: A Systematic Review and Dose-Response Meta-Analysis of Prospective Cohort Studies," *Ageing Research Reviews* 72 (December 2021): 101467, doi: 10.1016/j.arr.2021.101467.
52. S. Terés et al., "Oleic Acid Content Is Responsible for the Reduction in Blood Pressure Induced by Olive Oil," *Proceedings of the National Academy of Sciences of the United States of America* 105, no. 37 (September 2008): 13,811–16, doi: 10.1073/pnas.0807500105.
53. Jennifer J. Manly et al., "Estimating the Prevalence of Dementia and Mild Cognitive Impairment in the US: The 2016 Health and Retirement Study Harmonized Cognitive Assessment Protocol Project," *JAMA Neurology* 79, no. 12 (December 2022): 1,242–49, doi: 10.1001/jamaneurol.2022.3543.
54. Tomasz Wysoczański et al., "Omega-3 Fatty Acids and Their Role in Central Nervous System—A Review," *Current Medicinal Chemistry* 23, no. 8 (2016): 816–31, doi: 10.2174/0929867323666160122114439.
55. Michelle Healy-Stoffel and Beth Levant, "N-3 (Omega-3) Fatty Acids: Effects on Brain Dopamine Systems and Potential Role in the Etiology and Treatment of Neuropsychiatric Disorders," *CNS & Neurological Disorders Drug Targets* 17, no. 3 (2018): 216–32, doi: 10.2174/1871527317666180412153612; and Carlo Agostoni et al., "The Role of Omega-3 Fatty Acids in Developmental Psychopathology: A Systematic Review on Early Psychosis, Autism, and ADHD," *International Journal of Molecular Sciences* 18, no. 12 (December 2017): 2608, doi: 10.3390/ijms18122608.
56. Parris M. Kidd, "Omega-3 DHA and EPA for Cognition, Behavior, and Mood: Clinical Findings and Structural-Functional Synergies with Cell Membrane Phospholipids," *Alternative Medicine Review* 12, no. 3 (September 2007): 207–27, https://pubmed.ncbi.nlm.nih.gov/18072818/.

57. Rajesh Narendran et al., "Improved Working Memory but No Effect on Striatal Vesicular Monoamine Transporter Type 2 after Omega-3 Polyunsaturated Fatty Acid Supplementation," *PloS One* 7, no. 10 (2012): e46832, doi: 10.1371/journal.pone.0046832.
58. Karin Yurko-Mauro, Dominik D. Alexander, and Mary E. Van Elswyk, "Docosahexaenoic Acid and Adult Memory: A Systematic Review and Meta-Analysis," *PloS One* 10, no. 3 (March 2015): e0120391, doi: 10.1371/journal.pone.0120391.
59. Che-Sheng Chu et al., "Higher Serum DHA and Slower Cognitive Decline in Patients with Alzheimer's Disease: Two-Year Follow-Up," *Nutrients* 14, no. 6 (March 2022): 1159, doi: 10.3390/nu14061159.
60. Cécilia Samieri et al., "Fish Intake, Genetic Predisposition to Alzheimer Disease, and Decline in Global Cognition and Memory in 5 Cohorts of Older Persons," *American Journal of Epidemiology* 187, no. 5 (May 2018): 933–40, doi: 10.1093/aje/kwx330.
61. Yu Zhang et al., "Intakes of Fish and Polyunsaturated Fatty Acids and Mild-to-Severe Cognitive Impairment Risks: A Dose-Response Meta-Analysis of 21 Cohort Studies," *American Journal of Clinical Nutrition* 103, no. 2 (February 2016): 330–40, doi: 10.3945/ajcn.115.124081.
62. Rena I. Kosti et al., "Fish Intake, n-3 Fatty Acid Body Status, and Risk of Cognitive Decline: A Systematic Review and a Dose-Response Meta-Analysis of Observational and Experimental Studies," *Nutrition Reviews* 80, no. 6 (May 2022): 1,445–58, doi: 10.1093/nutrit/nuab078.
63. Marie N. Teisen et al., "Effects of Oily Fish Intake on Cognitive and Socioemotional Function in Healthy 8-9-Year-Old Children: The FiSK Junior Randomized Trial," *American Journal of Clinical Nutrition* 112, no. 1 (July 2020): 74–83, doi: 10.1093/ajcn/nqaa050.
64. Charles D. Scales Jr. et al., "Prevalence of Kidney Stones in the United States," *European Urology* 62, no. 1 (July 2012): 160–65, doi: 10.1016/j.eururo.2012.03.052.
65. Pietro Manuel Ferraro et al., "Risk of Kidney Stones: Influence of Dietary Factors, Dietary Patterns, and Vegetarian-Vegan Diets," *Nutrients* 12, no. 3 (March 2020): 779, doi: 10.3390/nu12030779.
66. E. Jéquier and F. Constant, "Water as an Essential Nutrient: The Physiological Basis of Hydration," *European Journal of Clinical Nutrition* 64, no. 2 (February 2010): 115–23, doi: 10.1038/ejcn.2009.111.
67. Tue H. Hansen et al., "The Effect of Drinking Water pH on the Human Gut Microbiota and Glucose Regulation: Results of a Randomized Controlled Cross-Over Intervention," *Scientific Reports* 8, no. 1 (November 2018): 16626, doi: 10.1038/s41598-018-34761-5.
68. Carol Boushey et al., *Dietary Patterns and All-Cause Mortality: A Systematic Review* (Alexandria, VA: USDA Nutrition Evidence Systematic Review, 2020).
69. Kevin D. Hall et al., "Energy Expenditure and Body Composition Changes after an Isocaloric Ketogenic Diet in Overweight and Obese Men," *American Journal of Clinical Nutrition* 104, no. 2 (August 2016): 324–33, doi: 10.3945/ajcn.116.133561; and Kevin D. Hall and Stephanie T. Chung, "Low-

Carbohydrate Diets for the Treatment of Obesity and Type 2 Diabetes," *Current Opinion in Clinical Nutrition and Metabolic Care* 21, no. 4 (July 2018): 308–12, doi: 10.1097/MCO.0000000000000470.

70. Sigrid Gibson et al., "The Effects of Sucrose on Metabolic Health: A Systematic Review of Human Intervention Studies in Healthy Adults," *Critical Reviews in Food Science and Nutrition* 53, no. 6 (2013): 591–614, doi: 10.1080/10408398.2012.691574.
71. Marie Lindefeldt et al., "The Ketogenic Diet Influences Taxonomic and Functional Composition of the Gut Microbiota in Children with Severe Epilepsy," *NPJ Biofilms and Microbiomes* 5, no. 1 (2019): 5, doi: 10.1038/s41522-018-0073-2.
72. Angela Genoni et al., "Long-Term Paleolithic Diet Is Associated with Lower Resistant Starch Intake, Different Gut Microbiota Composition and Increased Serum TMAO Concentrations," *European Journal of Nutrition* 59, no. 5 (August 2020): 1,845–58, doi: 10.1007/s00394-019-02036-y.
73. Claudio Hidalgo-Cantabrana et al., "Bifidobacteria and Their Health-Promoting Effects," *Microbiology Spectrum* 5, no. 3 (June 2017), doi: 10.1128/microbiolspec. BAD-0010-2016; and Li-Hao Cheng et al., "Psychobiotics in Mental Health, Neurodegenerative and Neurodevelopmental Disorders," *Journal of Food and Drug Analysis* 27, no. 3 (July 2019): 632–48, doi: 10.1016/j.jfda.2019.01.002.
74. Zohreh Tamanai-Shacoori et al., "Roseburia spp.: A Marker of Health?" *Future Microbiology* 12 (February 2017): 157–70, doi: 10.2217/fmb-2016-0130.
75. Lukas Schwingshackl et al., "Total Dietary Fat Intake, Fat Quality, and Health Outcomes: A Scoping Review of Systematic Reviews of Prospective Studies," *Annals of Nutrition & Metabolism* 77, no. 1 (2021): 4–15, doi: 10.1159/000515058.
76. Priyanka Bhandari and Amit Sapra, "Low Fat Diet," in *StatPearls* (Treasure Island, FL: StatPearls Publishing, 2023).
77. Ronald M. Krauss and Penny M. Kris-Etherton, "Public Health Guidelines Should Recommend Reducing Saturated Fat Consumption as Much as Possible: Debate Consensus," *American Journal of Clinical Nutrition* 112, no. 1 (July 2020): 25–26, doi: 10.1093/ajcn/nqaa134; and Nina Teicholz, "A Short History of Saturated Fat: The Making and Unmaking of a Scientific Consensus," *Current Opinion in Endocrinology, Diabetes, and Obesity* 30, no. 1 (February 2023): 65–71, doi: 10.1097/MED.0000000000000791.
78. Russell J. de Souza et al., "Intake of Saturated and Trans Unsaturated Fatty Acids and Risk of All Cause Mortality, Cardiovascular Disease, and Type 2 Diabetes: Systematic Review and Meta-Analysis of Observational Studies," *BMJ (Clinical Research Ed.)* 351 (2015): h3978, doi: 10.1136/bmj.h3978; and Patty W. Siri-Tarino et al., "Meta-Analysis of Prospective Cohort Studies Evaluating the Association of Saturated Fat with Cardiovascular Disease," *American Journal of Clinical Nutrition* 91, no. 3 (March 2010): 535–46, doi: 10.3945/ajcn.2009.27725.
79. Lee Hooper et al., "Reduction in Saturated Fat Intake for Cardiovascular Disease," *Cochrane Database of Systematic Reviews* 8, no. 8 (August 2020): CD011737, doi: 10.1002/14651858.CD011737.pub3.
80. Arne Astrup et al., "Saturated Fats and Health: A Reassessment and Proposal for

Food-Based Recommendations: JACC State-of-the-Art Review," *Journal of the American College of Cardiology* 76, no. 7 (August 2020): 844–57, doi: 10.1016/j.jacc.2020.05.077.

81. Mary Weiler, Steven R. Hertzler, and Svyatoslav Dvoretskiy, "Is It Time to Reconsider the U.S. Recommendations for Dietary Protein and Amino Acid Intake?" *Nutrients* 15, no. 4 (February 2023): 838, doi: 10.3390/nu15040838.
82. Mathilde Simonson, Yves Boirie, and Christelle Guillet, "Protein, Amino Acids and Obesity Treatment," *Reviews in Endocrine & Metabolic Disorders* 21, no. 3 (September 2020): 341–53, doi: 10.1007/s11154-020-09574-5.
83. Samuel Mettler, Nigel Mitchell, and Kevin D. Tipton, "Increased Protein Intake Reduces Lean Body Mass Loss during Weight Loss in Athletes," *Medicine and Science in Sports and Exercise* 42, no. 2 (February 2010): 326–37, doi: 10.1249/MSS.0b013e3181b2ef8e.
84. Stefan M. Pasiakos et al., "Effects of High-Protein Diets on Fat-Free Mass and Muscle Protein Synthesis Following Weight Loss: A Randomized Controlled Trial," *FASEB Journal* 27, no. 9 (June 2013): 3,837–47, doi: 10.1096/fj.13-230227.
85. Stephan von Haehling, John E. Morley, and Stefan D. Anker, "An Overview of Sarcopenia: Facts and Numbers on Prevalence and Clinical Impact," *Journal of Cachexia, Sarcopenia and Muscle* 1, no. 2 (December 2010): 129–33, doi: 10.1007/s13539-010-0014-2.
86. Jupil Ko and Young-Min Park, "Menopause and the Loss of Skeletal Muscle Mass in Women," *Iranian Journal of Public Health* 50, no. 2 (February 2021): 413–14, doi: 10.18502/ijph.v50i2.5362.
87. Patricia S. Rogeri et al., "Strategies to Prevent Sarcopenia in the Aging Process: Role of Protein Intake and Exercise," *Nutrients* 14, no. 1 (December 2021): 52, doi: 10.3390/nu14010052.
88. L. Gregorio et al., "Adequate Dietary Protein Is Associated with Better Physical Performance among Post-Menopausal Women 60–90 Years," *Journal of Nutrition, Health & Aging* 18, no. 2 (2014): 155–60, doi: 10.1007/s12603-013-0391-2.
89. Denise K. Houston et al., "Dietary Protein Intake Is Associated with Lean Mass Change in Older, Community-Dwelling Adults: The Health, Aging, and Body Composition (Health ABC) Study," *American Journal of Clinical Nutrition* 87, no. 1 (January 2008): 150–55, doi: 10.1093/ajcn/87.1.150.

Chapter 6: Magnificent Minerals

1. Kenneth J. Carpenter, "A Short History of Nutritional Science: Part 1 (1785–1885)," *Journal of Nutrition* 133, no. 3 (March 2003): 638–45, doi: 10.1093/jn/133.3.638.
2. Louis Rosenfeld, "Discovery and Early Uses of Iodine," *Journal of Chemical Education* 77, no. 8 (2000): 984–87, doi: 10.1021/ed077p984.
3. Angela M. Leung, Lewis E. Braverman, and Elizabeth N. Pearce, "History of U.S. Iodine Fortification and Supplementation," *Nutrients* 4, no. 11 (November 2012): 1,740–46, doi: 10.3390/nu4111740; and Penjani Mkambula et al., "The Unfinished Agenda for Food Fortification in Low- and Middle-Income Countries: Quantifying Progress, Gaps and Potential Opportunities," *Nutrients* 12, no. 2 (2020): 354, doi: 10.3390/nu12020354.

4. Flavia Fayet-Moore et al., "An Analysis of the Mineral Composition of Pink Salt Available in Australia," *Foods (Basel, Switzerland)* 9, no. 10 (October 2020): 1490, doi: 10.3390/foods9101490.
5. M. Bouga and E. Combet, "Emergence of Seaweed and Seaweed-Containing Foods in the UK: Focus on Labeling, Iodine Content, Toxicity and Nutrition," *Foods (Basel, Switzerland)* 4, no. 2 (2015): 240–53, doi: 10.3390/foods4020240.
6. Rie Kishida et al., "Frequency of Seaweed Intake and Its Association with Cardiovascular Disease Mortality: The JACC Study," *Journal of Atherosclerosis and Thrombosis* 27, no. 12 (December 2020): 1,340–47, doi: 10.5551/jat.53447.
7. Sanae Matsuyama et al., "Association between Adherence to the Japanese Diet and All-Cause and Cause-Specific Mortality: The Japan Public Health Center–Based Prospective Study," *European Journal of Nutrition* 60, no. 3 (July 2020): 1,327–36, doi: 10.1007/s00394-020-02330-0.
8. Sharon A. Winer and Andrea J. Rapkin, "Premenstrual Disorders: Prevalence, Etiology and Impact," *Journal of Reproductive Medicine* 51, Supplement 4 (April 2006): 339–47, https://pubmed.ncbi.nlm.nih.gov/16734317/.
9. Arman Arab et al., "Beneficial Role of Calcium in Premenstrual Syndrome: A Systematic Review of Current Literature," *International Journal of Preventive Medicine* 11 (September 2020): 156, doi: 10.4103/ijpvm.IJPVM_243_19.
10. Elizabeth R. Bertone-Johnson et al., "Calcium and Vitamin D Intake and Risk of Incident Premenstrual Syndrome," *Archives of Internal Medicine* 165, no. 11 (June 2005): 1,246–52, doi: 10.1001/archinte.165.11.1246.
11. S. Thys-Jacobs et al., "Calcium Carbonate and the Premenstrual Syndrome: Effects on Premenstrual and Menstrual Symptoms. Premenstrual Syndrome Study Group," *American Journal of Obstetrics and Gynecology* 179, no. 2 (August 1998): 444–52, doi: 10.1016/s0002-9378(98)70377-1.
12. Fatemeh Abdi et al., "Role of Vitamin D and Calcium in the Relief of Primary Dysmenorrhea: A Systematic Review," *Obstetrics & Gynecology Science* 64, no. 1 (January 2021): 13–26, doi: 10.5468/ogs.20205.
13. Bertone-Johnson et al., "Calcium and Vitamin D Intake and Risk of Incident Premenstrual Syndrome."
14. Lars Jacob Stovner et al., "The Global Prevalence of Headache: An Update, with Analysis of the Influences of Methodological Factors on Prevalence Estimates," *Journal of Headache and Pain* 23, no. 1 (April 2022): 34, doi: 10.1186/s10194-022-01402-2.
15. Jeanette A. Maier et al., "Headaches and Magnesium: Mechanisms, Bioavailability, Therapeutic Efficacy and Potential Advantage of Magnesium Pidolate," *Nutrients* 12, no. 9 (2020): 2660, doi: 10.3390/nu12092660.
16. Olga Cozzolino et al., "Understanding Spreading Depression from Headache to Sudden Unexpected Death," *Frontiers in Neurology* 9 (February 2018): 19, doi: 10.3389/fneur.2018.00019.
17. Andrew C. Miller et al., "Intravenous Magnesium Sulfate to Treat Acute Headaches in the Emergency Department: A Systematic Review," *Headache* 59, no. 10 (November 2019): 1,674–86, doi: 10.1111/head.13648.
18. A. Peikert, C. Wilimzig, and R. Köhne-Volland, "Prophylaxis of Migraine with

Oral Magnesium: Results from a Prospective, Multi-Center, Placebo-Controlled and Double-Blind Randomized Study," *Cephalalgia* 16, no. 4 (June 1996): 257–63, doi: 10.1046/j.1468-2982.1996.1604257.x.

19. Yechiam Ostchega, PhD, RN, et al., "Hypertension Prevalence among Adults Aged 18 and Over: United States, 2017–2018," *NCHS Data Brief* no. 364 (April 2020): 1–8, https://www.cdc.gov/nchs/data/databriefs/db364-h.pdf.
20. William Insull Jr., "The Pathology of Atherosclerosis: Plaque Development and Plaque Responses to Medical Treatment," *American Journal of Medicine* 122, Supplement 1 (January 2009): S3–S14, doi: 10.1016/j.amjmed.2008.10.013.
21. Andrea Grillo et al., "Sodium Intake and Hypertension," *Nutrients* 11, no. 9 (August 2019): 1970, doi: 10.3390/nu11091970.
22. Feng J. He, Jiafu Li, and Graham A. MacGregor, "Effect of Longer Term Modest Salt Reduction on Blood Pressure: Cochrane Systematic Review and Meta-Analysis of Randomised Trials," *BMJ (Clinical Research Ed.)* 346 (2013): f1325, doi: 10.1136/bmj.f1325.
23. Connie M. Weaver, "Potassium and Health," *Advances in Nutrition (Bethesda, Md.)* 4, no. 3 (May 2013): 368S–77S, doi: 10.3945/an.112.003533.
24. Aristea Binia et al., "Daily Potassium Intake and Sodium-to-Potassium Ratio in the Reduction of Blood Pressure: A Meta-Analysis of Randomized Controlled Trials," *Journal of Hypertension* 33, no. 8 (August 2015): 1,509–20, doi: 10.1097/HJH.0000000000000611.
25. Christina D. Filippou et al., "Dietary Approaches to Stop Hypertension (DASH) Diet and Blood Pressure Reduction in Adults with and without Hypertension: A Systematic Review and Meta-Analysis of Randomized Controlled Trials," *Advances in Nutrition (Bethesda, Md.)* 11, no. 5 (September 2020): 1,150–60, doi: 10.1093/advances/nmaa041.
26. Natalie Blanch et al., "Effect of Sodium and Potassium Supplementation on Vascular and Endothelial Function: A Randomized Controlled Trial," *American Journal of Clinical Nutrition* 101, no. 5 (May 2015): 939–46, doi: 10.3945/ajcn.114.105197.
27. Michael S. Stone, Berdine R. Martin, and Connie M. Weaver, "Short-Term RCT of Increased Dietary Potassium from Potato or Potassium Gluconate: Effect on Blood Pressure, Microcirculation, and Potassium and Sodium Retention in Pre-Hypertensive-to-Hypertensive Adults," *Nutrients* 13, no. 5 (2021): 1610, doi: 10.3390/nu13051610.
28. Kholood M. Mugharbel and Mowaffaq A. Al-Mansouri, "Prevalence of Obesity among Type 2 Diabetic Patients in Al-Khobar Primary Health Care Centers," *Journal of Family & Community Medicine* 10, no. 2 (May 2003): 49–53, https://pubmed.ncbi.nlm.nih.gov/23011992/.
29. Unai Galicia-Garcia et al., "Pathophysiology of Type 2 Diabetes Mellitus," *International Journal of Molecular Sciences* 21, no. 17 (2020): 6275, doi: 10.3390/ijms21176275.
30. Yinan Hua et al., "Molecular Mechanisms of Chromium in Alleviating Insulin Resistance," *Journal of Nutritional Biochemistry* 23, no. 4 (April 2012): 313–19, doi: 10.1016/j.jnutbio.2011.11.001.

31. W. Mertz, "Chromium in Human Nutrition: A Review," *Journal of Nutrition* 123, no. 4 (April 1993): 626–33, doi: 10.1093/jn/123.4.626.
32. R. A. Anderson et al., "Elevated Intakes of Supplemental Chromium Improve Glucose and Insulin Variables in Individuals with Type 2 Diabetes," *Diabetes* 46, no. 11 (November 1997): 1,786–91, doi: 10.2337/diab.46.11.1786.
33. Sheng Yuan et al., "Chocolate Consumption and Risk of Coronary Heart Disease, Stroke, and Diabetes: A Meta-Analysis of Prospective Studies," *Nutrients* 9, no. 7 (July 2017): 688, doi: 10.3390/nu9070688.
34. Ali Rostami et al., "High-Cocoa Polyphenol-Rich Chocolate Improves Blood Pressure in Patients with Diabetes and Hypertension," *ARYA Atherosclerosis* 11, no. 1 (January 2015): 21–29, https://www.ncbi.nlm.nih.gov/pmc/articles/PMC4460349/.
35. Kathleen L. Wyne et al., "Hypothyroidism Prevalence in the United States: A Retrospective Study Combining National Health and Nutrition Examination Survey and Claims Data, 2009–2019," *Journal of the Endocrine Society* 7, no. 1 (November 2022): bvac172, doi: 10.1210/jendso/bvac172.
36. Ulrike Gottwald-Hostalek and Barbara Schulte, "Low Awareness and Under-Diagnosis of Hypothyroidism," *Current Medical Research and Opinion* 38, no. 1 (January 2022): 59–64, doi: 10.1080/03007995.2021.1997258.
37. Alessandra Quintino-Moro et al., "High Prevalence of Infertility among Women with Graves' Disease and Hashimoto's Thyroiditis," *International Journal of Endocrinology* 2014 (2014): 982705, doi: 10.1155/2014/982705.
38. Antonio C. Bianco et al., "Adaptive Activation of Thyroid Hormone and Energy Expenditure," *Bioscience Reports* 25, nos. 3–4 (June–August 2005): 191–208, doi: 10.1007/s10540-005-2885-6.
39. Mara Ventura, Miguel Melo, and Francisco Carrilho, "Selenium and Thyroid Disease: From Pathophysiology to Treatment." *International Journal of Endocrinology* 2017 (2017): 1297658, doi: 10.1155/2017/1297658.
40. Lutz Schomburg, "Selenium, Selenoproteins and the Thyroid Gland: Interactions in Health and Disease," *Nature Reviews. Endocrinology* 8, no. 3 (October 2011): 160–71, doi: 10.1038/nrendo.2011.174.
41. Fei Wang et al., "Selenium and Thyroid Diseases," *Frontiers in Endocrinology* 14 (2023): 1133000, doi: 10.3389/fendo.2023.1133000.
42. Ying Zuo et al., "The Correlation between Selenium Levels and Autoimmune Thyroid Disease: A Systematic Review and Meta-Analysis," *Annals of Palliative Medicine* 10, no. 4 (April 2021): 4,398–408, doi: 10.21037/apm-21-449; and Konstantinos A. Toulis et al., "Selenium Supplementation in the Treatment of Hashimoto's Thyroiditis: A Systematic Review and a Meta-Analysis," *Thyroid* 20, no. 10 (October 2010): 1,163–73, doi: 10.1089/thy.2009.0351.
43. Milena Barcza Stockler-Pinto et al., "Effect of Selenium Supplementation via Brazil Nut (*Bertholletia excelsa*, HBK) on Thyroid Hormones Levels in Hemodialysis Patients: A Pilot Study," *Nutricion hospitalaria* 32, no. 4 (October 2015): 1,808–12, doi: 10.3305/nh.2015.32.4.9384.
44. M. Lemire et al., "No Evidence of Selenosis from a Selenium-Rich Diet in the Brazilian Amazon," *Environment International* 40 (2012): 128–36, doi: 10.1016/j.envint.2011.07.005.

45. Ananda S. Prasad, "Discovery of Human Zinc Deficiency: Its Impact on Human Health and Disease," *Advances in Nutrition (Bethesda, Md.)* 4, no. 2 (March 2013): 176–90, doi: 10.3945/an.112.003210.
46. Maria Maares and Hajo Haase, "Zinc and Immunity: An Essential Interrelation," *Archives of Biochemistry and Biophysics* 611 (December 2016): 58–65, doi: 10.1016/j.abb.2016.03.022.
47. Harri Hemilä, "Zinc Lozenges and the Common Cold: A Meta-Analysis Comparing Zinc Acetate and Zinc Gluconate, and the Role of Zinc Dosage," *JRSM Open* 8, no. 5 (May 2017), doi: 10.1177/2054270417694291.
48. Harri Hemilä and Elizabeth Chalker, "The Effectiveness of High Dose Zinc Acetate Lozenges on Various Common Cold Symptoms: A Meta-Analysis," *BMC Family Practice* 16 (February 2015): 24, doi: 10.1186/s12875-015-0237-6.
49. Ibid.
50. S. Sazawal et al., "Zinc Supplementation Reduces the Incidence of Acute Lower Respiratory Infections in Infants and Preschool Children: A Double-Blind, Controlled Trial," *Pediatrics* 102, 1 Pt 1 (July 1998): 1–5, doi: 10.1542/peds.102.1.1.
51. Martina Maywald and Lothar Rink, "Zinc in Human Health and Infectious Diseases," *Biomolecules* 12, no. 12 (2022): 1748, doi: 10.3390/biom12121748.
52. Christa Fischer Walker and Robert E. Black, "Zinc and the Risk for Infectious Disease," *Annual Review of Nutrition* 24 (2004): 255–75, doi: 10.1146/annurev.nutr.23.011702.073054.

Chapter 7: Vital Vitamins

1. Richard D. Semba, "Paris in the Time of François Magendie," *World Review of Nutrition and Dietetics* 104 (2012): 20–40, doi: 10.1159/000338584.
2. Richard D. Semba, "The Discovery of the Vitamins," *International Journal for Vitamin and Nutrition Research* 82, no. 5 (October 2012): 310–15, doi: 10.1024/0300-9831/a000124.
3. Richard D. Semba, "On the 'Discovery' of Vitamin A," *Annals of Nutrition & Metabolism* 61, no. 3 (2012): 192–98, doi: 10.1159/000343124.
4. Kenneth J. Carpenter, "A Short History of Nutritional Science: Part 1 (1785–1885)," *Journal of Nutrition* 133, no. 3 (March 2003): 638–45, doi: 10.1093/jn/133.3.638.
5. Sermin Timur and Nevin Hotun Sahin, "The Prevalence of Depression Symptoms and Influencing Factors among Perimenopausal and Postmenopausal Women," *Menopause (New York, N.Y.)* 17, no. 3 (May–June 2010): 545–51, doi: 10.1097/gme.0b013e3181cf8997.
6. Hadine Joffe, Anda Massler, and Katherine M. Sharkey, "Evaluation and Management of Sleep Disturbance during the Menopause Transition," *Seminars in Reproductive Medicine* 28, no. 5 (September 2010): 404–21, doi: 10.1055/s-0030-1262900.
7. Lin Ge et al., "Association of Pyridoxal 5'-Phosphate with Sleep-Related Problems in a General Population," *Nutrients* 14, no. 17 (August 2022): 3516, doi: 10.3390/nu14173516.

8. Carolina García-García and Inkyung Baik, "Effects of Poly-Gamma-Glutamic Acid and Vitamin B6 Supplements on Sleep Status: A Randomized Intervention Study," *Nutrition Research and Practice* 15, no. 3 (June 2021): 309–18, doi: 10.4162/nrp.2021.15.3.309.
9. Patrick Lemoine, Jena-Christophe Bablon, and Christèle Da Silva, "A Combination of Melatonin, Vitamin B6 and Medicinal Plants in the Treatment of Mild-to-Moderate Insomnia: A Prospective Pilot Study," *Complementary Therapies in Medicine* 45 (August 2019): 104–8, doi: 10.1016/j.ctim.2019.05.024; and Gorica Djokic et al., "The Effects of Magnesium–Melatonin–Vit B Complex Supplementation in Treatment of Insomnia," *Open Access Macedonian Journal of Medical Sciences* 7, no. 18 (August 2019): 3,101–5, doi: 10.3889/oamjms.2019.771.
10. Tamami Odai et al., "Depressive Symptoms in Middle-Aged and Elderly Women Are Associated with a Low Intake of Vitamin B6: A Cross-Sectional Study," *Nutrients* 12, no. 11 (2020): 3437, doi: 10.3390/nu12113437.
11. David T. Field et al., "High-Dose Vitamin B6 Supplementation Reduces Anxiety and Strengthens Visual Surround Suppression," *Human Psychopharmacology* 37, no. 6 (November 2022): e2852, doi: 10.1002/hup.2852.
12. A. H. Maclennan et al., "Oral Oestrogen and Combined Oestrogen/Progestogen Therapy versus Placebo for Hot Flushes," *Cochrane Database of Systematic Reviews* 2004, no. 4 (October 2004): CD002978, doi: 10.1002/14651858.CD002978.pub2.
13. John Paciuc, "Hormone Therapy in Menopause," *Advances in Experimental Medicine and Biology* 1242 (2020): 89–120, doi: 10.1007/978-3-030-38474-6_6; and Annalisa Geraci et al., "Sarcopenia and Menopause: The Role of Estradiol," *Frontiers in Endocrinology* 12 (May 2021): 682012, doi: 10.3389/fendo.2021.682012.
14. Howard N. Hodis and Wendy J. Mack, "Menopausal Hormone Replacement Therapy and Reduction of All-Cause Mortality and Cardiovascular Disease: It Is about Time and Timing," *Cancer Journal (Sudbury, Mass.)* 28, no. 3 (May/June 2022): 208–23, https://doi.org/10.1097/PPO.0000000000000591.
15. Katherine A. Guthrie et al., "Effects of Pharmacologic and Nonpharmacologic Interventions on Insomnia Symptoms and Self-Reported Sleep Quality in Women with Hot Flashes: A Pooled Analysis of Individual Participant Data from Four MsFLASH Trials," *Sleep* 41, no. 1 (January 2018): zsx190, doi: 10.1093/sleep/zsx190; and M. W. L. Morssinkhof et al., "Associations between Sex Hormones, Sleep Problems and Depression: A Systematic Review," *Neuroscience and Biobehavioral Reviews* 118 (November 2020): 669–80, doi: 10.1016/j.neubiorev.2020.08.006.
16. Andrew E. Czeizel et al., "Folate Deficiency and Folic Acid Supplementation: The Prevention of Neural-Tube Defects and Congenital Heart Defects," *Nutrients* 5, no. 11 (November 2013): 4,760–75, doi: 10.3390/nu5114760.
17. Zohra S. Lassi et al., "Folic Acid Supplementation during Pregnancy for Maternal Health and Pregnancy Outcomes," *Cochrane Database of Systematic Reviews* 2013, no. 3 (March 2013): CD006896, doi: 10.1002/14651858.CD006896.pub2.
18. Lynn L. Moore et al., "Folate Intake and the Risk of Neural Tube Defects: An

Estimation of Dose-Response," *Epidemiology (Cambridge, Mass.)* 14, no. 2 (March 2003): 200–205, doi: 10.1097/01.EDE.0000040253.12446.B2.

19. Krista S. Crider et al., "Folate and DNA Methylation: A Review of Molecular Mechanisms and the Evidence for Folate's Role," *Advances in Nutrition (Bethesda, Md.)* 3, no. 1 (January 2012): 21–38, doi: 10.3945/an.111.000992.
20. S. Voutilainen et al., "Low Dietary Folate Intake Is Associated with an Excess Incidence of Acute Coronary Events: The Kuopio Ischemic Heart Disease Risk Factor Study," *Circulation* 103, no. 22 (June 2001): 2,674–80, doi: 10.1161/01.cir.103.22.2674.
21. Dong-Hyun Kim et al., "Pooled Analyses of 13 Prospective Cohort Studies on Folate Intake and Colon Cancer," *Cancer Causes & Control* 21, no. 11 (November 2010): 1,919–30, doi: 10.1007/s10552-010-9620-8.
22. Noel G. Faux et al., "Homocysteine, Vitamin B12, and Folic Acid Levels in Alzheimer's Disease, Mild Cognitive Impairment, and Healthy Elderly: Baseline Characteristics in Subjects of the Australian Imaging Biomarker Lifestyle Study," *Journal of Alzheimer's Disease* 27, no. 4 (2011): 909–22, doi: 10.3233/JAD-2011-110752.
23. Marie A. Caudill, "Folate Bioavailability: Implications for Establishing Dietary Recommendations and Optimizing Status," *American Journal of Clinical Nutrition* 91, no. 5 (May 2010): 1,455S–60S, doi: 10.3945/ajcn.2010.28674E.
24. Doerte U. Junghaenel et al., "Demographic Correlates of Fatigue in the US General Population: Results from the Patient-Reported Outcomes Measurement Information System (PROMIS) Initiative," *Journal of Psychosomatic Research* 71, no. 3 (September 2011): 117–23, doi: 10.1016/j.jpsychores.2011.04.007.
25. Mayssam Nehme et al., "The Prevalence, Severity, and Impact of Post-COVID Persistent Fatigue, Post-Exertional Malaise, and Chronic Fatigue Syndrome," *Journal of General Internal Medicine* 38, no. 3 (February 2023): 835–39, doi: 10.1007/s11606-022-07882-x.
26. Ralph Carmel, "Subclinical Cobalamin Deficiency," *Current Opinion in Gastroenterology* 28, no. 2 (March 2012): 151–58, doi: 10.1097/MOG.0b013e3283505852.
27. Alessandra Vincenti et al., "Perspective: Practical Approach to Preventing Subclinical B12 Deficiency in Elderly Population," *Nutrients* 13, no. 6 (June 2021): 1913, doi: 10.3390/nu13061913.
28. U. Schlichtiger, K. Rettig, and S. Kauermann, "Effects of a Vitamin B6, B12, Folic Acid Combination on the Quality of Life and Vitality of Elderly People," *Geriatrie Forschung* 6 (1996): 185–96.
29. Fiona O'Leary, Margaret Allman-Farinelli, and Samir Samman, "Vitamin B12 Status, Cognitive Decline and Dementia: A Systematic Review of Prospective Cohort Studies," *British Journal of Nutrition* 108, no. 11 (December 2012): 1,948–61, doi: 10.1017/S0007114512004175.
30. Stefan Markun et al., "Effects of Vitamin B12 Supplementation on Cognitive Function, Depressive Symptoms, and Fatigue: A Systematic Review, Meta-Analysis, and Meta-Regression," *Nutrients* 13, no. 3 (March 2021): 923, doi: 10.3390/nu13030923.

31. Sudha Venkatramanan et al., "Vitamin B12 and Cognition in Children," *Advances in Nutrition (Bethesda, Md.)* 7, no. 5 (September 2016): 879–88, doi: 10.3945/an.115.012021; and M. W. Louwman et al., "Signs of Impaired Cognitive Function in Adolescents with Marginal Cobalamin Status," *American Journal of Clinical Nutrition* 72, no. 3 (September 2000): 762–69, doi: 10.1093/ajcn/72.3.762.
32. Hatice Altun et al., "Homocysteine, Pyridoxine, Folate and Vitamin B12 Levels in Children with Attention Deficit Hyperactivity Disorder," *Psychiatria Danubina* 30, no. 3 (September 2018): 310–16, doi: 10.24869/psyd.2018.310.
33. Çigdem Yektaş, Merve Alpay, and Ali Evren Tufan, "Comparison of Serum B12, Folate and Homocysteine Concentrations in Children with Autism Spectrum Disorder or Attention Deficit Hyperactivity Disorder and Healthy Controls," *Neuropsychiatric Disease and Treatment* 15 (August 2019): 2,213–19, doi: 10.2147/NDT.S212361.
34. Kamila S. Batista et al., "The Role of Vitamin B12 in Viral Infections: A Comprehensive Review of Its Relationship with the Muscle-Gut-Brain Axis and Implications for SARS-CoV-2 Infection," *Nutrition Reviews* 80, no. 3 (February 2022): 561–78, doi: 10.1093/nutrit/nuab092.
35. Andrew Kien Han Wee, "COVID-19's Toll on the Elderly and Those with Diabetes Mellitus—Is Vitamin B12 Deficiency an Accomplice?" *Medical Hypotheses* 146 (January 2021): 110374, doi: 10.1016/j.mehy.2020.110374.
36. Silke Luttenberger, Sigrid Wimmer, and Manuela Paechter, "Spotlight on Math Anxiety," *Psychology Research and Behavior Management* 2018, no. 11 (August 2018): 311–22, doi: 10.2147/PRBM.S141421.
37. Stuart Brody et al., "A Randomized Controlled Trial of High Dose Ascorbic Acid for Reduction of Blood Pressure, Cortisol, and Subjective Responses to Psychological Stress," *Psychopharmacology* 159, no. 3 (January 2002): 319–24, doi: 10.1007/s00213-001-0929-6.
38. Juliet M. Pullar, Anitra C. Carr, and Margreet C. M. Vissers, "The Roles of Vitamin C in Skin Health," *Nutrients* 9, no. 8 (August 2017): 866, doi: 10.3390/nu9080866.
39. Harri Hemilä and Elizabeth Chalker, "Vitamin C for Preventing and Treating the Common Cold," *Cochrane Database of Systematic Reviews* 2013, no. 1 (January 2013): CD000980, doi: 10.1002/14651858.CD000980.pub4.
40. Bettina Moritz et al., "The Role of Vitamin C in Stress-Related Disorders," *Journal of Nutritional Biochemistry* 85 (November 2020): 108459, doi: 10.1016/j.jnutbio.2020.108459.
41. Minju Sim et al., "Vitamin C Supplementation Promotes Mental Vitality in Healthy Young Adults: Results from a Cross-Sectional Analysis and a Randomized, Double-Blind, Placebo-Controlled Trial," *European Journal of Nutrition* 61, no. 1 (February 2022): 447–59, doi: 10.1007/s00394-021-02656-3.
42. Anitra C. Carr and Margreet C. M. Vissers, "Synthetic or Food-Derived Vitamin C—Are They Equally Bioavailable?" *Nutrients* 5, no. 11 (October 2013): 4,284–304, doi: 10.3390/nu5114284.
43. Shun-Chiao Chang et al., "Dietary Flavonoid Intake and Risk of Incident

Depression in Midlife and Older Women," *American Journal of Clinical Nutrition* 104, no. 3 (September 2016): 704–14, doi: 10.3945/ajcn.115.124545.

44. Tomoyo Yamada et al., "Frequency of Citrus Fruit Intake Is Associated with the Incidence of Cardiovascular Disease: The Jichi Medical School Cohort Study," *Journal of Epidemiology* 21, no. 3 (2011): 169–75, doi: 10.2188/jea.je20100084.
45. Manas K. Akmatov et al., "Secular Trends and Rural-Urban Differences in Diagnostic Prevalence of Hay Fever: A Claims-Based Study in Germany," *Journal of Asthma and Allergy* 15 (August 2022): 1,205–15, doi: 10.2147/JAA.S371791.
46. L. Tettamanti et al., "Different Signals Induce Mast Cell Inflammatory Activity: Inhibitory Effect of Vitamin E," *Journal of Biological Regulators and Homeostatic Agents* 32, no. 1 (January–February 2018): 13–19.
47. Shi-Yi Wang et al., "Serum Level and Clinical Significance of Vitamin E in Children with Allergic Rhinitis," *BMC Pediatrics* 20, no. 1 (July 2020): 362, doi: 10.1186/s12887-020-02248-w; and Sihai Wu and Aiping Wang, "Serum Level and Clinical Significance of Vitamin E in Pregnant Women with Allergic Rhinitis," *Journal of the Chinese Medical Association* 85, no. 5 (May 2022): 597–602, doi: 10.1097/JCMA.0000000000000723.
48. Aimee Hoskins et al., "Natural-Source d-α-Tocopheryl Acetate Inhibits Oxidant Stress and Modulates Atopic Asthma in Humans In Vivo," *Allergy* 67, no. 5 (May 2012): 676–82, doi: 10.1111/j.1398-9995.2012.02810.x; and Stephanie P. Kurti et al., "Improved Lung Function Following Dietary Antioxidant Supplementation in Exercise-Induced Asthmatics," *Respiratory Physiology & Neurobiology* 220 (January 2016): 95–101, doi: 10.1016/j.resp.2015.09.012.
49. Mohammad Hassan Javanbakht et al., "Randomized Controlled Trial Using Vitamins E and D Supplementation in Atopic Dermatitis," *Journal of Dermatological Treatment* 22, no. 3 (June 2011): 144–50, doi: 10.3109/09546630903578566.
50. Eduardo Shahar, Gamal Hassoun, and Shimon Pollack, "Effect of Vitamin E Supplementation on the Regular Treatment of Seasonal Allergic Rhinitis," *Annals of Allergy, Asthma & Immunology* 92, no. 6 (June 2004): 654–58, doi: 10.1016/S1081-1206(10)61432-9.
51. Mohammad-Hossein Shams et al., "Anti-Allergic Effects of Vitamin E in Allergic Diseases: An Updated Review," *International Immunopharmacology* 90 (January 2021): 107196, doi: 10.1016/j.intimp.2020.107196.
52. Abeer O. Elshaikh et al., "Influence of Vitamin K on Bone Mineral Density and Osteoporosis," *Cureus* 12, no. 10 (October 2020): e10816, doi: 10.7759/cureus.10816.
53. Tara Coughlan and Frances Dockery, "Osteoporosis and Fracture Risk in Older People," *Clinical Medicine (London, England)* 14, no. 2 (April 2014): 187–91, doi: 10.7861/clinmedicine.14-2-187.
54. P. Weber, "Vitamin K and Bone Health," *Nutrition (Burbank, Los Angeles County, Calif.)* 17, no. 10 (October 2001): 880–87, doi: 10.1016/s0899-9007(01)00709-2.
55. Marc Sim et al., "Dietary Vitamin K_1 Intake Is Associated with Lower Long-Term Fracture-Related Hospitalization Risk: The Perth Longitudinal Study of

Ageing Women," *Food & Function* 13, no. 20 (2022): 10,642–50, doi: 10.1039/d2fo02494b.

56. S. L. Booth et al., "Dietary Vitamin K Intakes Are Associated with Hip Fracture but Not with Bone Mineral Density in Elderly Men and Women," *American Journal of Clinical Nutrition* 71, no. 5 (May 2000): 1,201–8, doi: 10.1093/ajcn/71.5.1201.
57. M. H. J. Knapen et al., "Three-Year Low-Dose Menaquinone-7 Supplementation Helps Decrease Bone Loss in Healthy Postmenopausal Women," *Osteoporosis International* 24, no. 9 (September 2013): 2,499–507, doi: 10.1007/s00198-013-2325-6.
58. Ming-Ling Ma et al., "Efficacy of Vitamin K2 in the Prevention and Treatment of Postmenopausal Osteoporosis: A Systematic Review and Meta-Analysis of Randomized Controlled Trials," *Frontiers in Public Health* 10 (August 2022): 979649, doi: 10.3389/fpubh.2022.979649.

Chapter 8: Phenomenal Phytonutrients

1. Nicolas Monjotin et al., "Clinical Evidence of the Benefits of Phytonutrients in Human Healthcare," *Nutrients* 14, no. 9 (2022): 1712, doi: 10.3390/nu14091712.
2. David S. Seigler et al., "Do Certain Flavonoid IMPS Have a Vital Function?" *Frontiers in Nutrition* 8 (December 2021): 762753, doi: 10.3389/fnut.2021.762753.
3. Johanna M. Geleijnse and Peter Ch. Hollman, "Flavonoids and Cardiovascular Health: Which Compounds, What Mechanisms?" *American Journal of Clinical Nutrition* 88, no. 1 (July 2008): 12–13, doi: 10.1093/ajcn/88.1.12.
4. Maria Celeste Dias, Diana C. G. A. Pinto, and Artur M. S. Silva, "Plant Flavonoids: Chemical Characteristics and Biological Activity," *Molecules (Basel, Switzerland)* 26, no. 17 (2021): 5377, doi: 10.3390/molecules26175377.
5. Helmut Sies and Dean P. Jones, "Reactive Oxygen Species (ROS) as Pleiotropic Physiological Signalling Agents," *Nature Reviews. Molecular Cell Biology* 21, no. 7 (March 2020): 363–83, doi: 10.1038/s41580-020-0230-3.
6. James Dahlhamer, PhD, et al., "Prevalence of Chronic Pain and High-Impact Chronic Pain among Adults—United States, 2016," *Morbidity and Mortality Weekly Report* 67, no. 36 (September 2018): 1,001–6, doi: 10.15585/mmwr.mm6736a2.
7. Simona Dragan et al., "Dietary Patterns and Interventions to Alleviate Chronic Pain," *Nutrients* 12, no. 9 (August 2020): 2510, doi: 10.3390/nu12092510.
8. Bahare Salehi et al., "The Therapeutic Potential of Anthocyanins: Current Approaches Based on Their Molecular Mechanism of Action," *Frontiers in Pharmacology* 11 (2020): 1300, doi: 10.3389/fphar.2020.01300.
9. Vanisree Mulabagal et al., "Anthocyanin Content, Lipid Peroxidation and Cyclooxygenase Enzyme Inhibitory Activities of Sweet and Sour Cherries," *Journal of Agricultural and Food Chemistry* 57, no. 4 (2009): 1,239–46, doi: 10.1021/jf8032039.
10. Rachel Kimble, Katherine Jones, and Glyn Howatson, "The Effect of Dietary Anthocyanins on Biochemical, Physiological, and Subjective Exercise Recovery: A Systematic Review and Meta-Analysis," *Critical Reviews in Food Science and Nutrition* 63, no. 9 (2023): 1,262–76, doi: 10.1080/10408398.2021.1963208.

11. Arpita Basu, Jace Schell, and R. Hal Scofield, "Dietary Fruits and Arthritis," *Food & Function* 9, no. 1 (2018): 70–77, doi: 10.1039/c7fo01435j.
12. Jace Schell et al., "Strawberries Improve Pain and Inflammation in Obese Adults with Radiographic Evidence of Knee Osteoarthritis," *Nutrients* 9, no. 9 (2017): 949, doi: 10.3390/nu9090949.
13. Nasrin Ghoochani et al., "The Effect of Pomegranate Juice on Clinical Signs, Matrix Metalloproteinases and Antioxidant Status in Patients with Knee Osteoarthritis," *Journal of the Science of Food and Agriculture* 96, no. 13 (October 2016): 4,377–81, doi: 10.1002/jsfa.7647.
14. M. Ghavipour et al., "Pomegranate Extract Alleviates Disease Activity and Some Blood Biomarkers of Inflammation and Oxidative Stress in Rheumatoid Arthritis Patients," *European Journal of Clinical Nutrition* 71, no. 1 (January 2017): 92–96, doi: 10.1038/ejcn.2016.151.
15. Glinda S. Cooper, Milele L. K. Bynum, and Emily C. Somers, "Recent Insights in the Epidemiology of Autoimmune Diseases: Improved Prevalence Estimates and Understanding of Clustering of Diseases," *Journal of Autoimmunity* 33, nos. 3–4 (November–December 2009): 197–207, doi: 10.1016/j.jaut.2009.09.008.
16. Shuzhen Wang et al., "Immunomodulatory Effects of Green Tea Polyphenols," *Molecules (Basel, Switzerland)* 26, no. 12 (June 2021): 3755, doi: 10.3390/molecules26123755.
17. Dayong Wu et al., "Green Tea EGCG, T Cells, and T Cell–Mediated Autoimmune Diseases," *Molecular Aspects of Medicine* 33, no. 1 (February 2012): 107–18, doi: 10.1016/j.mam.2011.10.001.
18. Brahma N. Singh, Sharmila Shankar, and Rakesh K. Srivastava, "Green Tea Catechin, Epigallocatechin-3-Gallate (EGCG): Mechanisms, Perspectives and Clinical Applications," *Biochemical Pharmacology* 82, no. 12 (December 2011): 1,807–21, doi: 10.1016/j.bcp.2011.07.093.
19. Corina Serban et al., "Effects of Supplementation with Green Tea Catechins on Plasma C-Reactive Protein Concentrations: A Systematic Review and Meta-Analysis of Randomized Controlled Trials," *Nutrition (Burbank, Los Angeles County, Calif.)* 31, no. 9 (September 2015): 1,061–71, doi: 10.1016/j.nut.2015.02.004.
20. Jiayang Jin et al., "Tea Consumption Is Associated with Decreased Disease Activity of Rheumatoid Arthritis in a Real-World, Large-Scale Study," *Annals of Nutrition & Metabolism* 76, no. 1 (2020): 54–61, doi: 10.1159/000505952.
21. Z. Shamekhi et al., "A Randomized, Double-Blind, Placebo-Controlled Clinical Trial Examining the Effects of Green Tea Extract on Systemic Lupus Erythematosus Disease Activity and Quality of Life," *Phytotherapy Research* 31, no. 7 (July 2017): 1,063–71, doi: 10.1002/ptr.5827.
22. María Cuerda-Ballester et al., "Improvements in Gait and Balance in Patients with Multiple Sclerosis after Treatment with Coconut Oil and Epigallocatechin Gallate. A Pilot Study," *Food & Function* 14, no. 2 (January 2023): 1,062–71, doi: 10.1039/d2fo02207a.
23. Andrei Ivashynka et al., "The Impact of Lifetime Coffee and Tea Loads on

Multiple Sclerosis Severity," *Clinical Nutrition ESPEN* 47 (February 2022): 199–205, doi: 10.1016/j.clnesp.2021.12.014.

24. Diman Lamichhane et al., "Coffee and Tea Consumption in Relation to Risk of Rheumatoid Arthritis in the Women's Health Initiative Observational Cohort," *Journal of Clinical Rheumatology* 25, no. 3 (April 2019): 127–32, doi: 10.1097/RHU.0000000000000788.
25. Daniele Piovani et al., "Environmental Risk Factors for Inflammatory Bowel Diseases: An Umbrella Review of Meta-Analyses," *Gastroenterology* 157, no. 3 (September 2019): 647–59.e4, doi: 10.1053/j.gastro.2019.04.016.
26. Maryam Dastoorpoor et al., "A Case-Control Study of Drinking Beverages and the Risk of Multiple Sclerosis in Iran," *Journal of Health, Population, and Nutrition* 42, no. 1 (March 2023): 22, doi: 10.1186/s41043-023-00364-8.
27. Naghma Khan and Hasan Mukhtar, "Tea and Health: Studies in Humans," *Current Pharmaceutical Design* 19, no. 34 (2013): 6,141–47, doi: 10.2174/1381612811319340008.
28. Robin Poole et al., "Coffee Consumption and Health: Umbrella Review of Meta-Analyses of Multiple Health Outcomes," *BMJ (Clinical Research Ed.)* 359 (2017): j5024, doi: 10.1136/bmj.j5024.
29. Ian Clark and Hans Peter Landolt, "Coffee, Caffeine, and Sleep: A Systematic Review of Epidemiological Studies and Randomized Controlled Trials," *Sleep Medicine Reviews* 31 (February 2017): 70–78, doi: 10.1016/j.smrv.2016.01.006.
30. Sylva M. Schaefer et al., "Association of Alcohol Types, Coffee and Tea Intake with Mortality: Prospective Cohort Study of UK Biobank Participants," *British Journal of Nutrition* 129, no. 1 (January 2023): 115–25, doi: 10.1017/S000711452200040X.
31. Kyung Mi Yoo, In-Kyeong Hwang, and BoKyung Moon, "Comparative Flavonoids Contents of Selected Herbs and Associations of Their Radical Scavenging Activity with Antiproliferative Actions in V79-4 Cells," *Journal of Food Science* 74, no. 6 (August 2009): C419–C425, doi: 10.1111/j.1750-3841.2009.01191.x.
32. Elaheh Madadi et al., "Therapeutic Application of Betalains: A Review," *Plants (Basel, Switzerland)* 9, no. 9 (2020): 1219, doi: 10.3390/plants9091219.
33. Holy Brown, Isaac N. Natuanya, and Ojoye Ngoye Briggs, "Post-Prandial Effect of Beetroot (*Beta vulgaris*) Juice on Glucose and Lipids Levels of Apparently Healthy Subjects," *European Journal of Pharmaceutical and Medical Research* 4, no. 5 (June 2018): 60–62.
34. Ana Paula Ribeiro Barcelos de Castro et al., "Effect of Freeze-Dried Red Beet (*Beta vulgaris* L.) Leaf Supplementation on Biochemical and Anthropometrical Parameters in Overweight and Obese Individuals: A Pilot Study," *Plant Foods for Human Nutrition (Dordrecht, Netherlands)* 74, no. 2 (June 2019): 232–34, doi: 10.1007/s11130-019-00730-0.
35. Raúl Domínguez et al., "Effects of Beetroot Juice Supplementation on Cardiorespiratory Endurance in Athletes. A Systematic Review," *Nutrients* 9, no. 1 (January 2017): 43, doi: 10.3390/nu9010043.
36. Cristhian F. Montenegro et al., "Betalain-Rich Concentrate Supplementation

Improves Exercise Performance and Recovery in Competitive Triathletes," *Applied Physiology, Nutrition, and Metabolism* 42, no. 2 (February 2017): 166–72, doi: 10.1139/apnm-2016-0452.

37. Justin S. Van Hoorebeke et al., "Betalain-Rich Concentrate Supplementation Improves Exercise Performance in Competitive Runners," *Sports (Basel, Switzerland)* 4, no. 3 (July 2016): 40, doi: 10.3390/sports4030040.
38. Talitha Fernandes de Castro et al., "Effect of Beetroot Juice Supplementation on 10-km Performance in Recreational Runners," *Applied Physiology, Nutrition, and Metabolism* 44, no. 1 (January 2019): 90–94, doi: 10.1139/apnm-2018-0277.
39. Petey W. Mumford et al., "Effect of 1-Week Betalain-Rich Beetroot Concentrate Supplementation on Cycling Performance and Select Physiological Parameters," *European Journal of Applied Physiology* 118, no. 11 (November 2018): 2,465–76, doi: 10.1007/s00421-018-3973-1.
40. Lee J. Wylie et al., "Influence of Beetroot Juice Supplementation on Intermittent Exercise Performance," *European Journal of Applied Physiology* 116, no. 2 (February 2016): 415–25, doi: 10.1007/s00421-015-3296-4.
41. Jose Manuel Jurado-Castro et al., "Acute Effects of Beetroot Juice Supplements on Lower-Body Strength in Female Athletes: Double-Blind Crossover Randomized Trial," *Sports Health* 14, no. 6 (November–December 2022): 812–21, doi: 10.1177/19417381221083590.
42. Antonio Ranchal-Sanchez et al., "Acute Effects of Beetroot Juice Supplements on Resistance Training: A Randomized Double-Blind Crossover," *Nutrients* 12, no. 7 (June 2020): 1912, doi: 10.3390/nu12071912.
43. Tyler D. Williams et al., "Effect of Acute Beetroot Juice Supplementation on Bench Press Power, Velocity, and Repetition Volume," *Journal of Strength and Conditioning Research* 34, no. 4 (April 2020): 924–28, doi: 10.1519/JSC.0000000000003509.
44. Tania Reyes-Izquierdo et al., "Effect of Betalain-Rich Concentrate on Exercise Performance in Young, Healthy, Sedentary Individuals: A Double-Blind, Crossover, Placebo-Controlled Pilot Study," *Journal of Nutraceuticals and Food Science* 2, no. 3 (2017): 17.
45. Kay Scilley et al., "Early Age-Related Maculopathy and Self-Reported Visual Difficulty in Daily Life," *Ophthalmology* 109, no. 7 (July 2002): 1,235–42, doi: 10.1016/s0161-6420(02)01060-6; and Eva Mönestam and Britta Lundqvist, "Long-Time Results and Associations between Subjective Visual Difficulties with Car Driving and Objective Visual Function 5 Years after Cataract Surgery," *Journal of Cataract and Refractive Surgery* 32, no. 1 (January 2006): 50–55, doi: 10.1016/j.jcrs.2005.06.052.
46. Rui Fang et al., "Global, Regional, National Burden and Gender Disparity of Cataract: Findings from the Global Burden of Disease Study 2019," *BMC Public Health* 22, no. 1 (November 2022): 2068, doi: 10.1186/s12889-022-14491-0.
47. David B. Rein et al., "Prevalence of Age-Related Macular Degeneration in the US in 2019," *JAMA Ophthalmology* 140, no. 12 (December 2022): 1,202–8, doi: 10.1001/jamaophthalmol.2022.4401.
48. Takshma Bhatt and Kirtan Patel, "Carotenoids: Potent to Prevent Diseases

Review," *Natural Products and Bioprospecting* 10, no. 3 (June 2020): 109–17, doi: 10.1007/s13659-020-00244-2.

49. Dagfinn Aune et al., "Dietary Intake and Blood Concentrations of Antioxidants and the Risk of Cardiovascular Disease, Total Cancer, and All-Cause Mortality: A Systematic Review and Dose-Response Meta-Analysis of Prospective Studies," *American Journal of Clinical Nutrition* 108, no. 5 (November 2018): 1,069–91, doi: 10.1093/ajcn/nqy097.
50. El-Sayed M. Abdel-Aal et al., "Dietary Sources of Lutein and Zeaxanthin Carotenoids and Their Role in Eye Health," *Nutrients* 5, no. 4 (April 2013): 1,169–85, doi: 10.3390/nu5041169.
51. Xiao-Hong Liu et al., "Association between Lutein and Zeaxanthin Status and the Risk of Cataract: A Meta-Analysis," *Nutrients* 6, no. 1 (2014): 452–65, doi: 10.3390/nu6010452.
52. Le Ma et al., "Lutein and Zeaxanthin Intake and the Risk of Age-Related Macular Degeneration: A Systematic Review and Meta-Analysis," *British Journal of Nutrition* 107, no. 3 (February 2012): 350–59, doi: 10.1017/S0007114511004260.
53. B. Olmedilla et al., "Lutein, but Not Alpha-Tocopherol, Supplementation Improves Visual Function in Patients with Age-Related Cataracts: A 2-Y Double-Blind, Placebo-Controlled Pilot Study," *Nutrition (Burbank, Los Angeles County, Calif.)* 19, no. 1 (January 2003): 21–24, doi: 10.1016/s0899-9007(02)00861-4.
54. Liwen Feng et al., "Effects of Lutein Supplementation in Age-Related Macular Degeneration," *PloS One* 14, no. 12 (December 2019): e0227048, doi: 10.1371/journal.pone.0227048.
55. Rebecca L. Siegel et al., "Cancer Statistics, 2022," *CA: A Cancer Journal for Clinicians* 72, no. 1 (January 2022): 7–33, doi: 10.3322/caac.21708.
56. Skyler B. Johnson et al., "Use of Alternative Medicine for Cancer and Its Impact on Survival," *Journal of the National Cancer Institute* 110, no. 1 (January 2018), doi: 10.1093/jnci/djx145.
57. John D. Hayes, Michael O. Kelleher, and Ian M. Eggleston, "The Cancer Chemopreventive Actions of Phytochemicals Derived from Glucosinolates," *European Journal of Nutrition* 47, Supplement 2 (May 2008): 73–88, doi: 10.1007/s00394-008-2009-8.
58. Gölge Sarikamis, "Glucosinolates in Crucifers and Their Potential Effects against Cancer: Review," *Canadian Journal of Plant Science* 89, no. 5 (September 2009): 953–59, doi: 10.4141/CJPS08125.
59. Dagfinn Aune et al., "Fruit and Vegetable Intake and the Risk of Cardiovascular Disease, Total Cancer and All-Cause Mortality—A Systematic Review and Dose-Response Meta-Analysis of Prospective Studies," *International Journal of Epidemiology* 46, no. 3 (June 2017): 1,029–56, doi: 10.1093/ije/dyw319.
60. Ben Liu et al., "The Association of Cruciferous Vegetables Intake and Risk of Bladder Cancer: A Meta-Analysis," *World Journal of Urology* 31, no. 1 (February 2013): 127–33, doi: 10.1007/s00345-012-0850-0.
61. Xiaojiao Liu and Kezhen Lv, "Cruciferous Vegetables Intake Is Inversely Associated with Risk of Breast Cancer: A Meta-Analysis," *Breast (Edinburgh, Scotland)* 22, no. 3 (June 2013): 309–13, doi: 10.1016/j.breast.2012.07.013.

62. Q. J. Wu et al., "Cruciferous Vegetables Intake and the Risk of Colorectal Cancer: A Meta-Analysis of Observational Studies," *Annals of Oncology* 24, no. 4 (April 2013): 1,079–87, doi: 10.1093/annonc/mds601.
63. Elisa V. Bandera et al., "Fruits and Vegetables and Endometrial Cancer Risk: A Systematic Literature Review and Meta-Analysis," *Nutrition and Cancer* 58, no. 1 (2007): 6–21, doi: 10.1080/01635580701307929.
64. Qi-Jun Wu et al., "Cruciferous Vegetable Consumption and Gastric Cancer Risk: A Meta-Analysis of Epidemiological Studies," *Cancer Science* 104, no. 8 (August 2013): 1,067–73, doi: 10.1111/cas.12195.
65. Victoria A. Kirsh et al., "Prospective Study of Fruit and Vegetable Intake and Risk of Prostate Cancer," *Journal of the National Cancer Institute* 99, no. 15 (August 2007): 1,200–209, doi: 10.1093/jnci/djm065.
66. Bo Han, Xuepeng Li, and Tao Yu, "Cruciferous Vegetables Consumption and the Risk of Ovarian Cancer: A Meta-Analysis of Observational Studies," *Diagnostic Pathology* 9 (2014): 7, doi: 10.1186/1746-1596-9-7.
67. Li-yi Li et al., "Cruciferous Vegetable Consumption and the Risk of Pancreatic Cancer: A Meta-Analysis," *World Journal of Surgical Oncology* 13 (2015): 44, doi: 10.1186/s12957-015-0454-4.
68. Ben Liu et al., "Cruciferous Vegetables Intake and Risk of Prostate Cancer: A Meta-Analysis," *International Journal of Urology* 19, no. 2 (February 2012): 134–41, doi: 10.1111/j.1442-2042.2011.02906.x.
69. Cristina Bosetti et al., "A Pooled Analysis of Case-Control Studies of Thyroid Cancer. VII. Cruciferous and Other Vegetables (International)," *Cancer Causes & Control* 13, no. 8 (October 2002): 765–75, doi: 10.1023/a:1020243527152.
70. Elena Catanzaro et al., "Anticancer Potential of Allicin: A Review," *Pharmacological Research* 177 (March 2022): 106118, doi: 10.1016/j.phrs.2022.106118.
71. Enrique Guillamón et al., "In Vitro Antitumor and Anti-Inflammatory Activities of *Allium*-Derived Compounds Propyl Propane Thiosulfonate (PTSO) and Propyl Propane Thiosulfinate (PTS)," *Nutrients* 15, no. 6 (March 2023): 1363, doi: 10.3390/nu15061363.
72. Holly L. Nicastro, Sharon A. Ross, and John A. Milner, "Garlic and Onions: Their Cancer Prevention Properties," *Cancer Prevention Research (Philadelphia, Pa.)* 8, no. 3 (March 2015): 181–89, doi: 10.1158/1940-6207.CAPR-14-0172.
73. Yong Zhou et al., "Consumption of Large Amounts of Allium Vegetables Reduces Risk for Gastric Cancer in a Meta-Analysis," *Gastroenterology* 141, no. 1 (July 2011): 80–89, doi: 10.1053/j.gastro.2011.03.057.
74. Carlotta Galeone et al., "Onion and Garlic Use and Human Cancer," *American Journal of Clinical Nutrition* 84, no. 5 (November 2006): 1,027–32, doi: 10.1093/ajcn/84.5.1027.
75. Alena Vanduchova, Pavel Anzenbacher, and Eva Anzenbacherova, "Isothiocyanate from Broccoli, Sulforaphane, and Its Properties," *Journal of Medicinal Food* 22, no. 2 (February 2019): 121–26, doi: 10.1089/jmf.2018.0024.
76. H. Fakhar and A. Hashemi Tayer, "Effect of the Garlic Pill in Comparison with Plavix on Platelet Aggregation and Bleeding Time," *Iranian Journal of Pediatric Hematology and Oncology* 2, no. 4 (2012): 146–52, https://pubmed.ncbi.nlm.nih.gov/24575255/.

77. Gaber El-Saber Batiha et al., "Chemical Constituents and Pharmacological Activities of Garlic (*Allium sativum* L.): A Review," *Nutrients* 12, no. 3 (March 2020): 872, doi: 10.3390/nu12030872.
78. Azam Borzoei, Maryam Rafraf, and Mohammad Asghari-Jafarabadi, "Cinnamon Improves Metabolic Factors without Detectable Effects on Adiponectin in Women with Polycystic Ovary Syndrome," *Asia Pacific Journal of Clinical Nutrition* 27, no. 3 (2018): 556–63, doi: 10.6133/apjcn.062017.13.
79. E. Ernst and M. H. Pittler, "Efficacy of Ginger for Nausea and Vomiting: A Systematic Review of Randomized Clinical Trials," *British Journal of Anaesthesia* 84, no. 3 (March 2000): 367–71, doi: 10.1093/oxfordjournals.bja.a013442.
80. Pouya Nematolahi et al., "Effects of *Rosmarinus officinalis* L. on Memory Performance, Anxiety, Depression, and Sleep Quality in University Students: A Randomized Clinical Trial," *Complementary Therapies in Clinical Practice* 30 (February 2018): 24–28, doi: 10.1016/j.ctcp.2017.11.004.
81. Kristina S. Petersen et al., "Herbs and Spices Modulate Gut Bacterial Composition in Adults at Risk for CVD: Results of a Prespecified Exploratory Analysis from a Randomized, Crossover, Controlled-Feeding Study," *Journal of Nutrition* 152, no. 11 (November 2022): 2,461–70, doi: 10.1093/jn/nxac201.
82. Kristina S. Petersen et al., "Herbs and Spices at a Relatively High Culinary Dosage Improves 24-Hour Ambulatory Blood Pressure in Adults at Risk of Cardiometabolic Diseases: A Randomized, Crossover, Controlled-Feeding Study," *American Journal of Clinical Nutrition* 114, no. 6 (December 2021): 1,936–48, doi: 10.1093/ajcn/nqab291.
83. Ester S. Oh et al., "Four Weeks of Spice Consumption Lowers Plasma Proinflammatory Cytokines and Alters the Function of Monocytes in Adults at Risk of Cardiometabolic Disease: Secondary Outcome Analysis in a 3-Period, Randomized, Crossover, Controlled Feeding Trial," *American Journal of Clinical Nutrition* 115, no. 1 (January 2022): 61–72, doi: 10.1093/ajcn/nqab331.

Chapter 9: Nutrivore Foundational Foods

1. Xia Wang et al., "Fruit and Vegetable Consumption and Mortality from All Causes, Cardiovascular Disease, and Cancer: Systematic Review and Dose-Response Meta-Analysis of Prospective Cohort Studies," *BMJ (Clinical Research Ed.)* 349 (2014): g4490, doi: 10.1136/bmj.g4490.
2. Dagfinn Aune et al., "Fruit and Vegetable Intake and the Risk of Cardiovascular Disease, Total Cancer and All-Cause Mortality—A Systematic Review and Dose-Response Meta-Analysis of Prospective Studies," *International Journal of Epidemiology* 46, no. 3 (June 2017): 1,029–56, doi: 10.1093/ije/dyw319.
3. Jeffrey D. Stanaway et al., "Health Effects Associated with Vegetable Consumption: A Burden of Proof Study," *Nature Medicine* 28, no. 10 (2022): 2,066–74, doi: 10.1038/s41591-022-01970-5.
4 Seung Hee Lee, PhD, et al., "Adults Meeting Fruit and Vegetable Intake Recommendations—United States, 2019," *Morbidity and Mortality Weekly Report (MMWR)* 71, no. 1 (January 2022): 1–9, doi: 10.15585/mmwr.mm7101a1.
5. Aune et al., "Fruit and Vegetable Intake."
6. Chun Shing Kwok et al., "Dietary Components and Risk of Cardiovascular

Disease and All-Cause Mortality: A Review of Evidence from Meta-Analyses," *European Journal of Preventive Cardiology* 26, no. 13 (September 2019): 1,415–29, doi: 10.1177/2047487319843667.

7. Martha Clare Morris et al., "Nutrients and Bioactives in Green Leafy Vegetables and Cognitive Decline: Prospective Study," *Neurology* 90, no. 3 (January 2018): e214–e222, doi: 10.1212/WNL.0000000000004815.
8. Shilpa N. Bhupathiraju et al., "Quantity and Variety in Fruit and Vegetable Intake and Risk of Coronary Heart Disease," *American Journal of Clinical Nutrition* 98, no. 6 (December 2013): 1,514–23, doi: 10.3945/ajcn.113.066381.
9. Giovanna Masala et al., "Fruit and Vegetables Consumption and Breast Cancer Risk: The EPIC Italy Study," *Breast Cancer Research and Treatment* 132, no. 3 (2012): 1,127–36, doi: 10.1007/s10549-011-1939-7.
10. D. E. Williams et al., "Frequent Salad Vegetable Consumption Is Associated with a Reduction in the Risk of Diabetes Mellitus," *Journal of Clinical Epidemiology* 52, no. 4 (April 1999): 329–35, doi: 10.1016/s0895-4356(99)00006-2.
11. Kwok et al., "Dietary Components and Risk."
12. Ibid.
13. A. J. Cooper et al., "Fruit and Vegetable Intake and Type 2 Diabetes: EPIC-InterAct Prospective Study and Meta-Analysis," *European Journal of Clinical Nutrition* 66, no. 10 (October 2012): 1,082–92, doi: 10.1038/ejcn.2012.85.
14. Kwok et al., "Dietary Components and Risk."
15. Andreea Zurbau et al., "Relation of Different Fruit and Vegetable Sources with Incident Cardiovascular Outcomes: A Systematic Review and Meta-Analysis of Prospective Cohort Studies," *Journal of the American Heart Association* 9, no. 19 (October 2020): e017728, doi: 10.1161/JAHA.120.017728.
16. Ann W. Hsing et al., "Allium Vegetables and Risk of Prostate Cancer: A Population-Based Study," *Journal of the National Cancer Institute* 94, no. 21 (November 2002): 1,648–51, doi: 10.1093/jnci/94.21.1648.
17. Kwok et al., "Dietary Components and Risk."
18. Djibril M. Ba et al., "Prospective Study of Dietary Mushroom Intake and Risk of Mortality: Results from Continuous National Health and Nutrition Examination Survey (NHANES) 2003–2014 and a Meta-Analysis," *Nutrition Journal* 20, no. 1 (September 2021): 80, doi: 10.1186/s12937-021-00738-w.
19. Diane E. Threapleton et al., "Dietary Fibre Intake and Risk of Cardiovascular Disease: Systematic Review and Meta-Analysis," *BMJ (Clinical Research Ed.)* 347 (2013): f6879, doi: 10.1136/bmj.f6879.
20. Lukas Schwingshackl et al., "Food Groups and Risk of All-Cause Mortality: A Systematic Review and Meta-Analysis of Prospective Studies," *American Journal of Clinical Nutrition* 105, no. 6 (June 2017): 1,462–73, doi: 10.3945/ajcn.117.153148.
21. Mark L. Dreher, "Whole Fruits and Fruit Fiber Emerging Health Effects," *Nutrients* 10, no. 12 (November 2018): 1833, doi: 10.3390/nu10121833.
22. Shu Zhang et al., "Citrus Consumption and Incident Dementia in Elderly Japanese: The Ohsaki Cohort 2006 Study," *British Journal of Nutrition* 117, no. 8 (2017): 1,174–80, doi: 10.1017/S000711451700109X.

23. Aune et al., "Fruit and Vegetable Intake."
24. Kwok et al., "Dietary Components and Risk."
25. Ângelo Luís, Fernanda Domingues, and Luísa Pereira, "Association between Berries Intake and Cardiovascular Diseases Risk Factors: A Systematic Review with Meta-Analysis and Trial Sequential Analysis of Randomized Controlled Trials," *Food & Function* 9, no. 2 (February 2018): 740–57, doi: 10.1039/c7fo01551h.
26. Paul Knekt et al., "Flavonoid Intake and Risk of Chronic Diseases," *American Journal of Clinical Nutrition* 76, no. 3 (September 2002): 560–68, doi: 10.1093/ajcn/76.3.560.
27. X. Gao et al., "Habitual Intake of Dietary Flavonoids and Risk of Parkinson Disease," *Neurology* 78, no. 15 (April 2012): 1,138–45, doi: 10.1212/WNL.0b013e31824f7fc4.
28. Weida Liu et al., "Fruit, Vegetable, and Legume Intake and the Risk of All-Cause, Cardiovascular, and Cancer Mortality: A Prospective Study," *Clinical Nutrition (Edinburgh, Scotland)* 40, no. 6 (June 2021): 4,316–23, doi: 10.1016/j.clnu.2021.01.016.
29. L. A. Bazzano et al., "Legume Consumption and Risk of Coronary Heart Disease in US Men and Women: NHANES I Epidemiologic Follow-Up Study," *Archives of Internal Medicine* 161, no. 21 (November 2001): 2,573–78, doi: 10.1001/archinte.161.21.2573.
30. Ashkan Afshin et al., "Consumption of Nuts and Legumes and Risk of Incident Ischemic Heart Disease, Stroke, and Diabetes: A Systematic Review and Meta-Analysis," *American Journal of Clinical Nutrition* 100, no. 1 (July 2014): 278–88, doi: 10.3945/ajcn.113.076901.
31. Dagfinn Aune et al., "Nut Consumption and Risk of Cardiovascular Disease, Total Cancer, All-Cause and Cause-Specific Mortality: A Systematic Review and Dose-Response Meta-Analysis of Prospective Studies," *BMC Medicine* 14, no. 1 (2016): 207, doi: 10.1186/s12916-016-0730-3.
32. Giuseppe Grosso et al., "Nut Consumption on All-Cause, Cardiovascular, and Cancer Mortality Risk: A Systematic Review and Meta-Analysis of Epidemiologic Studies," *American Journal of Clinical Nutrition* 101, no. 4 (April 2015): 783–93, doi: 10.3945/ajcn.114.099515.
33. Lan Jiang et al., "Intake of Fish and Marine n-3 Polyunsaturated Fatty Acids and Risk of Cardiovascular Disease Mortality: A Meta-Analysis of Prospective Cohort Studies," *Nutrients* 13, no. 7 (2021): 2342, doi: 10.3390/nu13072342.
34. Kwok et al., "Dietary Components and Risk."
35. Yi Wan et al., "Fish, Long Chain Omega-3 Polyunsaturated Fatty Acids Consumption, and Risk of All-Cause Mortality: A Systematic Review and Dose-Response Meta-Analysis from 23 Independent Prospective Cohort Studies," *Asia Pacific Journal of Clinical Nutrition* 26, no. 5 (2017): 939–56, doi: 10.6133/apjcn.072017.01.
36. Iain A. Brownlee et al., "Markers of Cardiovascular Risk Are Not Changed by Increased Whole-Grain Intake: The WHOLEheart Study, a Randomised, Controlled Dietary Intervention," *British Journal of Nutrition* 104, no. 1 (July 2010): 125–34, doi: 10.1017/S0007114510000644.
37. Jabir Khan et al., "Overview of the Composition of Whole Grains' Phenolic

Acids and Dietary Fibre and Their Effect on Chronic Non-Communicable Diseases," *International Journal of Environmental Research and Public Health* 19, no. 5 (March 2022): 3042, doi: 10.3390/ijerph19053042.

38. Candida J. Rebello, Frank L. Greenway, and John W. Finley, "Whole Grains and Pulses: A Comparison of the Nutritional and Health Benefits," *Journal of Agricultural and Food Chemistry* 62, no. 29 (2014): 7,029–49, doi: 10.1021/jf500932z.
39. Schwingshackl et al., "Food Groups and Risk of All-Cause Mortality."
40. Myriam M.-L. Grundy et al., "Processing of Oat: The Impact on Oat's Cholesterol Lowering Effect," *Food & Function* 9, no. 3 (February 2018): 1,328–43, doi: 10.1039/c7fo02006f; and Anne Whitehead et al., "Cholesterol-Lowering Effects of Oat β-Glucan: A Meta-Analysis of Randomized Controlled Trials," *American Journal of Clinical Nutrition* 100, no. 6 (December 2014): 1,413–21, doi: 10.3945/ajcn.114.086108.
41. Qingtao Hou et al., "The Metabolic Effects of Oats Intake in Patients with Type 2 Diabetes: A Systematic Review and Meta-Analysis," *Nutrients* 7, no. 12 (2015): 10,369–87, doi: 10.3390/nu7125536.
42. C. A. Blais et al., "Effect of Dietary Sodium Restriction on Taste Responses to Sodium Chloride: A Longitudinal Study," *American Journal of Clinical Nutrition* 44, no. 2 (August 1986): 232–43, doi: 10.1093/ajcn/44.2.232; J. E. Stewart and R. S. J. Keast, "Recent Fat Intake Modulates Fat Taste Sensitivity in Lean and Overweight Subjects," *International Journal of Obesity (2005)* 36, no. 6 (June 2012): 834–42, doi: 10.1038/ijo.2011.155; and Paul M. Wise et al., "Reduced Dietary Intake of Simple Sugars Alters Perceived Sweet Taste Intensity but Not Perceived Pleasantness," *American Journal of Clinical Nutrition* 103, no. 1 (January 2016): 50–60, doi: 10.3945/ajcn.115.112300.
43. Victoria Aldridge, Terence M. Dovey, and Jason C. G. Halford, "The Role of Familiarity in Dietary Development," *Developmental Review* 29, no. 1 (March 2009): 32–44, doi: 10.1016/j.dr.2008.11.001.
44. Valentina De Cosmi, Silvia Scaglioni, and Carlo Agostoni, "Early Taste Experiences and Later Food Choices," *Nutrients* 9, no. 2 (February 2017): 107, doi: 10.3390/nu9020107.
45. Elizabeth D. Capaldi-Phillips and Devina Wadhera, "Associative Conditioning Can Increase Liking for and Consumption of Brussels Sprouts in Children Aged 3 to 5 Years," *Journal of the Academy of Nutrition and Dietetics* 114, no. 8 (August 2014): 1,236–41, doi: 10.1016/j.jand.2013.11.014.

Chapter 10: Busting Myths About What, When, and How to Eat

1. Ji-Sun Shin et al., "α-Solanine Isolated from *Solanum tuberosum* L. cv Jayoung Abrogates LPS-Induced Inflammatory Responses via NF-κB Inactivation in RAW 264.7 Macrophages and Endotoxin-Induced Shock Model in Mice," *Journal of Cellular Biochemistry* 117, no. 10 (October 2016): 2,327–39, doi: 10.1002/jcb.25530.
2. Mahsa Ghavipour et al., "Tomato Juice Consumption Reduces Systemic Inflammation in Overweight and Obese Females," *British Journal of Nutrition* 109, no. 11 (June 2013): 2,031–35, doi: 10.1017/S0007114512004278; and Gunawan Widjaja et al., "Effect of Tomato Consumption on Inflammatory

Markers in Health and Disease Status: A Systematic Review and Meta-Analysis of Clinical Trials," *Clinical Nutrition ESPEN* 50 (August 2022): 93–100, doi: 10.1016/j.clnesp.2022.04.019.

3. Mohsen Mazidi et al., "Tomato and Lycopene Consumption Is Inversely Associated with Total and Cause-Specific Mortality: A Population-Based Cohort Study, on Behalf of the International Lipid Expert Panel (ILEP)," *British Journal of Nutrition* 124, no. 12 (December 2020): 1,303–10, doi: 10.1017/S0007114519002150.
4. K. Barry Delclos et al., "Toxicity Evaluation of Bisphenol A Administered by Gavage to Sprague Dawley Rats from Gestation Day 6 through Postnatal Day 90," *Toxicological Sciences* 139, no. 1 (May 2014): 174–97, doi: 10.1093/toxsci/kfu022.
5. Lindsay D. Rogers, "What Does CLARITY-BPA Mean for Canadians?" *International Journal of Environmental Research and Public Health* 18, no. 13 (June 2021): 7001, doi: 10.3390/ijerph18137001.
6. Judy S. Lakind and Daniel Q. Naiman, "Daily Intake of Bisphenol A and Potential Sources of Exposure: 2005–2006 National Health and Nutrition Examination Survey," *Journal of Exposure Science & Environmental Epidemiology* 21, no. 3 (May–June 2011): 272–79, doi: 10.1038/jes.2010.9.
7. Matthew Lorber et al., "Exposure Assessment of Adult Intake of Bisphenol A (BPA) with Emphasis on Canned Food Dietary Exposures," *Environment International* 77 (April 2015): 55–62, doi: 10.1016/j.envint.2015.01.008.
8. Justin G. Teeguarden et al., "Twenty-Four Hour Human Urine and Serum Profiles of Bisphenol A during High-Dietary Exposure," *Toxicological Sciences* 123, no. 1 (September 2011): 48–57, doi: 10.1093/toxsci/kfr160.
9. Michael J. Orlich et al., "Ultra-Processed Food Intake and Animal-Based Food Intake and Mortality in the Adventist Health Study-2," *American Journal of Clinical Nutrition* 115, no. 6 (June 2022): 1,589–601, doi: 10.1093/ajcn/nqac043.
10. Paul N. Appleby et al., "Mortality in Vegetarians and Comparable Nonvegetarians in the United Kingdom," *American Journal of Clinical Nutrition* 103, no. 1 (January 2016): 218–30, doi: 10.3945/ajcn.115.119461.
11. Angela Bechthold et al., "Food Groups and Risk of Coronary Heart Disease, Stroke and Heart Failure: A Systematic Review and Dose-Response Meta-Analysis of Prospective Studies," *Critical Reviews in Food Science and Nutrition* 59, no. 7 (2019): 1,071–90, doi: 10.1080/10408398.2017.1392288.
12. Alison J. McAfee et al., "Red Meat Consumption: An Overview of the Risks and Benefits," *Meat Science* 84, no. 1 (January 2010): 1–13, doi: 10.1016/j.meatsci.2009.08.029.
13. Bradley C. Johnston et al., "Unprocessed Red Meat and Processed Meat Consumption: Dietary Guideline Recommendations from the Nutritional Recommendations (NutriRECS) Consortium," *Annals of Internal Medicine* 171, no. 10 (November 2019): 756–64, doi: 10.7326/M19-1621.
14. Vanessa Vigar et al., "A Systematic Review of Organic versus Conventional Food Consumption: Is There a Measurable Benefit on Human Health?" *Nutrients* 12, no. 1 (December 2019): 7, doi 10.3390/nu12010007.

15. Julia Baudry et al., "Health and Dietary Traits of Organic Food Consumers: Results from the NutriNet-Santé Study," *British Journal of Nutrition* 114, no. 12 (December 2015): 2,064–73, doi: 10.1017/S0007114515003761.
16. Crystal Smith-Spangler et al., "Are Organic Foods Safer or Healthier than Conventional Alternatives?: A Systematic Review," *Annals of Internal Medicine* 157, no. 5 (September 2012): 348–66, doi: 10.7326/0003-4819-157-5-201209040-00007; and Alan D. Dangour et al., "Nutrition-Related Health Effects of Organic Foods: A Systematic Review," *American Journal of Clinical Nutrition* 92, no. 1 (July 2010): 203–10, doi: 10.3945/ajcn.2010.29269.
17. Christine Hoefkens et al., "A Literature-Based Comparison of Nutrient and Contaminant Contents between Organic and Conventional Vegetables and Potatoes," *British Food Journal* 111 (2009): 1,078–97, doi: 10.1108/00070700910992934; V. Worthington, "Nutritional Quality of Organic versus Conventional Fruits, Vegetables, and Grains," *Journal of Alternative and Complementary Medicine (New York, N.Y.)* 7, no. 2 (April 2001): 161–73, doi: 10.1089/107555301750164244; Eunmi Koh, Suthawan Charoenprasert, and Alyson E. Mitchell, "Effect of Organic and Conventional Cropping Systems on Ascorbic Acid, Vitamin C, Flavonoids, Nitrate, and Oxalate in 27 Varieties of Spinach (*Spinacia oleracea* L.)," *Journal of Agricultural and Food Chemistry* 60, no. 12 (March 2012): 3,144–50, doi: 10.1021/jf300051f; and John P. Reganold et al., "Fruit and Soil Quality of Organic and Conventional Strawberry Agroecosystems," *PloS One* 5, no. 9 (September 2010): e12346, doi: 10.1371/journal.pone.0012346.
18. David R. Montgomery and Anne Biklé, "Soil Health and Nutrient Density: Beyond Organic vs. Conventional Farming," *Frontiers in Sustainable Food Systems* 5 (2021), doi: 10.3389/fsufs.2021.699147.
19. Donald R. Davis, Melvin D. Epp, and Hugh D. Riordan, "Changes in USDA Food Composition Data for 43 Garden Crops, 1950 to 1999," *Journal of the American College of Nutrition* 23, no. 6 (December 2004): 669–82, doi: 10.1080/07315724.2004.10719409.
20. Robin J. Marles, "Mineral Nutrient Composition of Vegetables, Fruits and Grains: The Context of Reports of Apparent Historical Declines," *Journal of Food Composition and Analysis* 56 (March 2017): 93–103, doi: 10.1016/j.jfca.2016.11.012.
21. S. K. Duckett et al., "Effects of Winter Stocker Growth Rate and Finishing System on: III. Tissue Proximate, Fatty Acid, Vitamin, and Cholesterol Content," *Journal of Animal Science* 87, no. 9 (September 2009): 2,961–70, doi: 10.2527/jas.2009-1850.
22. Mohammad Alothman et al., "The 'Grass-Fed' Milk Story: Understanding the Impact of Pasture Feeding on the Composition and Quality of Bovine Milk," *Foods (Basel, Switzerland)* 8, no. 8 (2019): 350, doi: 10.3390/foods8080350.
23. P. I. Ponte et al., "Influence of Pasture Intake on the Fatty Acid Composition, and Cholesterol, Tocopherols, and Tocotrienols Content in Meat from Free-Range Broilers," *Poultry Science* 87, no. 1 (January 2008): 80–88, doi: 10.3382/ps.2007-00148; and Bénédicte Lebret and Anne-Sophie Guillard, "Outdoor Rearing of

Cull Sows: Effects on Carcass, Tissue Composition and Meat Quality," *Meat Science* 70, no. 2 (June 2005): 247–57, doi: 10.1016/j.meatsci.2005.01.007.

24. Dominika Średnicka-Tober et al., "Composition Differences between Organic and Conventional Meat: A Systematic Literature Review and Meta-Analysis," *British Journal of Nutrition* 115, no. 6 (March 2016): 994–1,011, doi: 10.1017/S0007114515005073.
25. Cecilia Mugnai et al., "The Effects of Husbandry System on the Grass Intake and Egg Nutritive Characteristics of Laying Hens," *Journal of the Science of Food and Agriculture* 94, no. 3 (February 2014): 459–67, doi: 10.1002/jsfa.6269.
26. Lauren E. Macdonald et al., "A Systematic Review and Meta-Analysis of the Effects of Pasteurization on Milk Vitamins, and Evidence for Raw Milk Consumption and Other Health-Related Outcomes," *Journal of Food Protection* 74, no. 11 (November 2011): 1,814–32, doi: 10.4315/0362-028X.JFP-10-269.
27. Stephen P. Oliver et al., "Food Safety Hazards Associated with Consumption of Raw Milk," *Foodborne Pathogens and Disease* 6, no. 7 (September 2009): 793–806, doi: 10.1089/fpd.2009.0302.
28. Nicholas V. C. Ralston, J. John Kaneko, and Laura J. Raymond, "Selenium Health Benefit Values Provide a Reliable Index of Seafood Benefits vs. Risks," *Journal of Trace Elements in Medicine and Biology* 55 (September 2019): 50–57, doi: 10.1016/j.jtemb.2019.05.009.
29. Nicholas V. C. Ralston, "Selenium Health Benefit Values as Seafood Safety Criteria," *EcoHealth* 5, no. 4 (December 2008): 442–55, doi: 10.1007/s10393-008-0202-0.
30. A. Dick Vethaak and Juliette Legler, "Microplastics and Human Health," *Science (New York, N.Y.)* 371, no. 6530 (February 2021): 672–74, doi: 10.1126/science.abe5041.
31. Wendee Nicole, "Microplastics in Seafood: How Much Are People Eating?" *Environmental Health Perspectives* 129, no. 3 (March 2021): 34001, doi: 10.1289/EHP8936.
32. Kieran D. Cox et al., "Human Consumption of Microplastics," *Environmental Science & Technology* 53, no. 12 (June 2019): 7,068–74, doi: 10.1021/acs.est.9b01517.
33. Reuben Chukwuka Okocha, Isaac Olufemi Olatoye, and Olufemi Bolarinwa Adedeji, "Food Safety Impacts of Antimicrobial Use and Their Residues in Aquaculture," *Public Health Reviews* 39 (August 2018): 21, doi: 10.1186/s40985-018-0099-2.
34. Yi Wan et al., "Fish, Long Chain Omega-3 Polyunsaturated Fatty Acids Consumption, and Risk of All-Cause Mortality: A Systematic Review and Dose-Response Meta-Analysis from 23 Independent Prospective Cohort Studies," *Asia Pacific Journal of Clinical Nutrition* 26, no. 5 (2017): 939–56, doi: 10.6133/apjcn.072017.01.
35. Didem Peren Aykas et al., "Non-Targeted Authentication Approach for Extra Virgin Olive Oil," *Foods (Basel, Switzerland)* 9, no. 2 (2020): 221, doi: 10.3390/foods9020221.
36. Maryam S. Farvid et al., "Dietary Linoleic Acid and Risk of Coronary Heart Disease: A Systematic Review and Meta-Analysis of Prospective Cohort

Studies," *Circulation* 130, no. 18 (October 2014): 1,568–78, doi: 10.1161/CIRCULATIONAHA.114.010236.

37. Jun Li et al., "Dietary Intake and Biomarkers of Linoleic Acid and Mortality: Systematic Review and Meta-Analysis of Prospective Cohort Studies," *American Journal of Clinical Nutrition* 112, no. 1 (July 2020): 150–67, doi: 10.1093/ajcn/nqz349.
38. Guy H. Johnson and Kevin Fritsche, "Effect of Dietary Linoleic Acid on Markers of Inflammation in Healthy Persons: A Systematic Review of Randomized Controlled Trials," *Journal of the Academy of Nutrition and Dietetics* 112, no. 7 (July 2012): 1,029–41, doi: 10.1016/j.jand.2012.03.029.
39. Yu Zhang et al., "Cooking Oil/Fat Consumption and Deaths from Cardiometabolic Diseases and Other Causes: Prospective Analysis of 521,120 Individuals," *BMC Medicine* 19, no. 1 (April 2021): 92, doi: 10.1186/s12916-021-01961-2.
40. Yosra Allouche et al., "How Heating Affects Extra Virgin Olive Oil Quality Indexes and Chemical Composition," *Journal of Agricultural and Food Chemistry* 55, no. 23 (November 2007): 9,646–54, doi: 10.1021/jf070628u.
41. Lea Klein et al., "Selenium, Zinc, and Copper Status of Vegetarians and Vegans in Comparison to Omnivores in the Nutritional Evaluation (NuEva) Study," *Nutrients* 15, no. 16 (2023): 3538, doi: 10.3390/nu15163538.
42. Weston Petroski and Deanna M. Minich, "Is There Such a Thing as 'Anti-Nutrients'? A Narrative Review of Perceived Problematic Plant Compounds," *Nutrients* 12, no. 10 (September 2020): 2929, doi: 10.3390/nu12102929.
43. P. Priyodip, P. Y. Prakash, and S. Balaji, "Phytases of Probiotic Bacteria: Characteristics and Beneficial Aspects," *Indian Journal of Microbiology* 57, no. 2 (June 2017): 148–54, doi: 10.1007/s12088-017-0647-3; and Dina Karamad et al., "Probiotic Oxalate-Degrading Bacteria: New Insight of Environmental Variables and Expression of the oxc and frc Genes on Oxalate Degradation Activity," *Foods (Basel, Switzerland)* 11, no. 18 (September 2022): 2876, doi: 10.3390/foods11182876.
44. Angel A. López-González et al., "Protective Effect of Myo-Inositol Hexaphosphate (Phytate) on Bone Mass Loss in Postmenopausal Women," *European Journal of Nutrition* 52, no. 2 (March 2013): 717–26, doi: 10.1007/s00394-012-0377-6.
45. Pilar Sanchis et al., "Phytate Decreases Formation of Advanced Glycation End-Products in Patients with Type II Diabetes: Randomized Crossover Trial," *Scientific Reports* 8, no. 1 (June 2018): 9619, doi: 10.1038/s41598-018-27853-9.
46. Takeshi Ikenaga et al., "Effect of Inositol Hexaphosphate (IP6) on Serum Uric Acid in Hyperuricemic Subjects: A Randomized, Double-Blind, Placebo-Controlled, Crossover Study," *Plant Foods for Human Nutrition (Dordrecht, Netherlands)* 74, no. 3 (September 2019): 316–21, doi: 10.1007/s11130-019-00735-9.
47. Eric N. Taylor and Gary C. Curhan, "Determinants of 24-Hour Urinary Oxalate Excretion," *Clinical Journal of the American Society of Nephrology* 3, no. 5 (September 2008): 1,453–60, doi: 10.2215/CJN.01410308.
48. Marisa Porrini, Patrizia Riso, and Giovannangelo Oriani, "Spinach and Tomato

Consumption Increases Lymphocyte DNA Resistance to Oxidative Stress but This Is Not Related to Cell Carotenoid Concentrations," *European Journal of Nutrition* 41, no. 3 (June 2002): 95–100, doi: 10.1007/s003940200014.

49. Kirpal Panacer and Peter J. Whorwell, "Dietary Lectin Exclusion: The Next Big Food Trend?" *World Journal of Gastroenterology* 25, no. 24 (June 2019): 2,973–76, doi: 10.3748/wjg.v25.i24.2973.
50. Fardowsa Abdi et al., "Nutritional Considerations in Celiac Disease and Non-Celiac Gluten/Wheat Sensitivity," *Nutrients* 15, no. 6 (March 2023): 1475, doi: 10.3390/nu15061475.
51. D. L. Freed, "Do Dietary Lectins Cause Disease?" *BMJ (Clinical Research Ed.)* 318, no. 7190 (April 1999): 1,023–24, doi: 10.1136/bmj.318.7190.1023.
52. M. López-Moreno, M. Garcés-Rimón, and M. Miguel, "Antinutrients: Lectins, Goitrogens, Phytates and Oxalates, Friends or Foe?" *Journal of Functional Foods* 89 (February 2022): 104938, doi: 10.1016/j.jff.2022.104938.
53. Lan Shi, Susan D. Arntfield, and Michael Nickerson, "Changes in Levels of Phytic Acid, Lectins and Oxalates during Soaking and Cooking of Canadian Pulses," *Food Research International (Ottawa, Ont.)* 107 (May 2018): 660–68, doi: 10.1016/j.foodres.2018.02.056.
54. Dionysios V. Chartoumpekis et al., "Broccoli Sprout Beverage Is Safe for Thyroid Hormonal and Autoimmune Status: Results of a 12-Week Randomized Trial," *Food and Chemical Toxicology* 126 (April 2019): 1–6, doi: 10.1016/j.fct.2019.02.004.
55. Mark Messina, "Soybean Isoflavone Exposure Does Not Have Feminizing Effects on Men: A Critical Examination of the Clinical Evidence," *Fertility and Sterility* 93, no. 7 (May 2010): 2,095–104, doi: 10.1016/j.fertnstert.2010.03.002.
56. Flávia Ramos Kazan Oliveira et al., "Association between a Soy-Based Infant Diet and the Onset of Puberty: A Systematic Review and Meta-Analysis," *PloS One* 16, no. 5 (May 2021): e0251241, doi: 10.1371/journal.pone.0251241.
57. Gianluca Rizzo et al., "The Role of Soy and Soy Isoflavones on Women's Fertility and Related Outcomes: An Update," *Journal of Nutritional Science* 11 (March 2022): e17, doi: 10.1017/jns.2022.15.
58. Ivonne M. C. M. Rietjens, Jochem Louisse, and Karsten Beekmann, "The Potential Health Effects of Dietary Phytoestrogens," *British Journal of Pharmacology* 174, no. 11 (June 2017): 1,263–80, doi: 10.1111/bph.13622; and Jéssica C. P. Petrine and Bruno Del Bianco-Borges, "The Influence of Phytoestrogens on Different Physiological and Pathological Processes: An Overview," *Phytotherapy Research* 35, no. 1 (January 2021): 180–97, doi: 10.1002/ptr.6816.
59. Philippe Grandjean, "Paracelsus Revisited: The Dose Concept in a Complex World," *Basic & Clinical Pharmacology & Toxicology* 119, no. 2 (August 2016): 126–32, doi: 10.1111/bcpt.12622.
60. Coco Ballantyne, "Strange but True: Drinking Too Much Water Can Kill," *Scientific American*, June 21, 2007.
61. Michalina Oplatowska-Stachowiak and Christopher T. Elliott, "Food Colors: Existing and Emerging Food Safety Concerns," *Critical Reviews*

in Food Science and Nutrition 57, no. 3 (February 2017): 524–48, doi: 10.1080/10408398.2014.889652.

62. Asa Bradman et al., "Dietary Exposure to United States Food and Drug Administration–Approved Synthetic Food Colors in Children, Pregnant Women, and Women of Childbearing Age Living in the United States," *International Journal of Environmental Research and Public Health* 19, no. 15 (August 2022): 9661, doi: 10.3390/ijerph19159661.
63. Ian Mosby, "'That Won-Ton Soup Headache': The Chinese Restaurant Syndrome, MSG and the Making of American Food, 1968–1980," *Social History of Medicine* 22, no. 1 (April 2009), 133–51, doi: 10.1093/shm/hkn098.
64. A. N. Williams and K. M. Woessner, "Monosodium Glutamate 'Allergy': Menace or Myth?" *Clinical and Experimental Allergy* 39, no. 5 (May 2009): 640–46, doi: 10.1111/j.1365-2222.2009.03221.x; and Yoko Obayashi and Yoichi Nagamura, "Does Monosodium Glutamate Really Cause Headache?: A Systematic Review of Human Studies," *Journal of Headache and Pain* 17 (2016): 54, doi: 10.1186/s10194-016-0639-4.
65. Hellen D. B. Maluly, Adriana P. Arisseto-Bragotto, and Felix G. R. Reyes, "Monosodium Glutamate as a Tool to Reduce Sodium in Foodstuffs: Technological and Safety Aspects," *Food Science & Nutrition* 5, no. 6 (July 2017): 1,039–48, doi: 10.1002/fsn3.499.
66. Ashley Roberts, Barry Lynch, and Ivonne M. C. M. Rietjens, "Risk Assessment Paradigm for Glutamate," *Annals of Nutrition & Metabolism* 73, Supplement 5 (2018): 53–64, doi: 10.1159/000494783.
67. Aurélie Ballon, Manuela Neuenschwander, and Sabrina Schlesinger, "Breakfast Skipping Is Associated with Increased Risk of Type 2 Diabetes among Adults: A Systematic Review and Meta-Analysis of Prospective Cohort Studies," *Journal of Nutrition* 149, no. 1 (January 2019): 106–13, doi: 10.1093/jn/nxy194.
68. Richard Ofori-Asenso, Alice J. Owen, and Danny Liew, "Skipping Breakfast and the Risk of Cardiovascular Disease and Death: A Systematic Review of Prospective Cohort Studies in Primary Prevention Settings," *Journal of Cardiovascular Development and Disease* 6, no. 3 (August 2019): 30, doi: 10.3390/jcdd6030030.
69. Zhongyu Ren et al., "Association between Breakfast Consumption and Depressive Symptoms among Chinese College Students: A Cross-Sectional and Prospective Cohort Study," *International Journal of Environmental Research and Public Health* 17, no. 5 (February 2020): 1571, doi: 10.3390/ijerph17051571.
70. A. P. Smith, "Stress, Breakfast Cereal Consumption and Cortisol," *Nutritional Neuroscience* 5, no. 2 (April 2002): 141–44, doi: 10.1080/10284150290018946.
71. Megan Witbracht et al., "Female Breakfast Skippers Display a Disrupted Cortisol Rhythm and Elevated Blood Pressure," *Physiology & Behavior* 140 (March 2015): 215–21, doi: 10.1016/j.physbeh.2014.12.044.
72. Yangbo Sun et al., "Meal Skipping and Shorter Meal Intervals Are Associated with Increased Risk of All-Cause and Cardiovascular Disease Mortality among US Adults," *Journal of the Academy of Nutrition and Dietetics* 123, no. 3 (March 2023): 417–426.e3, doi: 10.1016/j.jand.2022.08.119.

73. Brad Jon Schoenfeld, Alan Albert Aragon, and James W. Krieger, "Effects of Meal Frequency on Weight Loss and Body Composition: A Meta-Analysis," *Nutrition Reviews* 73, no. 2 (February 2015): 69–82, doi: 10.1093/nutrit/nuu017.
74. Wei Wei et al., "Association of Meal and Snack Patterns with Mortality of All-Cause, Cardiovascular Disease, and Cancer: The US National Health and Nutrition Examination Survey, 2003 to 2014," *Journal of the American Heart Association* 10, no. 13 (July 2021): e020254, doi: 10.1161/JAHA.120.020254.
75. Seongeung Lee et al., "Effect of Different Cooking Methods on the Content of Vitamins and True Retention in Selected Vegetables," *Food Science and Biotechnology* 27, no. 2 (December 2017): 333–42, doi: 10.1007/s10068-017-0281-1.
76. Federica Ratto et al., "A Narrative Review on the Potential of Tomato and Lycopene for the Prevention of Alzheimer's Disease and Other Dementias," *Critical Reviews in Food Science and Nutrition* 62, no. 18 (2022): 4,970–81, doi: 10.1080/10408398.2021.1880363.
77. Michael L. Connolly, Julie A. Lovegrove, and Kieran M. Tuohy, "In Vitro Fermentation Characteristics of Whole Grain Wheat Flakes and the Effect of Toasting on Prebiotic Potential," *Journal of Medicinal Food* 15, no. 1 (January 2012): 33–43, doi: 10.1089/jmf.2011.0006; and Jae-Young Kim et al., "Effects of the Brown Seaweed *Laminaria japonica* Supplementation on Serum Concentrations of IgG, Triglycerides, and Cholesterol, and Intestinal Microbiota Composition in Rats," *Frontiers in Nutrition* 5 (April 2018): 23, doi: 10.3389/fnut.2018.00023.
78. Chun Shing Kwok et al., "Dietary Components and Risk of Cardiovascular Disease and All-Cause Mortality: A Review of Evidence from Meta-Analyses," *European Journal of Preventive Cardiology* 26, no. 13 (September 2019): 1,415–29, doi: 10.1177/2047487319843667.
79. Gao-feng Yuan et al., "Effects of Different Cooking Methods on Health-Promoting Compounds of Broccoli," *Journal of Zhejiang University. Science. B* 10, no. 8 (August 2009): 580–88, doi: 10.1631/jzus.B0920051.
80. Marilynn Schnepf and Judy Driskell, "Sensory Attributes and Nutrient Retention in Selected Vegetables Prepared by Conventional and Microwave Methods," *Journal of Food Quality* 17, no. 2 (April 1994): 87–99, doi: 10.1111/j.1745-4557.1994.tb00135.x.
81. Lauren C. Bylsma and Dominik D. Alexander, "A Review and Meta-Analysis of Prospective Studies of Red and Processed Meat, Meat Cooking Methods, Heme Iron, Heterocyclic Amines and Prostate Cancer," *Nutrition Journal* 14 (December 2015): 125, doi: 10.1186/s12937-015-0111-3.
82. Jungwon Kwon et al., "The Effects of Different Cooking Methods and Spices on the Formation of 11 HCAs in Chicken Wing and Pork Belly," *Food Control* 147 (May 2023): 109572, doi: 10.1016/j.foodcont.2022.109572.
83. Kanithaporn Puangsombat, Wannee Jirapakkul, and J. Scott Smith, "Inhibitory Activity of Asian Spices on Heterocyclic Amines Formation in Cooked Beef Patties," *Journal of Food Science* 76, no. 8 (October 2011): T174–T180, doi: 10.1111/j.1750-3841.2011.02338.x; and Hea Jin Kang et al., "Study on the

Reduction of Heterocyclic Amines by Marinated Natural Materials in Pork Belly," *Journal of Animal Science and Technology* 64, no. 6 (2022): 1,245–58, doi: 10.5187/jast.2022.e86.

84. S. Murray et al., "Effect of Cruciferous Vegetable Consumption on Heterocyclic Aromatic Amine Metabolism in Man," *Carcinogenesis* 22, no. 9 (September 2001): 1,413–20, doi: 10.1093/carcin/22.9.1413; and David G. Walters et al., "Cruciferous Vegetable Consumption Alters the Metabolism of the Dietary Carcinogen 2-Amino-1-Methyl-6-Phenylimidazo[4,5-b]Pyridine (PhIP) in Humans," *Carcinogenesis* 25, no. 9 (September 2004): 1,659–69, doi: 10.1093/carcin/bgh164.
85. Taraka V. Gadiraju et al., "Fried Food Consumption and Cardiovascular Health: A Review of Current Evidence," *Nutrients* 7, no. 10 (October 2015): 8,424–30, doi: 10.3390/nu7105404.
86. Pilar Guallar-Castillón et al., "Consumption of Fried Foods and Risk of Coronary Heart Disease: Spanish Cohort of the European Prospective Investigation into Cancer and Nutrition Study," *BMJ (Clinical Research Ed.)* 344 (January 2012): e363, doi: 10.1136/bmj.e363.
87. Leah E. Cahill et al., "Fried-Food Consumption and Risk of Type 2 Diabetes and Coronary Artery Disease: A Prospective Study in 2 Cohorts of US Women and Men," *American Journal of Clinical Nutrition* 100, no. 2 (August 2014): 667–75, doi: 10.3945/ajcn.114.084129.
88. Bradley P. Turnwald et al., "Increasing Vegetable Intake by Emphasizing Tasty and Enjoyable Attributes: A Randomized Controlled Multisite Intervention for Taste-Focused Labeling," *Psychological Science* 30, no. 11 (November 2019): 1,603–15, doi: 10.1177/0956797619872191.

Chapter 11: Applying Nutrivore Principles

1. Rebecca A. Seguin et al., "Consumption Frequency of Foods Away from Home Linked with Higher Body Mass Index and Lower Fruit and Vegetable Intake among Adults: A Cross-Sectional Study," *Journal of Environmental and Public Health* 2016 (2016): 3074241, doi: 10.1155/2016/3074241.
2. Shauna Golper et al., "Frequency of Meals Prepared Away from Home and Nutrient Intakes among US Adolescents (NHANES 2011–2018)," *Nutrients* 13, no. 11 (2021): 4019, doi: 10.3390/nu13114019.
3. Sayaka Nagao-Sato and Marla Reicks, "Food Away from Home Frequency, Diet Quality, and Health: Cross-Sectional Analysis of NHANES Data 2011–2018," *Nutrients* 14, no. 16 (August 2022): 3386, doi: 10.3390/nu14163386.
4. Yang Du et al., "Association between Frequency of Eating Away-from-Home Meals and Risk of All-Cause and Cause-Specific Mortality," *Journal of the Academy of Nutrition and Dietetics* 121, no. 9 (September 2021): 1,741–1,749.e1, doi: 10.1016/j.jand.2021.01.012.
5. Arpita Tiwari et al., "Cooking at Home: A Strategy to Comply with U.S. Dietary Guidelines at No Extra Cost," *American Journal of Preventive Medicine* 52, no. 5 (May 2017): 616–24, doi: 10.1016/j.amepre.2017.01.017.
6. Giulia Menichetti et al., "Machine Learning Prediction of the Degree of Food

Processing," *Nature Communications* 14, no. 1 (April 2023): 2312, doi: 10.1038/s41467-023-37457-1.

7. Kevin D. Hall et al., "Ultra-Processed Diets Cause Excess Calorie Intake and Weight Gain: An Inpatient Randomized Controlled Trial of Ad Libitum Food Intake," *Cell Metabolism* 30, no. 1 (July 2019): 67–77.e3, doi: 10.1016/j.cmet.2019.05.008.
8. Rachel Pechey and Pablo Monsivais, "Socioeconomic Inequalities in the Healthiness of Food Choices: Exploring the Contributions of Food Expenditures," *Preventive Medicine* 88 (July 2016): 203–9, doi: 10.1016/j.ypmed.2016.04.012.
9. Liangkui Li et al., "Effects of Quinoa (*Chenopodium quinoa* Willd.) Consumption on Markers of CVD Risk," *Nutrients* 10, no. 6 (June 2018): 777, doi: 10.3390/nu10060777.
10. Zach Conrad et al., "Higher-Diet Quality Is Associated with Higher Diet Costs When Eating at Home and Away from Home: National Health and Nutrition Examination Survey, 2005–2016," *Public Health Nutrition* 24, no. 15 (October 2021): 5,047–57, doi: 10.1017/S1368980021002810.
11. David T. Neal, Wendy Wood, and Jeffrey M. Quinn, "Habits—A Repeat Performance," *Current Directions in Psychological Science* 15, no. 4 (August 2006): 198–202, doi: 10.1111/j.1467-8721.2006.00435.x.

Index